A GUIDE TO CANINE
FELINE ORTHOPAEDIC S[

A Guide to Canine and Feline Orthopaedic Surgery

HAMISH R.DENNY

MA, VetMB, PhD, DSAO, FRCVS

THIRD EDITION

OXFORD

BLACKWELL SCIENTIFIC PUBLICATIONS

LONDON EDINBURGH BOSTON

MELBOURNE PARIS BERLIN VIENNA

© 1980, 1985, 1993 by
Blackwell Scientific Publications
Editorial Offices:
Osney Mead, Oxford OX2 OEL
25 John Street, London WC1N 2BL
23 Ainslie Place, Edinburgh EH3 6AJ
238 Main Street, Cambridge
  Massachusetts 02142, USA
54 University Street, Carlton
  Victoria 3053, Australia

Other Editorial Offices:
Librairie Arnette SA
2, rue Casimir-Delavigne
75006 Paris
France

Blackwell Wissenschafts-Verlag
Meinekestrasse 4
D-1000 Berlin 15
Germany

Blackwell MZV
Feldgasse 13
A-1238 Wien
Austria

First published 1980
Second edition 1985
Reprinted 1989, 1991
Third edition 1993

Set by Setrite Typesetters, Hong Kong
Printed and bound in Great Britain
by Hartnolls Ltd, Bodmin, Cornwall

DISTRIBUTORS

Marston Book Services Ltd
PO Box 87
Oxford OX2 ODT
(*Orders*: Tel: 0865 791155
          Fax: 0865 791927
          Telex: 837515)

USA
Blackwell Scientific Publications, Inc.
238 Main Street
Cambridge, MA 02142
(*Orders*: Tel: 800 759–6102
          617 876–7000)

Canada
Times Mirror Professional
Publishing Ltd
130 Flaska Drive
Markham, Ontario L6G 1B8
(*Orders*: Tel: 800 268–4178
          416 470–6739)

Australia
Blackwell Scientific Publications
Pty Ltd
54 University Street
Carlton, Victoria 3053
(*Orders*: Tel: 03 347–5552)

A catalogue record for this title
is available from the British Library

ISBN 0–632–03357–6

Contents

3 THE SKULL AND SPINE, 111

Preface

The first edition of *A Guide to Canine Orthopaedic Surgery* was published in 1980. The book was intended to be a guide to canine orthopaedic surgery in which conditions were described on a regional basis, instruction was simple and freely illustrated with line drawings. Rapid advances have continued to be made in many areas of small animal orthopaedics, a second edition was published in 1985 and the third edition was completed in 1991. The format remains the same as the previous texts but the book has been updated and expanded to cover a wide range of orthopaedic problems encountered in both the dog and the cat. Although the emphasis is on orthopaedic surgery, medical problems are also considered. It is hoped that the format of the book will enable it to be used as a rapid reference guide both by students and busy practitioners trying to keep pace with current trends in veterinary orthopaedics.

I gratefully acknowledge the help of my colleagues both at Bristol University and in practice who have made this book possible.

Hamish R. Denny

Chapter 1
Orthopaedic Surgical Pathology

FRACTURES

A fracture may be defined as a disruption in the continuity of a bone. The majority of fracture are caused by direct injury in road accidents or falls, the fractures occurring at or near the point of impact. A fracture may also be caused by an indirect force transmitted through bone or muscle to a vulnerable area of bone which breaks in a predictable manner; for example, fractures of the tibial tuberosity, olecranon or lateral condyle of the humerus. An incoordinate movement or excessive muscle contraction can result in this type of fracture. Factors which predispose to a fracture include the shape and position of the bone; hence long relatively exposed bones such as the radius and ulna and the tibia are more prone to fracture than the short compact bones of the carpus or tarsus.

The mechanical strength of a bone may be reduced locally by bone tumour formation or, generally, by disease caused by dietary or hormonal imbalance so that even minor trauma causes a fracture; this is called a pathological fracture.

THE CLASSIFICATION OF FRACTURES

Fractures may be classified according to:
1 External wounds.
2 Extent of bone damage.
3 Anatomical location and direction of the fracture line.
4 Relative displacement of the bone fragments.
5 Stability.

External wounds
A closed or simple fracture is one in which the overlying skin remains intact (Fig. 1.1) whereas an open or compound fracture is one in which there is a communication between the fracture site and a skin wound (Fig. 1.2).

Extent of bone damage
A complete fracture is one in which there is total disruption in the continuity of the bone and usually marked displacement of the fragments.

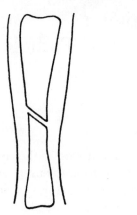

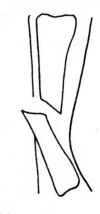

Fig. 1.2

Fig. 1.1

An incomplete fracture is one in which partial continuity of the bone is maintained as in the green stick (bending) fractures of young animals (Fig. 1.3) or fissure fractures in adults (Fig. 1.4).

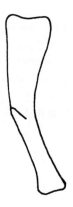
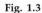
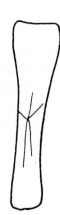

Fig. 1.3

Fig. 1.4

Anatomical location and direction of the fracture line
In classifying fractures by anatomical location, it is convenient to divide a typical long bone into three segments (Fig. 1.5).
1 The proximal epiphysis and the metaphysis consisting of cancellous bone.
2 The shaft consisting of cortical bone.
3 The distal metaphysis and epiphysis consisting of cancellous bone.
The fractures can then be described according to location — e.g. fracture of the proximal epiphysis or fracture of the shaft. Fractures of the epiphysis and growth plate injuries

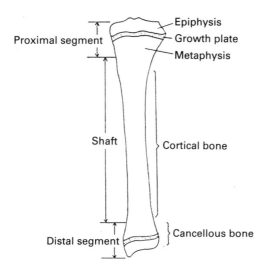

Fig. 1.5

are divided into six types (Salter & Harris 1963) and these
are described on page 106.

Shaft fractures can be further classified according to the
direction of the fracture line or the number of fragments.

Direction of fracture line
1 A transverse fracture is one in which the fracture line is
at right angles to the long axis of the bone (Fig. 1.6).
2 An oblique fracture is one at an angle to the long axis of
the bone (Fig. 1.7).

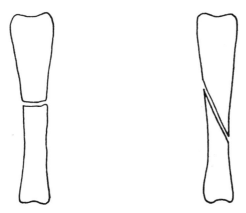

Fig. 1.6   Fig. 1.7

3 A spiral fracture curves around the bone (Fig. 1.8).
4 A comminuted fracture is one in which there are several
fragments (Fig. 1.9).
5 A segmental fracture is one in which the bone is broken
into three or more segments (Fig. 1.10).

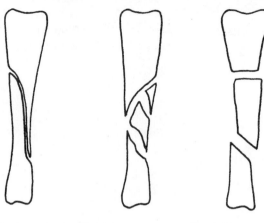

Fig. 1.8   Fig. 1.9   Fig. 1.10

Relative displacement of the fragments

1 A distraction or avulsion fracture is one in which a bone fragment is separated by the pull of the muscle, tendon or ligament which attaches to it, for example, fracture of the olecranon or avulsion of the tibial crest (Fig. 1.11).

2 An impacted fracture is one in which the fractured bone ends are driven into one another (Fig. 1.12).

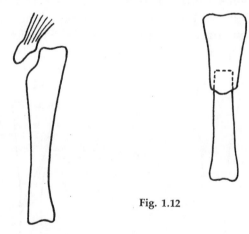

Fig. 1.12

Fig. 1.11

3 A compression fracture refers typically to fracture of a vertebra where a compressive force has resulted in shortening of a vertebra.

4 A depression fracture—this term is used to describe fractures of the skull in which the affected bone is 'pushed in', giving a concave deformity.

The stability of the fracture

A stable fracture is one in which the fragments interlock after reduction and resist shortening forces. The only fixation required in such a fracture is to prevent angular deformity. Most transverse fractures are in this category.

An unstable fracture is oblique or comminuted; here the fragments do not interlock following reduction and there is no resistance to shortening. Fixation is needed to maintain length, alignment and prevent rotation.

Classification of adult small animal fractures by numbers

A classification system for fractures of long bones in adult small animals was described by Prieur *et al.* in 1990. The system classifies:

1 The bone fractured.
2 The bone segment.
3 The fracture area.
4 The number of fragments.

The first two numbers of the classification system define the fracture location, the last two figures the fracture type. The system lends itself well to computerization and the international exchange of data.

The first number of the code indicates the bone fractured:

1 = humerus
2 = radius and ulna
3 = femur
4 = tibia.

The second number indicates the fractured bone segment:

−. 1 = proximal end
−. 2 = shaft
−. 3 = distal end.

The third number indicates the fracture area:

−. −. 1 = less than 5% of the bone length
−. −. 2 = between 5 and 25% of the bone length
−. −. 3 = more than 25% of the bone length.

The fourth number in the code corresponds with the number of fragments involved:

−. −. −. 2 = two fragment fracture
−. −. −. 3 = three fragment fracture
−. −. −. 4 = four or more fragments.

APPLICATION OF THE METHOD
A comminuted mid-shaft fracture of the femur is shown in

Fig. 1.13a; this would be classified as 3.2.2.4 (3 = femur, 2 = shaft, 2 = 5–25% of the bone length, and 4 = more than 4 fragments).

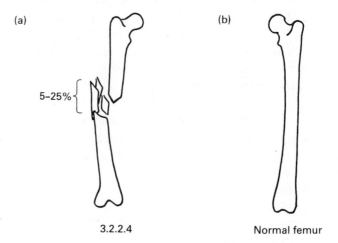

(a)

(b)

5–25%{

3.2.2.4

Normal femur

Fig. 1.13

For further information on this form of classification the reader is referred to Prieur *et al.* (1990).

FRACTURE HEALING

The use of radiographs in the assessment of fracture healing

Radiography is essential to supplement clinical assessment of fracture healing and the following routine examination is used:

A.P. (Fig. 1.14) and lateral (Fig. 1.15) views are taken preoperatively.

A.P. (Fig. 1.16) and lateral (Fig. 1.17) are taken postoperat-

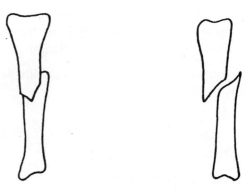

Fig. 1.14   **Fig. 1.15**

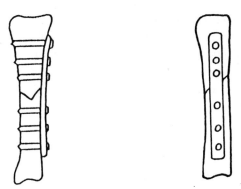

Fig. 1.16   Fig. 1.17

ively. When closed reduction is performed at least 50% of the fracture surfaces should be in contact if satisfactory healing is to occur (Fig. 1.18).

A.P. and lateral views are taken at 1 month.

A.P. and lateral views are taken at 2 months.

A.P. and lateral views are taken at 4 months when fracture healing is usually complete and implants can be removed as necessary (Figs 1.19, 1.20). For further information on implant removal see Table 1.1, page 9.

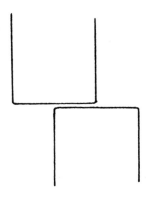

Fig. 1.18 Fifty per cent of fracture surface in contact.

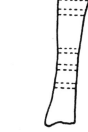

Fig. 1.19   Fig. 1.20

Normal fracture healing

The radiographic features of fracture healing are easy to follow, provided the normal sequence of events which occurs during healing is understood.

A fracture is primarily bridged by two advancing collars of cartilage and woven bone (callus) which arise from the osteogenic layers of the periosteum and the endosteum (see Figs 1.23, 1.24) (Ham & Harris 1956). In an unstable fracture the callus consists mainly of cartilage but in a stable fracture woven or immature bone predominates. The cartilage or woven bone is next invaded by capillaries headed by osteoclasts. At the same time osteoblasts lay down osteoid which matures to form bone, and collagen bundles are laid down in orderly lamellar fashion. In this way the initial scaffold of cartilage and woven bone which has stabilized the fracture is gradually replaced by mature lamellar bone. Remodelling by osteoclastic and osteoblastic activity is continued until the original shape of the bone is closely assumed again (Fig. 1.25). The final shape of the bone will conform to Wolff's law, i.e. 'that the internal architecture and external form of a bone are related to its function and change when the function is altered'.

Primary bone union

It is generally accepted that the function of callus is to stabilize the fragments and allow lamellar bone to grow and fill the fracture gap (Putnam & Pennock 1969); consequently, the size of the callus is related to the stability of the fracture (Hutzschemreuter *et al.* 1969), and usually the more unstable the fracture the greater the size of the callus. A completely stable fracture should therefore heal without callus formation; this situation was investigated experimentally by Muller (1963). He made a hole in a pig's radius and found that healing took place without the participation of either the periosteum or the endosteum, the defect being filled by direct ingrowth of cortical bone. This type of healing was called primary bone union.

Rigid immobilization of a fracture can be achieved by internal fixation and compression of the fracture site. The aim of compression treatment of fractures is to achieve primary bone union in which direct longitudinal reconstruction of the bone occurs without any radiologically visible periosteal or endosteal callus (Muller *et al.* 1970).

The rate of fracture healing

The rate of fracture healing is influenced by many factors.

The healing of fractures is more rapid in young animals; for example, in an immature dog union and remodelling of the fracture may be complete within 6 weeks, whereas in the mature dog it may be 4 months before remodelling is complete.

SPECIES OF ANIMAL
Clinically the rate of healing appears to vary with the species so that healing appears to be slower in horses and cattle than in cats and dogs, but this may well be due to the mechanical factors involved in that it is far easier to immobilize fractures in small animals than in large.

TYPE OF BONE INVOLVED
Cancellous bone has an abundant blood supply and heals more rapidly than compact bone. Consequently fractures involving metaphysis or the epiphysis of a bone heal faster than those of the diaphysis.

THE TYPE OF FRACTURE
Impacted fractures and long spiral or oblique fractures where the fracture surfaces are in close relation heal faster than those in which there is wide distraction of the fragments. Comminuted fractures, where there are multiple fragments, tend to heal more slowly because of inherent instability and disruption of blood supply to the fragments. Fracture healing is also delayed by the presence of infection.

Fracture healing time with different fixation devices
Brinker (1978) defined clinical union as that period in time during the recovery when fracture healing had progressed sufficiently for the fixation device to be removed. He produced a table giving the average anticipated healing time for simple fractures in dogs of different ages using different methods of fixation (Table 1.1).

Table 1.1 Time to reach clinical union (Brinker 1978.)

Age of animal	External fixation External fixator Intramedullary pin	Plate fixation
Under 3 months	2–3 weeks	4 weeks
3–6 months	4–6 weeks	2–3 months
6–12 months	5–8 weeks	3–5 months
Over 1 year	7–12 weeks	5 months–1 year

Radiographic changes during fracture healing
(Morgan 1972)
After reduction (Fig. 1.21) the first radiographic change at
the fracture site occurs at 10—14 days when the fracture
line becomes more distinct as a result of bone absorption
along the fracture edges (Fig. 1.22).

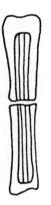   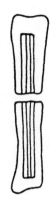

Fig. 1.21   Fig. 1.22

The initial callus is uncalcified and is therefore not visible
radiographically. The first reliable radiographic evidence
that bone healing has commenced is the appearance of
calcified periosteal callus (Fig. 1.23). Although the periosteal
callus tends to obscure the endosteal callus, radiographically
the endosteal callus contributes greatly to the disappearance
of the fracture line (Fig. 1.24).

The late radiographic signs of bony union are the restoration of the normal trabecular pattern which obscures the
original fracture line, and remodelling and restoration of the
continuity of the medullary cavity and cortex (Fig. 1.25).

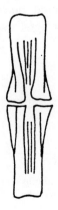   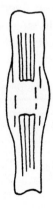   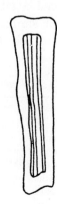

Fig. 1.23   Fig. 1.24   Fig. 1.25

These radiographic changes should be used to supplement clinical evidence of fracture union which may be briefly summarized as follows:

1 No pain on manipulation.

2 Stable fracture site.

3 Callus may be palpable depending on the method of fracture fixation.

COMPLICATIONS OF FRACTURE HEALING

The common complications of fracture healing include 'fracture disease', delayed and non-union, malunion, growth disturbances and osteomyelitis. *'Fracture disease'* is a term used by Muller (1963) to describe the syndrome of muscle wasting, joint stiffness and osteoporosis, which results from prolonged immobilization of a limb during the healing of a fracture. One of the important advantages of rigid internal fixation of a fracture is that early pain-free mobilization is possible and 'fracture disease' is avoided.

Delayed union and non-union

A frequent complication of fracture healing is delayed union. This is said to occur when a fracture has not healed in the time normally expected for that type of fracture. Delayed union may be superseded by the state of non-union, in which fracture healing stops and union will not occur without surgical intervention. The clinical signs of non-union include painful motion at the fracture site, progressive deformity, disuse of the limb and muscle atrophy. The causes of delayed and non-union are the same and are listed below.

1 Inadequate immobilization.

2 Gap between fragments due to:

  (a) Soft tissue interposition.

  (b) Malalignment of the fragments.

  (c) Distraction of the fragments by traction or the improper use of internal fixation devices.

3 Loss of blood supply by:

  (a) Damage to the nutrient vessels of the bone.

  (b) Excessive stripping or injury to the periosteum.

  (c) Severe comminution.

4 Infection.

5 General factors which delay wound healing.

The commonest cause of delayed union or non-union is inadequate immobilization of the fracture. Fracture healing will proceed in the presence of a certain amount of tension; a considerable amount of bending will also be tolerated but torsion or rotation impedes healing because it results in tearing of the fibroblastic network of the callus. The prime objective in the treatment of non-unions is to provide adequate fixation but this presupposes that bone is capable of a biological response. Accordingly, Weber and Cech (1976) have classified non-union fractures into two broad groups.

1 Biologically active or viable non-unions.

2 Biologically inactive or non-viable non-unions.

The biologically active group includes three types of non-union:

(a) The *hypertrophic type* is the commonest. This is seen as a complication of intramedullary pinning of humeral and femoral shaft fractures and is caused by rotation at the fracture site. Characteristically, a well-vascularized 'elephant-shaped' foot callus develops which does not bridge the fracture gap. The gap contains cartilage and fibrous tissue. There is sclerosis of the bone ends and later the medullary cavity becomes sealed (Fig. 1.26).

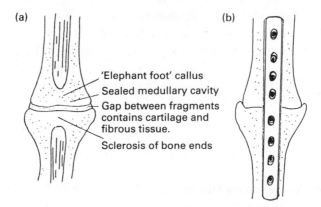

(a)

(b)

'Elephant foot' callus
Sealed medullary cavity
Gap between fragments contains cartilage and fibrous tissue.
Sclerosis of bone ends

Fig. 1.26

When this type of non-union is rigidly immobilized, preferably with a compression plate, then the cartilage and fibrous tissue in the gap between the bone ends rapidly ossifies (Fig. 1.26b). Therefore, unless there is malalignment of the fracture, it is not necessary to 'freshen up' the bone ends (see atrophic non-union, p. 14) or to use a bone graft to stimulate osteogenesis. An intramedullary pin, if still present, must of course be removed before application of a plate.

Other factors contributing to development of hypertrophic non-union are loose cerclage wire and/or sequestrae (necrotic bone fragments) at the fracture site (Fig. 1.27). The fracture must be opened to remove these; necrotic bone is quite distinct from normal bone, it is yellowish-white in appearance and the margins of the fragment tend to have a 'chewed out' appearance. Following the debridement of the fracture site, if the bone ends are uneven, it is generally worth cutting back the bone 2–3 mm with a saw to give two flat surfaces which can be apposed and compressed with a plate (Fig. 1.28). This gives optimal stability and the best chance for union to occur.

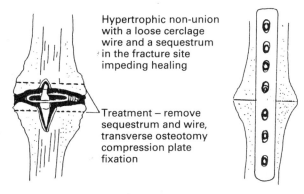

Hypertrophic non-union with a loose cerclage wire and a sequestrum in the fracture site impeding healing

Treatment – remove sequestrum and wire, transverse osteotomy compression plate fixation

Fig. 1.27   Fig. 1.28

(b) *Slightly hypertrophic type.* Instability following plate fixation may lead to this type of non-union in which there is minimal callus formation.

(c) *Oligotrophic type.* There is no callus formation and the fragments are usually widely separated and joined by fibrous tissue only. Failure to treat an avulsion fracture by internal fixation generally leads to an oligotrophic non-union.

All three types of biologically active non-union will usually heal provided rigid internal fixation is provided. The next group of non-unions, the biologically inactive or non-viable non-unions, are not so easy to deal with. There are four types:

1 The *dystrophic type* is seen as a complication of comminuted fractures where a poorly revascularized fragment or fragments impedes fracture healing.

2 The *necrotic type* is also seen in comminuted or infected fractures where non-viable fragments or sequestrae at the fracture site impede healing.

3 The *defect type.* Here a major defect in the bone caused by removal of fragments or sequestrae is too big to be bridged by the normal healing process.

4 The *atrophic type*. This is the commonest and most difficult type of non-union to deal with. It is seen as a complication of fractures of the radius and ulna in Toy Poodles and miniature breeds of dog. There is instability at the fracture site with loss of osteogenic activity, osteoporosis and eventually osteolysis (Fig. 1.29). Shearing forces

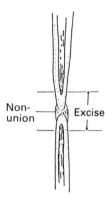

Fig. 1.29 Atrophic non-union.

at the fracture site (Sumner-Smith & Cawley 1970) are thought to predispose to the non-union of the radius and ulna and these occur if inadequate immobilization is achieved with a plaster cast. (Unless the cast is tight-fitting and extends from the foot to above the elbow, the dog is still able to rotate the upper forearm in the cast, causing shearing forces at the fracture site.) It is recommended that fresh fractures of the radius and ulna in toy and miniature breeds are treated by plate fixation whenever possible to avoid non-union and the ASIF mini-compression plates (Straumann Great Britain Ltd) are ideal for this purpose.

The prime objective in treating avascular non-unions is to stimulate osteogenesis. The fracture site is exposed, cartilage and fibrous tissue are excised and the bone ends are 'freshened up' by cutting back the bone 1−2 mm (Fig. 1.30). The fracture is stabilized with a plate and a cancellous bone graft is taken from the proximal humerus and packed around the fracture site to stimulate osteogenesis. If, despite these measures, non-union of the radius and ulna persists, then repeat operations are rarely successful in giving union and amputation should be considered.

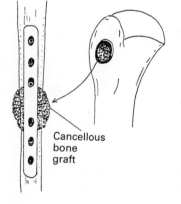

Cancellous
bone
graft

Fig. 1.30

Malunion
Malunion is defined as a fracture that has healed or is healing in an abnormal position. Causes are improper reduction and/or immobilization during healing (see radius and ulna fracture complications, p. 259).

Growth disturbance

Trauma to a growth plate with or without fracture may cause premature closure and result in shortening of the limb or angular deformity (see radius and ulna fracture complications).

OPEN (COMPOUND) FRACTURES AND OSTEOMYELITIS

An open fracture is one in which there is a communication between the fracture site and a skin wound. Open fractures may be classified as first, second or third degree according to the severity of tissue injury and contamination (Fig. 1.31a, b and c).

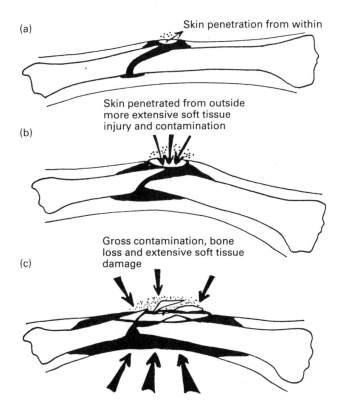

(a) Skin penetration from within

(b) Skin penetrated from outside more extensive soft tissue injury and contamination

(c) Gross contamination, bone loss and extensive soft tissue damage

Fig. 1.31 Open fractures: (a) 1st degree; (b) 2nd degree; (c) 3rd degree;

Basic principles of treatment of open fractures

Normal periosteum provides bone with an adequate defence against invading organisms, but when this protection is removed as a result of a fracture or surgery then the bone becomes extremely susceptible to infection (Peacock & Van Winkle 1970). The *ideal* treatment of open fractures should therefore be aimed at restoring the continuity of the periosteum and protecting it so that it may in turn defend the bone against infection; this can be achieved by perfect open reduction, rigid internal fixation, debridement and wide excision of the wound, followed by primary closure of the soft tissue.

Primary bacterial contamination occurs in only about a third of open fractures; any necrotic tissue which is left in the wound serves as a nidus for bacterial multiplication. Secondary bacterial infection of the wound occurs after 6–8 hours (Muller *et al.* 1970). Although the ideal method of treatment of compound fractures has been mentioned, there are risks, especially when metal implants are used in a potentially infected bone and so the cautious surgeon will vary the ideal method as necessary.

When the open fracture is less than 6–8 hours old, there is minimal soft tissue damage and no gross contamination of the wound with foreign material (first and second degree open fractures), then the wound may be safely excised and sutured. The fracture can be treated by internal fixation or external fixation at this stage depending on its location and type. If internal fixation is used the reduction of the fracture is best made through a clean surgical incision at some distance from the wound.

When an open fracture is over 8 hours old or there is gross contamination or soft tissue damage (third degree open fracture), then, following a thorough debridement and excision, the wound is left open and covered with a protective bandage. External fixation, or a Kirschner splint (see Fig. 1.31d–f, p. 18), is used to stabilize the fracture until union is complete, or internal fixation is subsequently carried out between 1 and 3 weeks provided that the original wound is healing with no evidence of infection. Open reduction and internal fixation is again carried out through a fresh surgical incision through healthy tissue. Primary internal fixation may be occasionally necessary in this second category of open fractures; if so, installation of a drainage tube is useful as it will allow continual drainage and also direct irrigation of the fracture site with the appropriate antibiotic solution. Irrigation drainage is maintained for a week post-operatively. Whatever method is used, parenteral antibiotic cover should be given.

Antibiotics and practical management of open fractures
(Fig. 1.31a–f)
Open fractures are regarded as contaminated and therefore

potentially infected. Second and third degree open fractures are more likely to become infected. These injuries should be treated as an emergency. In the first aid management the wound should be covered with a sterile dressing, a pressure bandage applied and external coaptation used where possible. Radiographs are taken to assess the extent of the fracture and decisions made on method of fixation that will be used.

Wound infection is eliminated by wound cleansing and debridement and prompt antibiotic therapy. Systemic administration of antibiotics is essential to achieve adequate concentrations in the fracture haematoma; the antibiotic is given initially as a single intravenous bolus as soon as possible after the injury (hours) to prevent bacterial proliferation. Swabs should be taken from the wound first for culture and sensitivity examination. The most commonly used antibiotic is a cephalosporin (Ceporex, Glaxo, 10 mg/kg twice daily); this antibiotic is bactericidal, broad spectrum, especially useful for staphylococcal infections and it achieves good levels in muscle and bone. The incidence of Gram-negative infections is higher in second and third degree open fractures and here a cephalosporin can be combined with an aminoglycoside, e.g. gentamicin (Gentovet, Arnolds, 2−5 mg/kg body weight/day divided into three equal doses).

Antibiotics are no substitute for inadequate wound debridement. In the preparation room any protective wound dressing is removed and swabs are taken from the wound for aerobic and anaerobic culture. K-Y Jelly (Johnson & Johnson) is applied to the wound surfaces to prevent contamination with hair and debris while the surrounding skin is clipped and the whole area prepared aseptically with dilute iodine solution (Betadine Surgical Scrub, Napp Laboratories). Gross debris is removed from the wound and initial lavage carried out by flushing the wound surfaces using lactated Ringer's solution (Hartmann's solution) and a syringe. The dog is then transferred to the operating theatre and sterile drapes are applied around the wound. Irrigation of the wound is continued with copious amounts of fluid. Water Pik-type cleansing is useful but if the system is not available a large syringe can be used to flush out the wound. Final irrigation can be done using an antibacterial solution, neomycin−polymyxin bacitracin solution (1 g neomycin, 500 000 units polymyxin, and 50 000 units bacitracin per litre of Ringer's solution); alternatively the wound can be irrigated with dilute povidone iodine (1 in 10). All non-viable tissue should be removed from the wound (if the tissue bleeds it is viable!). All large bone fragments which can be rigidly fixed (lag screw) should remain but smaller fragments which cannot be fixed, especially those which have lost their soft tissue attachments, are removed. The fracture should then be rigidly stabilized and as a general rule the safest way of doing this is by the use of an external fixator, placing the pins in healthy bone at some distance from the fracture site (Figs 1.31d, e, f). Primary wound closure should be avoided if the wound is over 6–8 hours old as this causes a significant rise in infection rates. Instead the wound is left open and protected with a bandage. Once the wound appears to be filling with healthy granulation tissue and is no longer discharging then closure can be safely undertaken. Alternatively the wound may be left to heal by second intention.

Prolonged antibiotic cover does not appear to reduce wound infection rates and consequently antibiotics are usually given for 5 days only following primary or secondary wound closure.

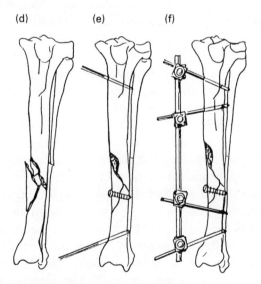

Fig. 1.31 (d) open fracture of the tibia (2nd degree); (e) wound debrided, small fragment removed, large fragment fixed with a lag screw; (f) external fixator used to stabilize the fracture.

Gas gangrene

Gas gangrene due to *Clostridium welchii* is an occasional complication of open fractures. Three cases were described by Denny *et al.* (1974). Two farm dogs sustained open femoral fractures; in each case the affected leg was grossly enlarged with emphysematous crackling evident on palpation. A marked elevation in body temperature was noted, maximum 106°F. Radiographic examination revealed pockets of gas in the soft tissues around the fracture site (Fig. 1.31g). In each case the soft tissues over the lateral side of the fracture was incised to allow drainage of large quantities of foul smelling purulent fluid. Pus, necrotic muscle and bone fragments were removed, and *Clostridium welchii* was cultured from the wound. The wound was irrigated with saline and crystalline penicillin and a drainage tube inserted prior to wound closure. The fracture site was irrigated with a solution of crystalline penicillin in saline twice daily for 5 days post-operatively and antibiotic cover with streptomycin and penicillin (Streptopen, Glaxo) was given during this period. The dogs' temperatures fell to normal within 3 days, drains were removed at 5 days and the fractures plated on the sixth day. Healing was uneventful in both cases.

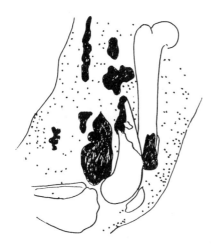

Fig. 1.31g Open fracture complicated by gas gangrene, pockets of gas (black shading) lie in the soft tissues around the fracture site.

Osteomyelitis

Osteomyelitis does however occur as a complication of open fractures and puncture wounds (Hickman 1967), and also unfortunately as one of the most common complications following the surgical treatment of fractures (Vaughan 1975). Organisms most frequently isolated from the infected bone in dogs include species of *Staphylococcus*, *Streptococcus*,

Pasteurella, Pseudomonas, Proteus and coliforms (Vaughan 1975).

Haematogenous spread of infection is rare; it may be seen in young animals when infection localizes in a damaged area of bone (usually the metaphysis) during the course of a bacteraemia.

When the focus of infection is within the medullary cavity there is rapid spread throughout it, pus penetrates the cortex, underruns the periosteum, breaks out and escapes through sinuses in the skin. Areas of cortical bone may lose their blood supply and become necrotic. The necrotic area of bone gradually separates as a sequestrum and becomes walled off by fibrous tissue and an area of dense new bone which is called an involucrum. Infection of the medullary cavity is known as osteomyelitis whereas localized infection of the periosteum or cortical bone are respectively known as periostitis and osteitis.

The clinical signs of osteomyelitis include soft tissue swelling, pain, sinus formation and intermittent pyrexia. Radiographic examination reveals areas of rarefaction in the bone, particularly in the metaphyses or around the metal implants such as pins, screws or plates which may have been used to stabilize a fracture (Fig. 1.32). Later there is periosteal new bone formation and if a sequestrum develops this will appear as an area of increased density in the bone surrounded by a zone of decreased density or osteolysis (Fig. 1.33).

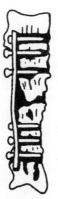
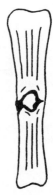

Fig. 1.32   Fig. 1.33

Low grade infection may be controlled by the administration of the appropriate antibiotic as determined by culture and sensitivity examination. Therapy should be continued for at least 3 weeks. In established cases of osteomyelitis adequate drainage must be provided and all sequestrae, necrotic bone and where necessary, metallic implants removed. Irrigation drainage is usually maintained for a week post-operatively.

Although infection delays healing of fractures union will occur provided the fracture is stable (Muller *et al.* 1970). Fractures complicated by osteomyelitis and non-union are best treated by thorough debridement of the infected bone followed by rigid immobilization of the fracture preferably with a plate (Vaughan 1975). Where there is active infection treatment can be carried out in two stages; firstly sequestrae and implants are removed and the appropriate antibiotic given for 7–10 days. At the second operation debridement is completed and the fracture stabilized with a plate. Large defects in the bone may be filled with a graft of chips of autogenous cancellous bone. Irrigation drainage of the fracture site is advisable in conjunction with a prolonged course of antibiotic therapy. Drains are not used if cancellous bone grafts have been inserted.

SELECTION OF ANTIBIOTICS IN THE
TREATMENT OF OSTEOMYELITIS

In cases of acute osteomyelitis following fracture repair there is usually drainage from the incision while in chronic cases sinus formation occurs. Swabs should be taken from the purulent discharge or from fluid aspirated from the fracture site. These are submitted for culture and sensitivity examination. While the results are awaited parenteral administration of a cephalosporin either alone or in combination with an aminoglycoside, e.g. gentamicin, is commenced. Two other antibiotics which are widely used in the treatment of osteomyelitis include clindamycin (Antirobe, Upjohn, 11 mg/kg body weight every 12 hours for a minimum of 28 days) and lincomycin (Lincocin, Upjohn, 11 mg/kg once every 12 hours). Clindamycin has a much wider spectrum of activity against both Gram-negative and Gram-positive organisms; lincomycin by comparison is not effective against Gram-negative organisms.

Once the appropriate antibiotic has been selected by culture and sensitivity examination then treatment should be continued for at least 3 weeks.

Pseudomonas infections can be treated with anti-pseudomonal penicillins such as carbenicillin and ticarcillin. These are relatively non-toxic compared with aminoglycosides such as gentamicin (ototoxic and nephrotoxic) and the peptides, polymyxin B and polymyxin E which are nephrotoxic and neurotoxic.

Gentamicin is a useful drug for the treatment of bone

infections which are resistant to other antibiotics. However gentamicin can only be given systemically for short periods because of its ototoxic and nephrotoxic side effects. This problem can be overcome by the use of polymethylmethacrylate beads impregnated with gentamicin (E. Merck in collaboration with Kultzer & Co.). A string of beads is implanted into the infected fracture site where they slowly release gentamicin creating a local concentration of the antibiotic with no undesirable systemic toxic effects. The beads are removed 2–3 weeks later.

BONE GRAFTS

Bone grafts are used to promote fracture healing in delayed union and non-union, to fill defects in bone resulting from fractures, osteomyelitis, cysts or tumours and they also have an important role in the arthrodesis of joints. The relevant literature on bone and cartilage transplantation was reviewed by Brown and Cruess (1982).

Bone grafts heal by a process of 'creeping substitution' (Ham & Leeson 1961). Most of the transplanted cells die and are gradually replaced by mesenchymal cells from the host bed which differentiate to form osteoblasts and osteoclasts. This process occurs more rapidly within the relatively porous structure of cancellous bone.

It is generally agreed that the healing process is most rapid when autogenous grafts are used, but although there is a delay in the healing rate of homogeneous grafts this is not significant enough to affect their use clinically (Vaughan 1972). Heterogeneous bone, however, is far less readily incorporated into the host site.

Bone grafts serve three main functions: they provide a scaffold in which new bone can be laid down, they provide a local source of calcium and minerals, and they cause increased osteogenesis because of their nature or by osseous metaplasia of the surrounding connective tissue.

There is considerable clinical and some experimental evidence that fresh autogenous cancellous bone grafts promote fracture healing, and this is probably due to the inductive properties of the matrix of the graft rather than the provision of cells with osteoblastic activity (Peacock & Van Winkle 1970). Cancellous bone grafts also 'survive well' in the presence of infection and are useful to promote healing of fractures complicated by osteomyelitis.

Cortical bone grafts possess rigidity and strength and can be used like a bone plate to restore the continuity of a bone. This type of graft acts purely as a scaffold and is gradually replaced by bone from the recipient site. Rigid immobilization of the graft is essential during this healing process. Cortical grafts seldom survive in the presence of infection and are rejected as sequestra.

Autografts

Autografts (bone transferred from one site to another in the same animal) of cancellous bone are rapidly vascularized and accepted at the recipient site even in the presence of infection. An autogenous cancellous bone graft stimulates bone formation through the transfer of viable bone cells and by the induction of osteogenesis at the recipient bed.

Sites commonly used for the collection of autogenous cancellous bone include the proximal humerus, the proximal femur, the proximal tibia and the crest of the ilium. Ideally the site of collection should be in the same leg as the recipient site. The proximal humerus is the most easily accessible and provides the largest quantities of cancellous bone.

A vertical skin incision is made directly over the lateral aspect of the greater tuberosity and extended down to the underlying bone. Using an orthopaedic hammer and gouge or chisel, a window is cut through the cortex (Fig. 1.34a). The gouge is used to loosen the underlying cancellous bone which is then scooped out with a curette and collected in a dry container. The graft should be transferred to the recipient site as soon as possible after collection. It is packed into a bone defect or around a fracture site and retained in position by careful suturing of the adjacent soft tissues.

Cancellous bone grafts taken from the proximal humerus are used most frequently in the following operations:

1 To stimulate osteogenesis in oligotrophic and atrophic non-union (Weber & Cech 1982). These types of non-union are a common complication of fractures of the radius and ulna in Toy Poodles and other miniature breeds of dog (Sumner-Smith & Cawley 1970). Cartilage and fibrous tissue at the fracture site is excised and the bone ends are cut back (Fig. 1.34b). Ideally, fixation should be achieved with a mini ASIF compression plate (Straumann Great Britain Ltd). A cancellous bone graft is packed around the fracture site and held in place by the surrounding soft tissues.

2 Cancellous bone grafts are essential for the successful early arthrodesis of the carpus and other joints (Vaughan 1972; Johnson 1980). After removal of the articular cartilage,

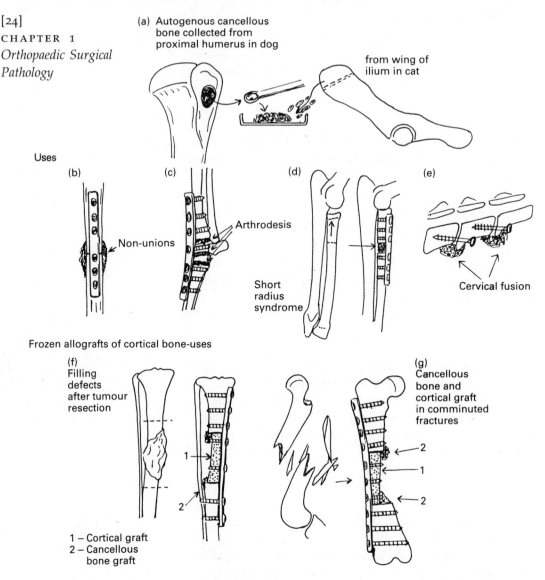

(a) Autogenous cancellous
bone collected from
proximal humerus in dog

from wing of
ilium in cat

Uses

(b)

Non-unions

(c)

Arthrodesis

(d)

Short
radius
syndrome

(e)

Cervical fusion

Frozen allografts of cortical bone-uses

(f)
Filling
defects
after tumour
resection

1
2

1 – Cortical graft
2 – Cancellous
bone graft

(g)
Cancellous
bone and
cortical graft
in comminuted
fractures

2
1
2

Fig. 1.34a–g

the joint spaces are packed with cancellous bone and rigid fixation is achieved with a plate. Once there is radiographic evidence of bone union across the joint spaces, the plate can be removed (Fig. 1.34c).

3 Bone grafts play a part in the treatment of growth disturbances caused by premature closure of the distal radial growth plate. Closure results in a short radius, an increase in the humeroradial joint space and elbow instability (Clayton-Jones & Vaughan 1970). In such cases, the radius can be lengthened by transverse osteotomy to allow the radial head to be moved proximally. Fixation is achieved with a plate and the defect in the radius is filled with a cancellous bone graft (Fig. 1.34d).

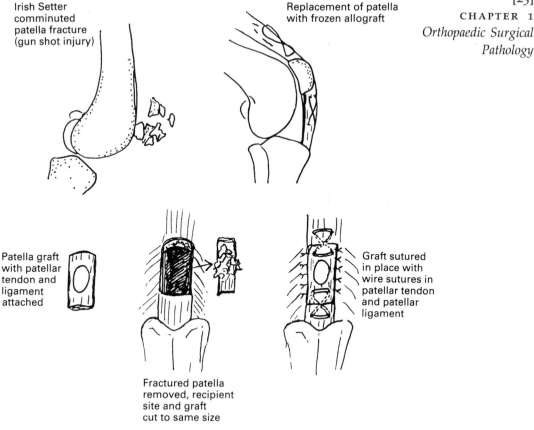

Irish Setter
comminuted
patella fracture
(gun shot injury)

Replacement of patella
with frozen allograft

Patella graft
with patellar
tendon and
ligament
attached

Fractured patella
removed, recipient
site and graft
cut to same size

Graft sutured
in place with
wire sutures in
patellar tendon
and patellar
ligament

Fig. 1.34h

4 The proximal humerus is a convenient site for collection of cancellous bone for cervical fusion. The main indication for the operation is treatment of cervical spondylopathy (canine wobbler syndrome) when cord compression is caused by vertebral instability. A wide disc fenestration is carried out between each unstable vertebra and lag screws are placed across the vertebral bodies. A cancellous bone graft is packed over the ventral aspect of the intervertebral disc spaces and held in place by closure of the longus colli muscle. The graft proliferates causing cervical fusion within 3 months (Fig. 1.34e).

Autogenous cortical bone grafts provide structural support but are more slowly incorporated at the recipient site than cancellous grafts. Most of the graft dies and is gradually removed and replaced by bone from the recipient site.

Allografts

A disadvantage of using autogenous cortical bone grafts is that two operations have to be performed on the same animal. The problem can be overcome simply by the use of allografts (bone from another animal of the same species). Although the allograft provokes an immunological response this does not prevent incorporation of the graft at the recipient site. The allograft dies and is gradually replaced. The cortical allograft does not provide cells which are capable of new bone formation, but allografts of cancellous bone will induce osteogenesis at the recipient site. Although there is a delay in the incorporation of allografts compared with autogenous grafts, this delay is not significant enough to affect the use of allografts in clinical cases. Thompson & Cocoon (1970) showed that there was little difference between the healing time using viable and frozen allografts, and it is probable that antigenicity of the graft is decreased by freezing.

Allografts of cancellous, cortical or corticocancellous bone can be collected from a donor animal immediately after euthanasia. The bone must be collected under conditions of strict asepsis and freed from periosteum and soft tissue. Bone stored in sterile containers at −20°C can be kept for years. The author has successfully used bone grafts which have been stored for between 1 and 3 years. If a large bone defect is to be filled then a tubular or hemicylindrical corticocancellous allograft taken from the metaphyseal region should be used. The graft consists mainly of cancellous bone which is rapidly vascularized while the thin layer of cortical bone provides structural support. This type of graft is more readily vascularized than a graft of compact bone taken from the diaphysis.

The frozen graft is allowed to thaw at room temperature for approximately 30 minutes before being inserted at the recipient site. If a cortical or corticocancellous graft is being used to bridge a defect, then it must be rigidly immobilized, preferably with a compression plate. In addition, some autogenous cancellous bone should be collected and packed around the proximal and distal ends of the graft as this will speed up its incorporation in the recipient site (Bacher & Schmidt 1980; Alexander 1983). Figures 1.34f, 1.34g illustrate the use of corticocancellous allografts to fill (a) a defect resulting from excision of a benign bone tumour and (b) a large defect in bone resulting from a severely comminuted fracture.

Extensive research has been carried out in the field of cartilage and joint transplantation. Fresh and frozen osteocartilaginous allografts tend to undergo extensive degeneration with destruction of cartilage which is thought to be due to lack of revascularization. Shell grafts consisting of articular cartilage and a relatively thin layer of subchondral bone stand a better chance of being revascularized. This type of graft may have a clinical application in the treatment of osteochondritis dissecans of the stifle when there has been extensive loss of articular cartilage.

The largest component of a joint which has been successfully transplanted without microvascular anastomosis is the patella (Vaughan & Formston 1973). Experimental studies have shown that patella allografts are completely revascularized and remodelled without serious anatomical deformity and limb function remains normal. Patellar transplantation provides an alternative to patellectomy in the management of severely comminuted fractures (Fig. 1.34h).

Bone grafts in cats
The basic principles of collection, storage and use of bone grafts in the cat are very similar to the dog. In the cat, however, collection of autogenous cancellous bone from the proximal humerus, femur or tibia may prove frustrating as only small quantities of cancellous bone can be obtained especially in adult cats. The crest of the ilium provides a much more satisfactory site for collection and the bone can be used either as a flat piece or it is cut into small pieces which are packed into the recipient site. If large defects have to be bridged with a bone graft then frozen allografts of cortical or corticocancellous bone are used.

CONCLUSION
In conclusion, the veterinary orthopaedic surgeon can use bone grafts in a wide variety of techniques. Fresh autogenous cancellous bone grafts should be used to stimulate bone formation while frozen cortical or corticocancellous bone allografts provide an excellent scaffold in reconstructive bone surgery.

NUTRITIONAL DISORDERS OF BONE
(Bennett 1976)

An adequate dietary intake of calcium, phosphorus and vitamin D is needed for the development and maintenance of normal bone. The requirements for dogs have been estimated (Krook 1971) as:

1 Calcium 265 mg/kg body weight/day.
2 Phosphorus 220 mg/kg body weight/day.
3 Vitamin D 7 iu/kg body weight/day.

These figures apply to adult dogs; puppies need twice this intake. It is important to feed the correct ratio of calcium to phosphorus otherwise a relative deficiency of one or other occurs. The calcium to phosphorus ratio should be 1:1. In most diets there tends to be an excess of phosphorus—for example in meat the ratio of phosphorus to calcium is 20:1. A diet of meat and water rapidly leads to calcium deficiency but carnivores in the wild avoid this problem by eating the bones of their victims which are a natural balanced source of calcium and phosphorus. The growing puppy will need about 50% meat in the diet initially which is gradually reduced to 30–40%—the rest is made up with carbohydrate and vegetable. If the puppy is receiving a balanced diet, the natural way of supplementing calcium and phosphorus is to give milk and bone meal. The latter is given at a rate of 15–20 g/kg dry weight of food (Abrams 1962). It should be stressed however, that bone meal will not correct an abnormal dietary calcium: phosphorus ratio. If the puppy is calcium deficient, then calcium lactate is given (available in 300 mg tablets—Evans).

Vitamin D is needed for the absorption of calcium from the bowel. Natural sources of the vitamin are meat, milk, eggs and sunlight. Supplements are given as necessary as cod liver oil capsules (5 ml cod liver oil/10 kg body weight for daily growth).

Dietary requirements in cats
(From *Nutrient Requirements of Cats* 1986)
The cat is a carnivore and as such its nutritional requirements differ from the dog which is an omnivore. The specialized carnivorous metabolism of the cat has resulted in some nutrients which are derived from animal tissue being essential for cats but not for dogs. The cat has insignificant or limited ability to synthesize nutrients such as vitamin A, arachidonic acid, arginine, taurine and niacin, but its specialized metabolism allows consumption of high protein meals at all times and consequently a higher protein intake is required than in dogs.

The cat is born with small stores of calcium and requires 200–400 mg calcium per day (6–8 g/kg diet) for good bone development. The ratio of calcium to phosphorus is important for both absorption and utilization of these minerals. The calcium:phosphorus ratio should be in the range 0.9:1 to 1.1:1. In the growing kitten dietary concentrations of 8 g calcium/kg and 6 g phosphorus/kg are recommended. Vitamin D is involved in the metabolism of calcium and phosphorus and for kittens the minimal requirement should be provided by 500 iu (12.5 pg) of vitamin D per kg diet.

Nutritional secondary hyperparathyroidism ('all meat syndrome', juvenile osteoporosis, osteogenesis imperfecta)
Nutritional secondary hyperparathyroidism results from calcium deficiency, either due to lack of dietary calcium or a relative deficiency due to excess dietary phosphorus. The condition is seen most frequently in puppies and kittens fed on all meat diets, in which calcium levels are low and phosphorus levels are high. Other causes are: inability to absorb or utilize dietary calcium (true osteogenesis imperfecta) which is seen in some lines of German Shepherd puppies, or reduced availability of dietary calcium as in vitamin D deficiency or renal insufficiency.

Calcium deficiency causes hypocalcaemia and parathyroid hormone release. Calcium is resorbed from the skeleton to maintain normal blood calcium levels (9–12 mg/100 ml serum). Clinical features of the condition include lameness, pain, difficulty in standing, bone deformity and pathological fractures. The fractures tend to involve the spine and hind limbs. Radiographic examination reveals generalized loss of bone density, thin cortices and pathological fractures.

TREATMENT
Obviously the meat-rich diet should be terminated and substituted with a nutritionally balanced diet supplemented with calcium lactate. Analgesics are given as necessary to control pain. Vitamin D supplementation should be avoided, especially in the early stages of treatment because it promotes further bone absorption and may aggravate the condition. Severely affected puppies, particularly those which are paraplegic or those with several pathological fractures, should be destroyed on humane grounds.

Hypertrophic osteodystrophy
(skeletal scurvy, Barlow's disease)
Hypertrophic osteodystrophy is seen in the larger breeds of dog between 4 and 6 months of age. The aetiology of the condition is uncertain but it tends to be seen in rapidly growing puppies that are having excessive vitamin and mineral supplements. Vitamin C deficiency has also been suggested as a cause but although vitamin C has proved useful in treatment it should be realized that dogs are capable of synthesizing their own vitamin C.

CLINICAL SIGNS

The metaphyses of the long bones, especially the distal radius and distal tibia, become enlarged, warm and painful. Affected animals are reluctant to move and an intermittent high fever is often noted. The radiographic changes associated with hypertrophic osteodystrophy are summarized in Fig. 1.35a.

Most animals recover in 1—2 months provided strict rest is given, the excess vitamin and mineral supplements are curtailed and a light diet is given. Campbell (1964) has found the administration of vitamin C (oral dose 0.5—1 g/day) useful in the treatment. Analgesics and anti-inflammatory drugs are used to relieve pain and pyrexia. Although dogs may have a complete remission of clinical signs, relapses do occasionally occur during the remaining growth period.

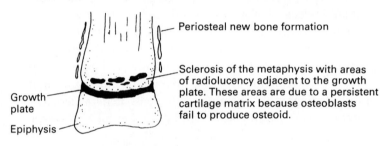

Periosteal new bone formation

Sclerosis of the metaphysis with areas of radiolucency adjacent to the growth plate. These areas are due to a persistent cartilage matrix because osteoblasts fail to produce osteoid.

Growth plate

Epiphysis

Fig. 1.35a Hypertrophic osteodystrophy.

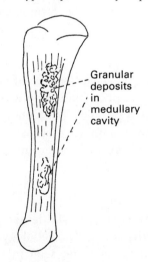

Granular deposits in medullary cavity

Fig. 1.35b Panosteitis.

Rickets (Campbell 1964)

Rickets is a name which is often loosely and wrongly used to describe nutritional bone disorders in young dogs and cats. Clinically, the disease is now very rare. It probably results from a dietary deficiency of vitamin D, calcium and/or phosphorus. Vitamin D deficiency results in a cartilage matrix that is highly stable and does not calcify. In young animals this results in thickened and irregular growth plates, mushrooming of the metaphyses, softening and bending of bones.

OTHER BONE DISEASES

Eosinophilic panosteitis (Bohning *et al*. 1970)
Although panosteitis is commonly seen in the United States, it is rare in this country (Tandy 1977). It affects the long bones of large breeds of dog, especially the German Shepherd. Lameness is sudden in onset, may last a few days or several weeks and tends to shift from leg to leg. The recurring bouts of lameness usually subside by the time the dog reaches 2 years of age. There is pain on palpation of affected bones and, on X-ray, granular deposits or sclerotic areas are seen in the medullary cavity (Fig. 1.35b). Treatment is symptomatic, analgesics or corticosteroids being given to relieve pain.

Hypertrophic pulmonary osteopathy (HPOA; Alexander *et al*. 1965)
Hypertrophic pulmonary osteopathy is seen as a complication of chronic pulmonary disease and results in periosteal proliferation. It is most frequently associated with pulmonary neoplasia. The distal parts of the limb become swollen and painful and there is obvious lameness. The classical radiographic signs consist of extensive, rough periosteal new bone formation beginning on the distal phalanges, metacarpal bones and metatarsal bones. Other bones may become involved. If the primary lesion in the lung can be removed, regression of symptoms will occur. Generally, however, treatment is not feasible.

Craniomandibular osteopathy (Riser *et al*. 1967)
This condition is seen particularly in West Highland Terriers and this has led to the name 'Westie's Disease'. Other Terrier breeds are also susceptible. The cause is not known but the lesion is essentially a periostitis with new bone formation on the ventral borders of the horizontal mandibular rami and around the tympanic bullae. There is obvious swelling of the jaws, inappetence, lethargy and pyrexia. Symptoms become apparent between 3 and 6 months of age. Puppies will show pain on palpation of the mandible

or on opening the jaws. The condition tends to run an undulant course and regress at about 1 year of age. Corticosteroids generally provide effective relief from symptoms.

Renal secondary hyperparathyroidism

Renal insufficiency with a reduction in glomerular filtration rate may cause retention of phosphorus with a reduction in blood calcium leading to hyperparathyroidism. Parathyroid hormone release causes osteoclastic resorption of bone to boost serum calcium levels. The process of demineralization affects all bones but the skull, particularly the mandible and maxilla are affected first. The mandible feels soft and 'rubbery'. The teeth are often loose and excessive salivation may be noted. Softening of the maxilla can result in respiratory obstruction. Radiographic examination of the skull shows demineralization but the teeth are very prominent because of loss of density of the surrounding bone. The aim of treatment is to correct renal function.

Dwarfism in dogs

Proportionate dwarfism is actively selected for in the establishment of miniature breeds of dog such as the Dachshund, Bulldog and Basset hound. There are few reports of true pathological skeletal dysplasias causing dwarfism in the dog, and these were reviewed by Whitbread *et al.* in 1983. The majority of reports concern the miniature poodle, but skeletal dysplasias have also been recorded in the Alaskan Malamute, Beagle and English Pointer. In the English Pointer the condition is described as an enchondrodystrophy with changes both in growth plate cartilage leading to dwarfism and articular cartilage causing lameness. In this breed there is a homozygous recessive mode of inheritance (Whitbread *et al.* 1983).

Hypervitaminosis A (feline osteodystrophy; Seawright *et al.* 1967; Clarke *et al.* 1970)

Vitamin A is necessary for normal enchondral ossification. However when the dietary intake of vitamin A is excessive, as in cats fed on large amounts of raw liver, then periosteal new bone formation occurs. The condition is seen most often in cats between 2 and 4 years of age. There is often evidence of spinal stiffness particularly in the cervical region and the cat may be lame or reluctant to move. In immature animals growth may be retarded. Radiographic examination in typical cases shows extensive new bone formation in the cervical and thoracic region with exostoses causing fusion of the vertebrae and spinous processes. New bone formation is often seen at the metaphyses of long bones and around joints. Treatment involves correcting the diet and eliminating the source of vitamin A. This will halt progression of the condition and there is usually some clinical improvement within a few weeks, however, exostoses and joint lesions remain. If lameness is a problem then treatment with prednisolone is helpful especially in cases which are identified early.

Osteopetrosis

Osteopetrosis, 'marble bone', is a term used to describe a generalized increase in skeletal mass (Marks 1984). In osteopetrotic bone there is a marked endosteal thickening of the cortex with irregular dense structures within the medullary cavity. The subchondral bone is extremely dense and cancellous bone structures are no longer visible.

Congenital osteopetrosis has been described in dogs and is reported to cause anaemia (Riser & Frankhauser 1970; Lees & Sautter 1979). Two cases have been described in adult cats (Kramers *et al.* 1988) and one of these developed anaemia.

Feline leukaemia virus-induced medullary sclerosis has also been reported in experimental kittens (Hoover & Kociba 1974).

BONE TUMOURS

Bone tumours in the dog can be classified as follows:

Benign bone tumours
Osteoma.
Osteochondroma.
Enchondroma.
Benign chondroblastoma.
Osteoclastoma.
Bone cyst.
Non-ossifying fibroma.

Malignant bone tumours
Osteosarcoma.
Chondrosarcoma.
Fibrosarcoma.
Malignant giant cell tumour.

Allied malignant lesions of bone
Reticulum cell sarcoma.
Multiple myeloma.
Haemangiosarcoma.
Haemopericytoma.

Metastatic bone tumours

OSTEOSARCOMA

It is important for the orthopaedic surgeon to be able to differentiate between benign and malignant bone tumours. Unfortunately the majority of bone tumours encountered in the dog are malignant and the osteosarcoma accounts for 80% of tumours of the skeletal system. Benign bone tumours and also metastatic bone tumours are uncommon in animals. Osteosarcomas are found in the large and giant breeds of dog and it is generally the older animal that is affected but cases have been recorded in dogs as young as 1 year of age. The primary tumour is usually found in the metaphyseal region of a long bone and the predilection sites are the proximal humerus, the distal radius, the distal femur and the proximal tibia, but any part of the skeleton can be affected. The tumour presents as a hard, often painful swelling. The radiographic changes associated with osteosarcomas have been described by Morgan (1972) and Gibbs *et al.* (1984) (see Figs 1.35c, d, e). These include destruction of cortical bone, growth of the tumour beyond the original confines of the bone development of a tumour mass that may become ossified or may contain calcified material. Osteosarcomas appear radiographically to be one of three types:
1 osteoblastic
2 osteoclastic, which is slightly more common, and
3 a mixture of osteoblastic and osteoclastic.

Approximately 50% of osteosarcomas give rise to a 'sunburst' effect which is a reaction of the periosteum to produce radiating spicules of new bone.

Osteosarcomas seldom invade joint spaces or adjacent bones. However, changes due to pressure deformity and periosteal reaction may be seen on radiographs. Osteosarcomas rarely follow trauma and it is probably coincidental that a tumour develops at an old fracture site.

Early radiographic diagnosis of osteosarcoma is not always easy. If there is any doubt about the radiographic diagnosis then the examination should be repeated approximately 4 weeks later when typical changes associated with the tumour should have become apparent.

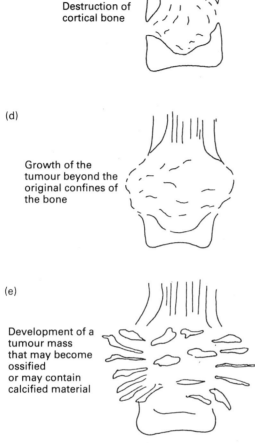

(c)

Destruction of
cortical bone

(d)

Growth of the
tumour beyond the
original confines of
the bone

(e)

Development of a
tumour mass
that may become
ossified
or may contain
calcified material

Fig. 1.35c,d,e Radiographic features of osteosarcoma.

The prognosis is generally hopeless because osteosarcomas are highly malignant and metastasize to the lungs. Chest radiographs should be taken, however very few cases have radiographic evidence of lung metastases when the primary tumour is identified. Euthanasia is usually recommended on diagnosis and treatment by amputation is seldom justified because affected animals inevitably have to be destroyed within 6 months of surgery because of lung metastases. However there are treatment options and these are listed below.

Treatment of malignant bone tumours
Although the prognosis for many malignant bone tumours is poor, treatment regimes are available and it is likely that major developments will be made in the next few years (McGlennon 1991). It is essential to have an accurate histo-

logical diagnosis based on examination of biopsy material from the tumour before treatment is commenced.

Pain relief is essential; non-steroidal anti-inflammatory agents such as phenylbutazone or piroxicam are used. In addition the administration of prednisolone, 0.5−1 mg/kg in divided doses, also helps to relieve pain, and improves the dog's appetite and sense of well being. If pain can be adequately controlled in this way then some owners may request this as the sole method of treatment giving the dog a few more weeks or perhaps months to enjoy life rather than putting the animal through amputation and perhaps chemotherapy. If pain cannot be adequately controlled with drugs or surgery then euthanasia must be recommended on humane grounds.

OSTEOSARCOMA

Treatment options:

1 Amputation alone: the median survival time following management by amputation alone is between 18 and 25 weeks with 10−21% of cases still alive at 1 year (Brodey & Abt 1976; Maudlin *et al.* 1988).

2 Amputation with chemotherapy. Two recent reports have produced encouraging results using cisplatin alone (Shapiro *et al.* 1989) or cisplatin combined with doxorubicin following amputation (Maudlin *et al.* 1988). The median survival time was 43 weeks with both protocols.

3 Limb salvage techniques. Occasionally osteosarcomas develop in the distal ulna (Fig. 1.35f) and here block resection of the tumour mass is possible with no effect on limb func-

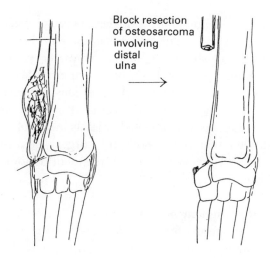

Fig. **1.35f**

tion. The ulna is transected through healthy bone proximal to the tumour mass and the entire distal ulna is dissected out with the tumour. The procedure does not seem to affect carpal stability or function. Although the procedure is simple and in most operated cases the tumour mass has apparently been completely excised, local recurrence rates are high and in a series of six cases treated by the author there was a recurrence of the tumour within 6 months. Block resection of osteosarcomas arising in the distal radius or tibia are also possible; the defect is replaced with a cortical allograft held in place with a compression plate. Arthrodesis of the carpus or hock is an essential part of the procedure (Fig. 1.35g). Used alone, the results of the limb salvage procedures are no better than amputation because of metastatic disease so the procedure must be used in conjunction with other forms of therapy; chemotherapy, using cisplatin, is currently the treatment of choice.

4 Radiotherapy. Radiation has a palliative effect on osteosarcomas and will initially reduce pain and swelling, how-

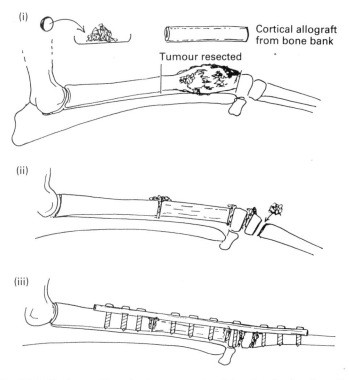

Fig. 1.35g Block resection of osteosarcoma involving the distal radius: (i) cancellous bonegraft taken from proximal humerus; (ii) articular cartilage removed from carpal joints, cancellous bone packed into joint spaces and at junction with allograft of cortical bone; (iii) fixation with a Dynamic Compression plate.

ever tumour regrowth and pain recur in most cases within 4–6 months of treatment. Prophylactic irradiation of the lungs has not been effective in preventing the development of lung metastases.

Osteosarcomas in the cat (Turrell & Pool 1982; Bitetto *et al*. 1987)
Amputation is the treatment of choice for osteosarcoma involving the appendicular skeleton and carries a much better prognosis than for dogs.

GIANT CELL TUMOURS OF BONE (OSTEOCLASTOMA)
Giant cell tumours are very rare in domestic animals. Occasional cases have been described in the cat and dog (Bennett & Duff 1983). The radiographic appearance of the tumour could be confused with a bone cyst or expanding non-osteogenic osteosarcoma. The tumour presents as an expansile well-circumscribed osteolytic area with thinning of the overlying cortices and no periosteal new bone formation. The osteoclastoma is usually slow growing but the degree of malignancy is variable; secondary spread to the lungs and kidneys has been reported. Successful treatment of a tumour involving the distal ulna in a cat by block resection was reported by Bennett & Duff (1983).

CHONDROSARCOMA
Chondrosarcomas do not metastasize as rapidly as osteosarcomas and some cases have been cured following early amputation or radical excision of rib tumours.

OSTEOCHONDROMA
Osteochondromas are cartilage-capped exostoses arising from any bone that develops from cartilage. They can be solitary or multiple; if multiple the condition is often called osteochondromatosis or multiple cartilaginous exostoses. Multiple cartilaginous exostoses are said to be an inherited defect in the dog (Pool 1978). Radiographically lesions appear as dense areas of bone interspersed with radiolucent areas of cartilage. These are seen in the metaphyseal regions of long bones but can also affect vertebrae, ribs, scapula and pelvis. If lesions cause pain or mechanical interference then surgical removal is indicated but in most cases this is unnecessary because growth of the tumour stops once the growth plates close.

In the cat solitary osteochondromas are rare and affect the axial skeleton only (Turrell & Pool 1982). Multiple lesions are more common and tend to be seen in adult cats arising mainly on the perichondrium of flat bones and occasionally on the appendicular skeleton.

SYNOVIAL OSTEOCHONDROMATOSIS

Synovial osteochondromatosis is a condition in which numerous foci of cartilage develop in the synovial membrane of a joint or occasionally of a bursa or tendon sheath. It is thought that metaplasia of the sublining connective tissue of the membrane occurs. The foci of cartilage detach and remain free in the joint space and frequently become ossified. The condition is uncommon in both man and dogs. Gregory & Pearson (1990) reviewed the literature and described a case involving the stifle in an 11-year-old Labrador. The condition has also been reported in the shoulder, hip and hock joints (Flo *et al.* 1987). It also occurs in cats (Kealy 1979). Cases tend to be mature animals of the larger breeds. There is chronic lameness, with swelling and discomfort evident on manipulation of the affected joint. Radiographs demonstrate extensive calcified deposits in and around the joint (Fig. 1.35h). The treatment of choice is total synovectomy with removal of loose bodies but this may prove difficult. Flo *et al.* (1987) reported dramatic results with this type of surgery in four cases. At the author's clinic one case of synovial osteochondromatosis was seen affecting the carpus in an 8-year-old Labrador. The dog already had a chronic subluxation of the radio-carpal joint so arthrodesis was used to relieve lameness.

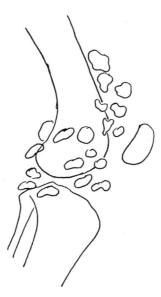

Fig. 1.35h Synovial osteochondromatosis, multiple calcified masses surround the joint.

Subsequent follow-up radiographs showed extensive re-modelling of the periarticular changes associated with the osteochondromatosis.

NON-OSTEOGENIC MALIGNANT TUMOURS OF BONE
(Gibbs *et al.* 1985)

Although osteosarcoma is by far the commonest malignant tumour to affect bone of the appendicular skeleton, a wide variety of neoplasms of other histological types, both primary and secondary, have also been reported. In a series of 34 dogs described by Gibbs *et al.* (1985), the commonest tumour types were fibrosarcoma (nine cases), metastatic tumours (eight cases) and haemangiosarcomas (five cases). These tumours are termed non-osteogenic because although they may stimulate production of new bone, it is not formed specifically by neoplastic cells. No distinctive radiological features could be related to histological type, but only one demonstrated radiological signs indistinguishable from the characteristic changes of osteosarcoma. Lung metastases were detected radiographically in 15% of cases. Eight dogs were treated either by amputation or surgical excision of the tumour mass and three of these dogs are known to have survived without recurrence for more than 2 years.

FIBROSARCOMA AND HAEMANGIOSARCOMA

When these tumour types arise in the appendicular skeleton the usual treatment is amputation. Fibrosarcomas carry a better prognosis than osteosarcomas, but the prognosis for haemangiosarcoma is very guarded in view of their potential to metastasize.

SQUAMOUS CELL CARCINOMAS
(Theilen & Madwell 1987)

These tumours often arise around the nail bed. There is swelling, ulceration and usually secondary infection. Radiographic examination shows lysis of the third and sometimes the second phalanx. These cases are often mis-diagnosed as simply nail bed infections and are treated with antibiotics initially. Radical amputation of the digit is the treatment of choice.

SYNOVIAL SARCOMAS (McGlennon *et al.* 1988)

Synovial sarcomas are uncommon. The tumour occurs most frequently in middle-aged dogs of medium to large breeds. There is a gradual onset of lameness with the development of a soft tissue mass around a joint. The tumour is locally invasive and radiographic examination will reveal varying degrees of bone and joint involvement. Amputation appears to be the most effective form of treatment but only some 25% of cases survive for more than a year following diagnosis. The most common sites of metastases are the lungs and local lymph nodes. Tilmant *et al.* (1986) described the successful chemotherapeutic treatment of one case using doxorubicin and cyclophosphamide.

MALIGNANT HISTIOCYTOSIS
This is an uncommon condition but is seen as a familial form of cancer (autosomal recessive) in the Bernese Mountain Dog. It can effect joints and has been recorded as a cause of chronic elbow lameness in a young adult dog (Miller 1991). Radiographic examination shows evidence of degenerative joint disease with erosions in the subchondral bone. The tumour invades the joint and is associated with marked soft tissue swelling. The prognosis is invariably hopeless in these cases.

Bone cysts
Bone cysts are occasionally encountered in the dog and the literature on these lesions has been reviewed by Carrig *et al.* (1975). The cyst is generally found in the metaphyseal region of either the distal radius or ulna, femur or tibia. Young dogs of the large breeds are affected, a painless bony swelling develops and radiographs show a radiolucent lesion with marked thinning of the overlying cortices (Fig. 1.35i). There is no evidence of an actively destructive process or of any reactive periosteal new bone present. Trabeculation within the cysts is minimal. The cyst should be drained, and the cavity curetted and then packed with a cancellous bone graft. The response to surgery is usually good and the cyst decreases in size while the bone cortices thicken.

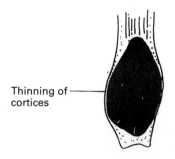

Thinning of cortices

Fig. 1.35i Bone cyst.

Calcinosis circumscripta

Calcinosis circumscripta is the name given to a granuloma-tous lesion which consists of chalky/putty-like masses embedded in fibrous tissue. The condition is seen most often in the German Shepherd and affected animals are under 1 year of age. Lesions may be single or multiple and can be found in a variety of sites, such as the foot, closely attached to the cervical vertebrae, the thorax, elbow, ischium and even under the tongue. The lesions are benign and they can be excised. However, surgical excision may be difficult because of the firm soft tissue attachments. Calcinosis circumscripta lesions in the neck are closely attached to the cervical vertebrae and excision carries a real risk of damage to the nerve roots of the brachial plexus. In this site, therefore, surgical treatment should be avoided. There is a tendency for the lesion to stop growing and, in fact, to regress by the time the dog reaches 1 year of age. The aetiology of calcinosis circumscripta is unknown but it has been described as an inherited local metabolic defect of connective tissue (Seawright & Grono 1961).

JOINT INJURY

A diarthrodial joint (Fig. 1.36) consists essentially of two opposing bone surfaces which are covered with hyaline cartilage and joined peripherally by a joint capsule. The articular surface of the bone is composed of compact bone covered with hyaline cartilage. The cartilage has no nerve or blood supply and it is generally accepted that it derives its nutrition from synovial fluid. The cartilage is well adapted to counter concussion and friction by means of its structure and lubrication by synovial fluid. Although microscopically chrondrocytes show no sign of activity, it has been demonstrated that the turnover of the matrix is rapid, indeed far greater than could possibly be required to replenish wear and tear over areas of high pressure (Mankin & Lippiello 1970). The matrix which is continuously produced by chondrocytes is broken down at the same time by proteolytic enzymes, in particular cathepsin D (Bassett 1966). This process of autolysis occurs in the substance of cartilage rather than on the surface and normally the balance between anabolism and catabolism is so precise that the thickness of the matrix varies little throughout life.

Repair of articular cartilage depends on the depth and position of the defect. Superficial defects in the cartilage never heal unless they are close to the attachment of the synovial membrane, whereas a wound which extends through cartilage to the sub-chondral bone is gradually filled with fibrocartilage (Meacham & Roberts 1971; Vaughan & Robins 1975). Joint instability results in fibrous tissue hypertrophy. This tissue is replaced by plaques of cartilage which later undergo endochondral ossification to form osteophytes. These changes occur particularly at the transitional zone of the joint which is the junction between periosteum, synovial membrane and articular cartilage. The area has a profuse blood supply.

The joint capsule consists of two layers (Fig. 1.36), the outer fibrous layer which is thickened in parts to form ligaments and the inner layer or synovial membrane which is responsible for the secretion and absorption of synovial fluid. The synovial membrane has a rich supply of arteries, lymphatics and nerves. Its surfaces are covered with fine villi which hypertrophy in disease.

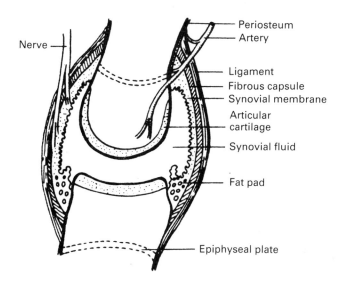

Fig. 1.36

The component structures of a joint may be torn or stretched when a joint is forced beyond its normal range of physiological movement, in a fall or incoordinate movement; alternatively injury may be precipitated by the abnormal structure and hence abnormal movement of the joint as in hip dysplasia, or by excessive wear and tear in the old or overweight animal. Whatever the initial cause a sequence of events follows which is called osteo-arthrosis or degenerative joint disease (Olsson 1971).

Injury to areas of articular cartilage results in loss of elasticity, softening and later fissure formation. Chondroitin sulphate is released from the damaged cartilage and this provokes an inflammatory response at the synovial membrane. Grossly the membrane becomes thickened and secretes increased amounts of synovial fluid. At the same time the fibrous joint capsule undergoes a normal inflammatory response with increased vascularity and swelling. Later there is fibrous thickening of the capsule and the development of osteophytes, particularly at the transitional zone of the joint.

The tissue changes, especially degeneration of the articular cartilage, are irreversible and treatment should be aimed at preventing the progression of the disease as soon as possible. This may be achieved by rest for at least a month. The administration of analgesics and anti-inflammatory drugs, such as corticosteroids, can be useful to control the pain associated with the disease but only when strict rest is enforced, otherwise premature use of the joint may result in further damage.

Corticosteroids remain one of the most effective groups of agent used for the relief of symptoms of joint disease because they inhibit all stages of inflammation. Short-term administration is usually well tolerated but the long-term systemic use of corticosteroids is associated with undesirable side effects. Repeated intra-articular corticosteroid injections may lead to cartilage destruction (Mankin 1974).

THE MANAGEMENT OF CHRONIC LAMENESS IN DOGS

Most chronic lameness is due to pain and the main aim of treatment is pain relief. Canine joint disease can be divided into:
1 Non-inflammatory joint disease.
2 Inflammatory joint disease.

Non-inflammatory joint disease
Non-inflammatory joint disease is usually described as degenerative joint disease (DJD) or osteo-arthrosis in which there is fragmentation and loss of articular cartilage, sclerosis of sub-chondral bone and periarticular osteophyte formation.

Degenerative joint disease can be primary; this is the most common articular problem in people over 40 years of age and most will have gross changes in weight-bearing articular surfaces. Similar changes are common in older overweight dogs although this is not always associated with lameness. The problem occurs because cartilage does not maintain its normal state during ageing.

Degenerative joint disease can also be secondary as a result of any condition which damages cartilage directly or causes joint instability or abnormal wear. Secondary DJD results from developmental conditions such as hip dysplasia, patellar luxations, osteochondrosis, and conformation faults, e.g. straight stifles. DJD can also occur secondary to acquired conditions such as rupture of the anterior cruciate ligament or articular fractures.

The clinical signs of DJD are initially stiffness and lameness after exercise. As the condition progresses the dog will be stiff and lame after rest but this tends to wear off as the dog 'warms up' with exercise. Later stiffness and lameness become a constant problem and may become noticeably worse in cold damp weather.

In the treatment of DJD adequate rest is important. Excessive use of damaged joints aggravates the clinical signs and accelerates joint destruction. Owners should be told that the changes are irreversible and that the dog cannot be expected to be as active as before. An exercise regime of 'a little and often' is the most beneficial, that is short frequent walks (10 minutes maximum) on a leash three or four times a day. With controlled exercise it should be possible to keep lameness to a minimum and reduce the need for analgesic or anti-inflammatory treatment. Owners should be encouraged to experiment with the amount of exercise, making changes gradually until an optimum is found for the dog. Certain activities should be avoided, for example the dog which has had cruciate ligament surgery or has osteo-arthrosis in the stifles should not be allowed to chase and retrieve balls or sticks because sudden turns will certainly place undue stresses on the stifle with acute flare-ups of lameness. Similarly jumping and stairs should be avoided in dogs with carpal arthritis. If there has been an acute flare-up of lameness then give the dog 4–6 weeks rest only allowing the animal out on a leash several times a day for toilet purposes. If the affected joint can be easily immobilized, e.g. the carpus, then apply a gutter splint for 4 weeks. Provided lameness appears to resolve with this rest period then the next stage is a regime of short frequent walks. It is also important to reduce stress on damaged joints by proper weight control; obese animals should be put on a strict diet (prescription diets, e.g. Hills RD and later WD are ideal for this). Adjuncts to treatment are the provision of warmth, massage and physiotherapy.

DRUG THERAPY

If the dog is only stiff on rising and lameness wears off with exercise and there is no obvious pain on joint manipulation then no treatment is prescribed except restricted exercise. Dogs with DJD tend to have their 'good days' and 'bad days' when there has been a flare-up of lameness. Working dogs seem to have more than their fair share of DJD and owners will often want something positive done to allow their animals to work. Under these circumstances non-steroidal anti-inflammatories are given on working days to keep the dog comfortable but it is important to allow the animal adequate rest inbetween times.

Non-steroidal anti-inflammatories

Non-steroidal anti-inflammatory drugs (NSAIDs) act by blocking biosynthesis of inflammatory mediators, particularly prostaglandins. This is achieved through inhibition of cyclo-oxygenase, an enzyme essential to the arachidonic acid pathway. NSAIDs are most suitable for the relief of mild or chronic low grade pain. All NSAIDs reduce pain by reducing inflammation; in addition they have a specific analgesic effect through their anti-prostaglandin activity. These drugs also reduce pyrexia. The major side effect of NSAIDs is gastric irritation with vomiting, diarrhoea and gastric haemorrhage. Blood dyscrasias can occur and occasionally there is liver and kidney toxicity. The cat is particularly susceptible to toxic effects as it lacks many of the metabolic pathways used by other species for drug excretion.

Drugs currently available (Short & Beadle 1978; Taylor 1985; Carmichael 1990)

Aspirin. Aspirin remains one of the most popular NSAIDs: 300 mg tablets; 25 mg/kg divided into two daily doses. Gastric irritation can be a problem and as cats are unable to excrete the drug effectively it should only occasionally be used in this species.

Paracetamol. 500 mg tablets; 25 mg/kg divided into four daily doses. Causes less gastric irritation than aspirin but does not give such good pain relief. Overdose causes liver toxicity and fatalities have occurred in cats.

Codeine (= opiate but often used in combination with NSAIDs). Alkaloid from natural opium; much weaker analgesic than opium; useful analgesic for low grade pain; dose 1–2 mg/kg, dogs and cats effective up to 12 hours. Although codeine is an opiate it is mentioned here as it is often used in combination with other drugs, e.g. Pardale V and Budale V (see below).

Pardale V (Arnolds). Combination of paracetamol, codeine phosphate and caffeine hydrate. 10 mg tablets; small dog 5 mg every 8 h, large dog 20–30 mg every 8 h.

Budale V (Dales Pharmaceuticals, similar to Pardale V).

Phenylbutazone (Buvetzone, Willows Francis). For chronic use 1–2 mg/kg divided into two or three daily doses. Higher doses for acute flare-ups of joint pain: 5 mg/kg divided into two or three daily doses for a few days and then reduce dose to chronic level. Causes less gastric irritation than aspirin but can cause blood dyscrasias and bone marrow suppression. It should not be used in dogs with cardiac or kidney disease. The lower dose rate should be used in cats and for the shortest possible period to avoid toxic effects.

Tomanol (Intervet). This is a combination of phenylbutazone and isopyrin.

Ibuprofen (Brufen, Boots). Brufen is a propionic acid derivative which some report as a safe NSAID for use in the dog at 20 mg/kg divided into three daily doses. Others report that as little as 8 mg/kg given over 30 days caused severe gastric ulceration in dogs (Adams *et al.* 1969) and therefore its use should be avoided in dogs if possible.

Naproxen (Naprosyn). This drug is reported to be useful for the relief of severe spinal pain (Carmichael 1990). Dose is 1 mg/kg every 48 h, however like ibuprofen naproxen is a propionic acid derivative and has been associated with vomiting and hepatic toxicity in dogs.

Carprofen. Appears to be a potent anti-inflammatory drug which will prove suitable for use in the dog (McKellar *et al.*

1990), dosage up to 4 mg/kg in a divided daily dose. The major advantage of the drug is its apparently lower gastro-intestinal toxicity in the dog.

Flunixin meglumine (Finadyne, Schering-Plough Animal Health). Appears to be a strong analgesic, however it is recommended that the drug is not used for more than 3 days at a time in the dog, dose 1.1 mg/kg. Useful drug for the treatment of acute pain of short duration, e.g. disc protrusions, fractures or following surgery.

Piroxicam (Feldene Pfizer). This drug is a potent NSAID, similar to aspirin in its efficacy. It is given at a dose rate of 0.3 mg/kg once every 48 h. Unlike other NSAIDs, piroxicam does not appear to inhibit production of proteoglycans and may stimulate chondrocyte function and consequently the drug has particular appeal for the management of osteo-arthrosis. In man the drug gives significant relief from pain associated with osteo-arthritis, and is more effective than either aspirin or codeine for the relief of post-operative pain. Piroxicam is well tolerated by dogs and may well prove to be the NSAID of choice.

Mefenamic acid (Ponstan Parke Davis). Mefenamic acid is given at a dose of 10 mg/kg, divided dose twice daily. Available in 250 mg capsules or syrup of 10 mg/ml, syrup has been used in cats but not widely so far. The side effects of the drug are similar to phenylbutazone. Some dogs tolerate the drug long term very well but others soon develop gastric irritation.

Pentosan polysulphate sodium (Cartrophen Vet, Univet). Pentosan polysulphate sodium is a semi-synthetic polymer possessing strong anti-inflammatory activity. It stimulates biosynthesis of normal synovial fluid and also inhibits the enzymes involved in the degradation of cartilage. By supporting chondrocyte activities, it increases cartilage matrix replacement. In addition it mobilizes thrombi and fibrin deposits in synovial tissues and sub-chondral vessels, restoring normal perfusion of the joints and sub-chondral structures. Cartrophen Vet is indicated for the treatment of non-inflammatory degenerative joint disease in dogs. The dosage is 3 mg of pentosan polysulphate per kg body weight by subcutaneous injection on four occasions with an interval of 5−7 days between each injection.

The choice of drugs is listed below.

Prednoleucotropin (PLT) (prednisolone + hexamine + cinchophen, BK Vet). This is a very useful preparation for the treatment of DJD. Cats: half a tablet twice daily, dogs weighing 30 kg: one tablet three times daily.

Prednisolone (Animalcare). Initial dose of prednisolone: 2 mg/kg once daily for 5 days, followed by a chronic maintenance dose of 1 mg/kg every other day.

Steroids hasten degenerative changes in joints and should only be used in cases that are unresponsive to NSAIDs.

Pentazocine (Fortral, Wyeth). This is a controlled opiate analgesic with one-third the potency of morphine. The dose in the dog and the cat is 2 mg/kg by injection. It is also available in 25 mg tablets and used at a dose rate of 25 mg b.i.d. has proved useful in control of chronic pain in Labrador-sized dogs.

Treatment of inflammatory joint disease (arthritis, infective, bacterial)

IMMUNE-BASED EROSIVE INFLAMMATORY JOINT DISEASE, E.G. RHEUMATOID ARTHRITIS

The condition carries a poor prognosis. Treatment is symptomatic; aspirin and prednisolone are used to provide pain relief.

SYSTEMIC LUPUS ERYTHEMATOSUS (SLE)

High doses of prednisolone are used to treat this condition — see p. 56.

SEPTIC/BACTERIAL ARTHRITIS

Prolonged (at least 3 weeks) antibiotic therapy usually with ampicillin has proved the most effective treatment for this condition — see p. 54. NSAIDs such as piroxicam are also given to help control joint pain.

Other methods of relieving chronic joint pain

INJECTION OF SODIUM HYALURONATE INTO THE DAMAGED JOINT

This technique is widely practised in equine orthopaedics

and has some application in the dog, particularly the animal which has chronic osteo-arthrosis, for example following an old cruciate ligament rupture. If there is an acute flare-up of lameness due to trauma to the affected stifle then intra-articular injection of sodium hyaluronate (the author has used 1 ml of Equron, Duphar, in medium sized dogs) tends to 'dampen down' the lameness within a few days.

Equron trial in dogs (Denny 1990)
Twelve dogs were treated for chronic osteoarthrosis of the stifle joint. The osteo-arthrosis was caused by rupture of the anterior cruciate ligament in 10 dogs, medial luxation of the patella in one dog and osteochrondritis dissecans in another.

The degree of osteo-arthrosis was assessed from radiographs of the stifle and was graded as slight, moderate or severe.

A single dose of sodium hyaluronate (Equron, Duphar) was injected into the stifle, 1 ml in 11 cases and 2 ml in a St. Bernard. The dogs were anaesthetized for the procedure and the injection was given under conditions of strict asepsis. A 20 gauge needle was used; this was introduced into the cranial compartment of the stifle from the lateral aspect just caudal to the straight patellar ligament. A sample of synovial fluid was aspirated before the Equron was injected.

The results were assessed by questionnaire sent to owners 6 months after treatment.

Joint swelling and pain 24−48 h following injection were noted in two dogs. An improvement in limb function was reported in seven dogs; there was no change in the others. The improvement was said to be immediate in three, occurred within 48 h in one, took 2−3 weeks in one, and 3 months in two other dogs. Five of the dogs were reported to have regained full limb function following treatment. Varying degrees of lameness persisted in the other seven dogs in the series.

Two owners were very pleased with the result. Equron seemed to be most effective in the dog with chronic osteo-arthrosis when an acute flare-up of lameness had occurred.

FENESTRATION TECHNIQUES AND OSTEOTOMIES
Fenestration techniques for the relief of joint pain were developed in humans when it was noticed that any osteotomy performed near an osteo-arthritic joint invariably resulted in relief of joint pain. It was thought that pain was

partly due to venous congestion in the ends of long bones and the osteotomy relieved this. So rather than doing an osteotomy surgeons began drilling holes transversely through the ends of long bones to relieve venous congestion and hopefully relieve joint pain. This fenestration operation can be readily performed in the dog with osteo-arthritis of the stifle as an adjunct to the routine removal of peri-articular osteophytes and damaged portions of the medial meniscus.

JOINT REPLACEMENT

This is the ultimate treatment for the relief of chronic hip pain and hip replacement operations are now being carried out in dogs at many clinics with increasing frequency.

SALVAGE PROCEDURES

Salvage procedures for the relief of chronic pain include:
1 Excision arthroplasty, commonly carried out on the hip and occasionally on the temporomandibular joint.
2 Arthrodesis: the surgical fusion of a joint will relieve pain. The shoulder, elbow, carpus, stifle, hock and digits are all joints which can be fused in dogs and cats. Arthrodesis of the shoulder, carpus, hock, or phalanges has little obvious affect on locomotion but a more profound change in gait is more obvious after elbow or stifle fusion.

AMPUTATION OR EUTHANASIA

These are the final options in the relief of chronic pain.

Infectious arthritis

Although haematogenous spread of infection to joints is common in young farm animals, the condition is rare in the dog. Direct infection as a complication of a penetrating wound, arthrotomy, or by extension of infection from a local purulent focus occurs more frequently. The sequence of pathological changes is similar to but far more marked than in osteo-arthrosis, with rapid and extensive destruction of areas of articular cartilage and sub-chondral bone. Later there is marked periarticular new bone formation which may eventually result in ankylosis of the joint.

Clinical examination reveals a hot, swollen, extremely painful joint and if the joint is open there will be a discharge of pus and synovial fluid. Treatment of infective arthritis involves removal of purulent material from the joint; this is done by aspiration through a needle in closed cases and by flushing the joint out with sterile normal saline in open cases. The joint is irrigated with aqueous penicillin or other appropriate antibiotic solution. Open cases are protected with a bandage and left to heal by granulation. Prolonged parenteral antibiotic therapy is essential. In chronic cases surgical debridement and synovectomy may be necessary to eradicate the infection. Even when infection has been eradicated pain may persist as a result of the extensive destruction of the joint surfaces, and this pain may only be relieved by arthrodesis of the joint or amputation of the limb.

TREATMENT OF SEPTIC ARTHRITIS
FOLLOWING JOINT SURGERY

Strict asepsis is essential for the prevention of joint infection following arthrotomy, nevertheless infections do occasionally occur and can usually be traced back to faults in asepsis, prolonged operating time or rough handling of the soft tissues.

In the acute case there is joint swelling, pain and pyrexia within a few days of surgery. Most cases will respond to antibiotic therapy, e.g. cephalosporin (Ceporex, Glaxo, 10 mg/kg twice daily). Joint immobilization helps to relieve pain and this can be done with a Robert Jones-type bandage.

Chronic infections are seen most often following anterior cruciate ligament surgeries, especially when synthetic materials such as braided nylon have been used as a prosthesis to replace the ligament. Lameness which is often severe persists for weeks or months following surgery; the stifle is thickened with pain and crepitus evident on manipulation. Sinus tracts appear and these will not heal until all remnants of the prosthesis have been removed. Radiographic examination will show soft tissue swelling, periarticular osteophyte formation and areas of bone destruction which involve not only the joint surfaces but extend into the bone tunnels making these larger and more distinct (Fig. 1.37).

Arthrotomy should be performed. It is imperative to remove any synthetic material that has been used as a cruciate ligament prosthesis. Portions of the synovial membrane should be taken for culture and sensitivity examination. The joint is thoroughly washed out with lactated Ringer's solution; if necessary a drainage tube can be left *in situ* to allow drainage and local irrigation with antibiotic solution (ampicillin) while the results of culture are awaited. The tube is removed after 3 or 4 days and the appropriate antibiotic should be given for at least 3 weeks.

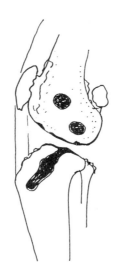

Fig. 1.37 Chronic infective arthritis following cruciate ligament replacement with braided nylon prosthesis.

If the organisms isolated from the joint are sensitive to gentamicin only then a string of polymethylmethacrylate beads impregnated with gentamicin (E. Merck in collaboration with Kultzer & Co.) can be placed in the joint for 3 weeks. The beads slowly release the gentamicin creating a local concentration of the antibiotic with no undesirable toxic side effects. The successful application of this method was described in the dog by Brown & Bennett in 1988.

Healing of a stifle which has been infected is invariably associated with the development of marked periarticular fibrosis which will stabilize the joint; there is no need therefore to attempt cruciate ligament replacement again after removal of the original prosthesis.

BACTERIAL INFECTIVE ARTHRITIS IN THE DOG

Bacterial infective arthritis is a relatively uncommon cause of lameness in dogs. Most cases appear to be due to haematogenous localization of bacteria in a joint and trauma may predispose a joint to infection. In 1988 Bennett & Taylor described 58 cases of confirmed bacterial arthritis. They recognized two syndromes, first the classic acute onset case and second those cases with a more chronic low grade infection syndrome. The condition occurs more commonly in large breeds of dog. The carpus is the joint most frequently affected but the shoulder, hip and stifle have also been involved. Affected joints are swollen or thickened and painful. Lameness is often severe. Few dogs show evidence of systemic illness and routine blood counts are usually normal. Synovial fluid from affected joints has a raised white cell count and most of these cells are polymorphonuclear leucocytes. Culture from synovial fluid may give false negatives and it is best to culture from the synovial membrane if possible. The organisms most frequently isolated are *Streptococcus* and *Staphylococcus intermedius*. Radiographic examination of the joint may reveal little initially except for soft tissue swelling but later destructive changes will be seen extending down into the sub-chondral bone and there will be varying degrees of periarticular new bone formation. Most cases respond successfully to prolonged antibiotic therapy (6–8 weeks). Selection of antibiotic is based on culture and sensitivity examination but the initial antibiotic of choice is ampicillin (Bennett & Taylor 1988).

Infective polyarthritis
Infective polyarthritis associated with *Erysipelothrix rhusiopathiae* is occasionally encountered in the dog. The condition has been reviewed by Houlton & Jefferies (1989); they described a case of a 7-month-old Irish Wolfhound with both polyarthritis and multiple discospondylitis lesions.

Lyme disease (arthritis) in dogs
Lyme disease is a multisystem inflammatory disorder associated with infection by the spirochaete *Borrelia burgdorferi* which is carried by ticks. In Europe the vector is the sheep tick *Ixodes ricinus*. Lyme disease was first recognized in the United States in humans and has been diagnosed in a number of domesticated animals during the past 10 years. The first case of Lyme disease in the dog in the United Kingdom was reported by May *et al*. in 1990. Diagnosis was based on contact with sheep ticks and a positive antibody titre to *B. burgdorferi*. The dog had a chronic foreleg lameness, pyrexia, localized lymphadenopathy and leucocytosis with neutrophilia and a shift to the left. Synovial fluid from the elbows had inflammatory characteristics. The lameness responded to antibiotic therapy with clavulanate potentiated amoxycillin (Synulox, Beecham Animal Health).

Rheumatoid arthritis (Newton & Lipowitz 1975; Biery & Newton 1975; Bennett 1987a)
Rheumatoid arthritis is comparatively rare in the dog. Immune complexes form in the joints and erosion of cartilage occurs causing severe and often progressive polyarthritis. The condition has been recorded most frequently in Shelties, Collies and Dachshunds. There is lameness, swelling and

pain associated with several joints. The carpus and hock are most frequently affected. The American Rheumatism Association use 11 criteria, listed below, to establish a diagnosis of rheumatoid arthritis and at least nine of these should be present to confirm the diagnosis in the dog.

1 Morning stiffness.
2 Pain or tenderness of joint motion.
3 Swelling of at least one joint (soft tissue or fluid).
4 Swelling of any other joint.
5 Symmetrical onset of joint swelling and symptoms.
6 Subcutaneous nodules.
7 Radiographic changes typical of rheumatoid arthritis.
8 Positive rheumatoid factor—by a reliable method.
9 Poor mucin precipitate of synovial fluid.
10 Characteristic histological synovial changes. Villous projection of the synovium with lymphoid and plasma cell infiltration.
11 Characteristic histological findings of nodules.

The classical radiographic changes associated with rheumatoid arthritis are flask-shaped destructive lesions in the sub-chondral bone. Treatment can only be palliative and salicylates (aspirin) provide the most effective relief.

Recent work by Bell *et al.* (1991) has shown that dogs with rheumatoid arthritis have significantly higher concentrations of antibodies to canine distemper virus in their synovial fluid compared with dogs with other forms of joint disease.

Systemic lupus erythematosus (Krum *et al.* 1977;
Bennett 1987b)
Systemic lupus erythematosus (SLE) is a complex disorder characterized by the development of one or all of the following clinical syndromes:
1 Haemolytic anaemia.
2 Thrombocytopenic purpura.
3 Glomerulonephritis.
4 Polyarthritis.

SLE is an autoimmune disease and diagnosis is based on the demonstration of antinuclear antibodies. Polyarthritis due to SLE should be differentiated from rheumatoid arthritis—erosions in the articular cartilage are not seen so frequently as in the latter. Another feature of SLE is joint instability, caused by degenerative changes in the supporting ligaments; this is seen particularly in the carpus and the stifle. Dogs with SLE are treated with high doses of prednisolone. The long-term prognosis is poor.

Bennett (1987b) recommends treatment with a combination of prednisolone (1 mg/kg body weight daily dose) and cyclophosphamide (dose varies with body weight, 2.0 mg/kg in dogs weighing 10–30 kg, used on four consecutive days each week). Cyclophosphamide treatment was discontinued after 2 months, steroids were used for another month after terminating cytotoxic drugs. Half the dogs treated in this way showed a marked improvement and remissions of 5 months to 2 years were recorded in a few cases.

Immune-based non-erosive inflammatory joint disease of the dog

POLYARTHRITIS/POLYMYOSITIS SYNDROME

Bennett & Kelly (1987) described a connective tissue disorder in six young adult dogs (five were Spaniel breeds) characterized by non-erosive polyarthritis and polymyositis. Diagnosis was based on clinical features of stiffness, joint swelling, joint pain, muscle atrophy, muscle pain and contracture and the presence of chronic active inflammation seen in biopsies of muscle and synovium. Only two of the six dogs made an apparent recovery following treatment with cyclophosphamide and prednisolone.

CANINE IDIOPATHIC POLYARTHRITIS

Idiopathic polyarthritis includes cases of non-infective polysynovitis which cannot be classified into more defined groups. Bennett described 67 cases (1987c). Most of the dogs in his series were young adults and exhibited lameness, pyrexia, inappetence and lethargy. Radiographic examination of the affected joints showed soft tissue changes only. Bennett divided cases into four types:

Type I Uncomplicated polyarthritis with none of the associations reported in the other types. Prednisolone was the treatment of choice in this group, 1–2 mg/kg in a daily divided dose. This was used for 2–3 weeks and then gradually reduced.

Type II Reactive arthritis, a polyarthritis associated with an infective disease process remote from the joints such as respiratory or urinary tract infection. Treatment as for type I, but in addition broad spectrum antibiotics were used.

Type III Enteropathic arthritis, polyarthritis associated with gastro-intestinal disease, e.g. gastro-enteritis or ulcerative colitis. Treatment as for type I but in addition antibiotics and kaolin preparations used.

In dogs which relapsed following withdrawal of prednisolone, the treatment was either repeated or the dose increased or cytotoxic drugs (cyclophosphamide or azathioprine) used.

Type IV Neoplastic-related polyarthritis, polyarthritis associated with neoplastic disease remote from the joints. No specific treatment was tried in these cases except for short-term steroid therapy to control joint inflammation.

The prognosis for dogs with idiopathic polyarthritis (except for those with type IV lesions) is generally better than that for other types of inflammatory joint disease such as rheumatoid, systemic lupus erythematosus and the polyarthritis/polymyositis syndrome.

Arthritis in cats

Apart from arthritis associated with cat bite sepsis, trauma, secondary hyperparathyroidism and hypervitaminosis A, joint disease is seldom recorded in the cat. Polyarthritis associated with pyrexia and regional lymphadenopathy has been described (Wilkinson & Robins 1979; Pedersen 1975). The aetiology of this condition was not determined but treatment with prednisolone on a reducing dosage schedule produced remission of clinical signs (Wilkinson & Robins 1979).

Feline calcivirus (FCV) is a well-recognized pathogen in cats and is responsible for the majority of cases of 'cat flu'. FCV has been associated with other clinical conditions besides upper respiratory tract disease; these include a chronic stomatitis and a lameness syndrome (Dawson 1991). Lameness has been seen in cats both following vaccination and following natural infection with FCV. Lameness is often accompanied by pyrexia and anorexia. The condition tends to be self-limiting and resolves in 24–48h. Lameness has been produced experimentally by Pedersen *et al.* (1983) using an FCV isolate from a lame cat.

THE HEALING OF TENDONS

Mature tendons consist essentially of tightly packed bundles of collagen in which fibrocytes are interspersed. The blood supply is poor and is derived mainly from the mesotendon which is a synovial membrane lying between the tendon and its sheath. Tendons heal slowly but healing of the sheath is much more rapid. When a tendon is severed, the resultant wound is invaded by fibroblasts derived from the paratenon (Skoog & Persson 1954). They defined the paratenon as the subcutaneous connective tissue, i.e. the fascia, surrounding a tendon. The fibroblasts lay down randomly orientated collagen fibrils. The collagen fibrils then become organized so that by 3 months post-injury they are found to be longitudinally orientated between the severed tendon ends and randomly orientated in the surrounding tissues (Peacock 1964). Macroscopically the scar filling the gap is difficult to distinguish from normal tendinous tissue. Mason & Allen (1961) investigated the tensile strength of tendons during the healing process and found that function of the tendon during the early stages of exudation, fibroplasia and fibrous union had a deleterious effect on healing whereas function of the tendon during the stage of maturation and organization accelerated the process. Consequently, following tendon repair complete immobilization is essential for 1 month post-operatively and then a gradual increase in movement is allowed during the following 2 months. In tendon repair, restoration of tensile strength is a prime objective, but at the same time gliding function should be maintained if normal limb movement is to continue. Gliding function of the tendon is commonly complicated by excessive scar tissue formation; this can be minimized by the surgical techniques employed in the repair and also by controlled exercise during the latter stages of healing.

Sprains and strains
A strain is an injury to a muscle tendon unit and can be classified as first degree (mild), second degree (moderate), or third degree (severe injury).

A sprain is a ligamentous injury and can be classified into three types in the same way as strains. A third-degree sprain is characterized by complete rupture of the ligament or avulsion of the ligament from bone.

THE HEALING OF MUSCLE

In general damaged muscle is replaced by scar tissue (Walter & Israel 1967). However, in voluntary striated muscle limited regeneration may occur so that although the continuity of a surgical incision is restored primarily by fibrous tissue, this may later be replaced by muscle if sarcolemmal proliferation occurs.

CANINE MYOPATHIES

Myopathies can be inflammatory or degenerative in origin. Inflammatory myopathies in the dog may have infectious causes such as *Toxoplasma gondii*, *Leptospira* spp. and *Clostridium welchii* (see p. 19).

Toxoplasma gondii

Toxoplasma gondii has a predilection for nervous tissue and muscle. When it affects these tissues it can cause three clinical entities:

1 A generalized central nervous form which can occur in conjunction with distemper.

2 A severe acute necrotizing myositis with some nervous involvement in adult dogs (Greene *et al.* 1985; Braund *et al.* 1988).

3 A polyradiculitis and polymyositis of young dogs usually 3–6 months of age (Core *et al.* 1982). This syndrome presents as a posterior paresis in the first few weeks of life which develops into a characteristic spastic hyperextension of the hindlegs.

Diagnosis is based on serum toxoplasma titre estimation and/or muscle biopsy. A combination of sulphonamides and pyrimethamine has been recommended for the treatment of cases of toxoplasmosis in dogs and cats (Oliver *et al.* 1987).

Non-infectious inflammatory myopathies include eosinophilic myositis and idiopathic polymyositis.

Eosinophilic myositis

The condition is seen most often in German Shepherds. The masticatory muscles are affected and two clinical syndromes are recognized: the acute syndrome in which animals are presented with pain and swelling of the temporal, masseter and pterygoid muscles, and the form where animals are presented with atrophy of the jaw muscles and a limited range of jaw movement. The cause of eosinophilic myositis is unknown but both the acute and chronic syndromes respond to steroid therapy (prednisolone).

Idiopathic polymyositis

Idiopathic polymyositis is probably the commonest polymyopathy seen in dogs and affects adult animals of the larger breeds (Christman & Averill 1983). Clinical signs include weakness either after rest or with exercise, stiff gait, muscle pain, and pyrexia. Muscle atrophy, trembling, dysphagia and regurgitation may also occur. Prednisolone is used to treat the condition, but this should not be commenced until muscle biopsy has ruled out toxoplasmosis or bacterial myositis.

Degenerative myopathies can be subdivided into hereditary and acquired myopathies.

Hereditary or breed-specific myopathies

MYOTONIA IN CHOW CHOWS (Farrow & Malik 1981)
Myotonia describes the state in which active contraction of a muscle persists after cessation of voluntary effort or stimulation. Signs become apparent from 2–3 months of age; these include stiff gait, bunny hopping, and difficulty in rising or climbing stairs. The pup's action improves with exercise but becomes worse with excitement or cold weather. If muscles are percussed with artery forceps a dimple is formed which persists for several seconds. This myotonic dimple can be produced both in the conscious and the anaesthetized animal. Procainamide (500 mg orally every 6 h) may reduce signs of myotonia in affected dogs.

HEREDITARY MYOPATHY IN LABRADOR RETRIEVERS
(Kramer *et al.* 1981; McKerrell & Braund 1987)
In the UK this condition appears to be confined to Labrador Retrievers from working strains. Clinical signs become apparent at 3–5 months of age and include weakness that becomes worse with exercise, limb stiffness and a hopping gait. The condition is made worse by excitement and cold weather. Megalo-oesophagus has been reported as a complicating feature in one case (McKerrell & Braund 1987). Rest and the administration of diazepam help alleviate the signs. The condition stabilizes at about 6 months of age, however muscle atrophy persists and there is poor exercise tolerance which makes affected animals unsuitable for work, but they can be kept as house pets.

GOLDEN RETRIEVER MYOPATHY
This myopathy affects male animals from 6–8 weeks of age and is characterized by severe stiffness and weakness. There is progressive muscle atrophy and the jaw muscles may be affected as well as the limbs (DeLahunta 1983).

IRISH TERRIER MYOPATHY
A myopathy affecting male Irish terriers from 8 weeks of age has been described by Wentink *et al.* (1972).

Acquired degenerative myopathies

ATROPHIC MYOPATHY

Examples are disuse atrophy or neurogenic atrophy following peripheral nerve injury.

ISCHAEMIC MYOPATHY

Examples are bacterial endocarditis or *Dirofilaria* infection.

NUTRITIONAL MYOPATHY

A myopathy associated with diets deficient in vitamin E or selenium has been produced experimentally in dogs but is unlikely to occur in clinical cases.

METABOLIC MYOPATHY

Muscle atrophy and weakness are well-recognized features in dogs with hyperadrenocorticism but some cases have more marked abnormalities indicative of myopathy, i.e. stiff gait with increased resistance to limb flexion.

EXERCISE-INDUCED MYOPATHY

Exercise-induced myopathy is seen most often in the racing Greyhound. Ischaemic changes occur in muscle with consequent rhabdomyolysis and haemoglobinuria. The dog is distressed and the affected muscles are swollen and painful. Severely affected dogs may collapse and die while others can die 2 or 3 days later because of renal failure associated with myoglobinuria. Intravenous fluids and sodium bicarbonate are essential to correct the hypovolaemia and metabolic disturbance.

Swimmers

Occasionally one or more puppies in a litter is affected by the swimmer syndrome. Affected puppies are unable to stand and make swimming movements with their limbs in abduction when they attempt to move. They often have flat chests and if allowed to survive may develop permanent joint deformity. The pups are strong and alert and no neurological deficits are usually apparent. The pathogenesis of the condition is not understood; it is described as a musculoskeletal growth abnormality.

Breeders who recognize the condition can sometimes improve or correct the deformity by hobbling the legs, splinting the chest and keeping the pups on soft litter.

Abrams J.T. (1962) *The Feeding of Dogs*. W. Green & Sons, Edinburgh.

Adams S.S., Bough R.G. & Cliffe E.E. (1969) Absorption distribution and toxicity of ibuprofen. *Toxicol. Appl. Pharmacol.* **15**, 310−22.

Alexander J.E., Keown G.H. & Patolay J.L. (1965) Granular cell myoblastoma with hypertrophic osteopathy in a mare. *J. Am. Vet. Med. Assoc.* **146**, 703.

Alexander J.W. (1983) Use of a combination of cortical bone allografts and cancellous bone autografts to replace massive bone loss in fresh fractures and selected non-unions. *J. Am. Anim. Hosp. Assoc.* **19**, 671.

Bacher J.D. & Schmidt R.E. (1980) Effects of autogenous cancellous bone on healing of homogeneous cortical bone grafts. *J. Small Anim. Pract.* **21**, 235.

Bassett C.A.C. (1966) *Cartilage Degradation and Repair*. Proceedings of a Workshop, Washington, DC. National Academy of Sciences, National Research Council.

Bell S.C., Carter S.D. & Bennett D. (1991) Distemper and rheumatoid arthritis in dogs. *Res. Vet. Sci.* **50**, 64.

Bennett D. (1976) Nutrition and bone disease in the dog and cat. *Vet. Rec.* **98**, 313.

Bennett D. (1987a) Immune-based erosive inflammatory joint disease of the dog: canine rheumatoid arthritis. *J. Small Anim. Pract.* **28**, 779−819.

Bennett D. (1987b) Immune-based non-erosive inflammatory joint disease of the dog. 1. Canine systemic lupus erythematosus. *J. Small Anim. Pract.* **28**, 871−89.

Bennett D. (1987c) Immune-based non-erosive inflammatory joint disease of the dog. 3. Canine idiopathic polyarthritis. *J. Small Anim. Pract.* **28**, 909−28.

Bennett D. & Duff R.S.I. (1983) Giant cell tumour of the ulna of the cat. *J. Small Anim. Pract.* **24**, 341−5.

Bennett D. & Kelly D.F. (1987) Immune-based non-erosive inflammatory joint disease of the dog. 2. Polyarthritis/polymyositis syndrome. *J. Small Anim. Pract.* **28**, 891−908.

Bennett D. & Taylor D.J. (1988) Bacterial infective arthritis in the dog. *J. Small Anim. Pract.* **29**, 207−30.

Biery D.N. & Newton C.D. (1975) Radiographic appearance of rheumatoid arthritis in the dog. *J. Am. Anim. Hosp. Assoc.* **11**, 607.

Bitetto W.V., Schrader A.K. & Mooney S.C. (1987) Osteosarcoma in cats, 22 cases (1974−1984). *J. Am. Vet. Med. Assoc.* **190**, 91.

Bohning R., Suter P., Hohn R.B. & Marshall J. (1970) Clinical and radiological survey of canine panosteitis. *J. Am. Vet. Med. Assoc.* **156**, 870−84.

Braund K.G., Blagburn B.L., Toivo-Kinnuion M., Amling K.A. & Pidgeon G.L. (1988) Toxoplasma polymyositis/polymyopathy, a new variant in two mature dogs. *J. Am. Anim. Hosp. Assoc.* **24**, 93−7.

Brinker W.O. (1978) *Small Animal Fractures*. East Lansing, Michigan Department of Continuing Education Services, Michigan State University Press.

Brodey R.S. & Abt D.A. (1976) Results of surgical treatment in 65 dogs with osteosarcoma. *J. Am. Vet. Med. Assoc.* **168**, 1032.

Brown A. & Bennett D. (1988) Gentamicin-impregnated polymethylmethacrylate for the treatment of septic arthritis. *Vet. Rec.* **123**, 625−6.

Brown K.L.B. and Cruess R.L. (1982) Bone and cartilage transplantation in orthopaedic surgery. *J. Bone Joint Surg.* **64A**, 270.

Campbell J.R. (1964) The effect of low calcium intake and vitamin D supplements on bone structure in young growing dogs. *J. Small Anim. Pract.* **5**, 229.

Carmichael S. (1990) Management of the lame dog. *The Veterinary Annual* **30**, 233−41.

Carrig L.B., Pool R.R. & McElroy J.M. (1975) Polyostatic cystic bone lesions in a dog. *J. Small Anim. Pract.* **16**, 495.

Christman C.L. & Averill D.R. (1983) Diseases of peripheral nerves and muscles. In: S.J. Ettinger (ed.) *Textbook of Veterinary Internal Medicine*, 2nd edn. W.B. Saunders & Co., Philadelphia.

Clarke L., Seawright A.A. & Ardlicka J. (1970) Extoses in hypervitaminosis A cats with optimal calcium–phosphorus intakes. *J. Small Anim. Pract.* **11**, 553.

Clayton-Jones D.G. & Vaughan L.C. (1970) Disturbances in the growth of the radius in dogs. *J. Small Anim. Pract.* **11**, 453.

Core D.M., Hoff E.J. & Milton J.L. (1982) Hindlimb extension as a result of *Toxoplasma gondii* polyradiculoneuritis. *J. Am. Anim. Hosp. Assoc.* **19**, 713–16.

Dawson S. (1991) *Feline Calicivirus and Arthritis.* Paper Synopses of BSAVA Congress 1991. Wakefield, p. 108.

DeLahunta A. (1983) *Veterinary Neuroanatomy and Clinical Neurology*, 2nd edn. W.B. Saunders & Co., Philadelphia.

Denny H.R. (1990) Unpublished.

Denny H.R., Minter H. & Osborne A.D. (1974) Gas gangrene in the dog. *J. Small Anim. Pract.* **15**, 523–7.

Farrow B.R.H. & Malik R. (1981) Hereditary myotonia in the Chow Chow. *J. Small Anim. Pract.* **22**, 451–65.

Flo G.L., Stickle R.L. & Dunstan R.W. (1987) Synovial chondrometaplasia in 5 dogs. *J. Am. Vet. Med. Assoc.* **191**, 1417–22.

Gibbs C., Denny H.R. & Kelly D.F. (1984) The radiological features of osteosarcoma of the appendicular skeleton in dogs, a review of 74 cases. *J. Small Anim. Pract.* **25**, 177–92.

Gibbs C., Denny H.R. & Lucke V.M. (1985) The radiological features of non-osteogenic malignant tumours of bone in the appendicular skeleton of the dog: a review of 34 cases. *J. Small Anim. Pract.* **26**, 537–53.

Greene C.G., Cook J.R. & Mahaffey E.A. (1985) Clindamycin for treatment of toxoplasma polymyositis in a dog. *J. Am. Vet. Med. Assoc.* **187**, 631–4.

Gregory S.P. & Pearson G.R. (1990) Synovial osteochondromatosis in a Labrador retriever bitch. *J. Small Anim. Pract.* **31**, 580–3.

Ham A.W. & Harris W.R. (1956) Repair and transplantation of bone. In: *The Biochemistry and Physiology of Bone*, Academic Press, New York.

Ham A.W. & Leeson T.S. (1961) *Histology*, 4th edn. J.B. Lipincott Co., Philadelphia and Montreal.

Hickman J. (1967) *Veterinary Orthopaedics.* Oliver & Boyd Ltd, London.

Hoover E.A. & Kociba G.J. (1974) Bone lesions in cats with anaemia induced by feline leukaemia virus. *J. Nat. Cancer Inst.* **53**, 1277–84.

Houlton J.E.F. & Jefferies A.R. (1989) Infective polyarthritis and multiple discospondylitis in a dog due to *Erysipelothrix rhusiopathiae*. *J. Small Anim. Pract.* **30**, 35–8.

Hutzschenreuter P., Perren S.M. & Steinemann S. (1969) Some effects of rigidity of internal fixation on the healing pattern of osteotomies. *Injury* **1**, 77.

Johnson K.A. (1980) Carpal arthrodesis in dogs. *Aust. Vet. J.* **56**, 565–73.

Kealy J.K. (1979) *Diagnostic Radiology of the Dog and Cat.* W.B. Saunders & Co., Philadelphia, p. 371.

Kramer J.W., Hegreberg G.A. & Hamilton M.J. (1981) Inheritance of a neuromuscular disorder of Labrador Retriever dogs. *J. Am. Vet. Med. Assoc.* **179**, 380.

Kramers P., Fluckiger M.A., Rahn B.A. & Cordey J. (1988) Osteopetrosis in cats. *J. Small Anim. Pract.* **29**, 153–64.

Krook L.L., Lutwak P. & Henrikson F. (1971) Reversability of nutritional osteoporosis. *J. Nutr.* **101**, 233.

Krum S.H., Cardinet G.H., Anderson B.C. & Holliday T.A. (1977) Polymyositis and polyarthritis associated with systemic lupus erythematosus in the dog. *J. Am. Vet. Med. Assoc.* **170**, 61.

Lees G.E. & Sautter J.H. (1979) Anaemia and osteopetrosis in a dog. *J. Am. Vet. Med. Assoc.* **175**, 820–4.

McGlennon N.J. (1991) In: *Manual of Small Animal Oncology*. The British Small Animal Veterinary Association, London.

McGlennon N.J., Houlton J.E.F. & Gorman N.T. (1988) Synovial sarcoma in the dog—a review. *J. Small Anim. Pract.* **29**, 139–52.

McKellar Q.A., Pearson T., Bogan J.A. *et al.* (1990) Pharmacokinetics, tolerance and serum thromboxane inhibition of carprofen in the dog. *J. Small Anim. Pract.* **31**, 443–8.

McKerrell R.E. & Braund K.G. (1987) Hereditary myopathy in Labrador retrievers: clinical variations. *J. Small Anim. Pract.* **28**, 479–89.

Mankin H.J. (1969) The reaction of articular cartilage to injury and osteoarthritis. *N. Engl. J. Med.* **291**, 1285.

Mankin H.J. & Lippiello L. (1970) Biochemical and metabolic abnormalities in articular cartilage from osteoarthritic human hips. *J. Bone Joint Surg.* **52A**, 424.

Marks S.C. (1984) Congenital osteopetrotic mutations as probes of the origin, structure and function of osteoclasts. *Clin. Orthop.* **189**, 239–64.

Mason M.L. & Allen H.C. (1961) Rate of healing in tendon—an experimental study of tensile strength. *Ann. Surg.* **113**, 424.

Maudlin G.M., Matus R.E., Withrow S.J. & Patnaik A.K. (1988) Canine osteosarcoma: treatment by amputation versus amputation and adjuvant chemotherapy using doxorubicin and cisplatin. *J. Vet. Intern. Med.* **2**, 177.

May C., Bennett D. & Carter S.C. (1990) Lyme Disease in the dog. *Vet. Rec.* **126**, 293.

Meacham G. & Roberts C. (1971) Repair of the joint surface from subarticular tissue in the rabbit knee. *J. Anat.* **109**, 317.

Miller A. (1991) *A Case of Malignant Histiocytosis Affecting the Elbow of a Bernese Mountain Dog*. Presented at the British Veterinary Orthopaedic Association Meeting, Birmingham.

Morgan J.P. (1972) *Radiology in Veterinary Orthopedics*. Lea & Febiger, Philadelphia.

Muller M.E. (1963) Internal fixation for fresh fractures and for non-union. *Proc. Roy. Soc. Med.* **56**, 455.

Muller M.E., Allgower M. & Willeneger H. (1970) *Manual of Internal Fixation*. Springer Verlag, Berlin, Heidelberg, New York.

Newton C.D. & Lipowitz A.J. (1975) Canine rheumatoid arthritis: a brief review. *J. Am. Anim. Hosp. Assoc.* **11**, 595.

Nutrient Requirements of Cats, rev. edn. (1986) National Academy Press, Washington D.C.

Oliver J.E., Hoerlein B.F. & Mayhew I.G. (1987) *Veterinary Neurology*. W.B. Saunders & Co., Philadelphia, pp. 235–6.

Olsson Sten-Erik (1971) Degenerative joint disease (osteoarthrosis): a review with special reference to the dog. *J. Small Anim. Pract.* **12**, 333.

Peacock E.A. (1964) Fundamental aspects of wound repair relating to the reconstruction of gliding function after tendon repair. *Surg. Gynec. Obstet.* **119**, 241.

Peacock E. & Van Winkel W. (1970) *The Surgery and Biology of Wound Repair*. W.B. Saunders & Co., Philadelphia, London & Toronto.

Pedersen N.C. (1975) Feline leukaemia virus and progressive polyarthritis. *Feline Pract.* **5**, 8.

Pedersen N.C., Laliberte L. & Ekman S. (1983) A transient febrile 'limping' syndrome of kittens caused by two different strains of feline calcivirus. *Feline Pract.* **13**, 26–35.

Pool R.R. (1978) In: J.E. Moulton (ed.) *Tumours in Domestic Animals*, 2nd edn. University of California Press, Berkeley, pp. 89–149.

Prieur W.D., Braden T.D. & von Rechenberg B. (1990) A suggested classification of adult small animal fractures. *Vet. Comp. Orthop. Traumatol.* **3**, 111–16.

Putnam R.W. & Pennock E.W. (1969) Compression plating in veterinary orthopaedics. *Mod. Vet. Pract.* **50**, 28.

Riser W.H. & Frankhauser R. (1970) Osteopetrosis in the dog, a report of 3 cases. *J. Am. Vet. Med. Radiol. Soc.* **11**, 29–34.

Riser W.F., Parkes L.J. & Shirer J.F. (1967) Canine craniomandibular osteopathy. *J. Am. Vet. Radiol. Soc.* **8**, 23.

Salter R.B. & Harris W.R. (1963) Injuries involving the epiphyseal plate. *J. Bone Joint Surgery* **45A**, 587.

Seawright A.A. and Grono L.R. (1961) Calcinosis circumscripta in dogs. *Aust. Vet. J.* **37**, 421.

Seawright A.A., English P.B. & Gartner R.J.W. (1967) Hypervitaminosis A and deforming cervical spondylosis in the cat. *J. Comp. Pathol.* **77**, 29.

Shapiro W., Fossum T.W., Kitchell B.E., Couto C.G. & Theilan G.H. (1988) Use of cisplatin for treatment of appendicular osteosarcoma in dogs. *J. Am. Vet. Med. Assoc.* **192**, 507.

Short P.R. & Beadle R.E. (1978) Pharmacology of anti-arthritic drugs. *Vet. Clin. North Am.* **8**, 401.

Skoog T. & Persson B.H. (1954) An experimental study of early healing of tendons. *Plast. Reconstruct Surg.* **13**, 384.

Sumner-Smith G. & Cawley A.J. (1970) Non-union of fractures in the dog. *J. Small Anim. Pract.* **11**, 311.

Tandy J. (1977) A case of panosteitis. *Vet. Rec.* **100**, 287.

Taylor P. (1985) Analgesia in the dog and cat. *In Practice* **January**, 5–13.

Theilen G.H. & Madewell B.R. (1987) In: *Veterinary Cancer Medicine*, 2nd edn. Lea & Febiger, Philadelphia.

Thompson N. & Cocoon J.A. (1970) Experience with onlay grafts to the jaws. A preliminary study in dogs. *Plastic Reconstr. Surg.* **46**, 341.

Tilmant L.L., Gorman N.T., Ackerman N., Calderwood May M.B. & Parker R. (1986) Chemotherapy of synovial sarcoma in a dog. *J. Am. Vet. Med. Assoc.* **188**, 530.

Turrell J.M. & Pool R.R. (1982) Primary bone tumours in the cat: a retrospective study of 15 cats and a literature review. *Vet. Radiol.* **23**, 152.

Vaughan L.C. (1972) The use of bone autografts in canine orthopaedic surgery. *J. Small Anim. Pract.* **13**, 455.

Vaughan L.C. (1975) Complications associated with the internal fixation of fractures in dogs. *J. Small Anim. Pract.* **16**, 415.

Vaughan L.C. & Formston C. (1973) Experimental transplantation of the patella in dogs. *J. Small Anim. Pract.* **14**, 267.

Vaughan L.C. & Robins G.M. (1975) Surgical remodelling of the femoral trochlea: an experimental study. *Vet. Rec.* **96**, 447.

Walter J.B. & Israel M.S. (1967) *General Pathology.* J. & A. Churchill Ltd, London, Toronto.

Weber H. & Cech O. (1976) *Pseudoarthrosis.* Bern, H. Huber, Verlag.

Weber H. & Cech O. (1982) Classification of non-unions. In: Sumner-Smith G. (ed.) *Bone in Clinical Orthopaedics*. Philadelphia, Saunders, p. 401.

Wentink G.H., Linde-Sidman J.S., Van der Meijer A.E.F.H. *et al.* (1972) Myopathy with a possible recessive X-linked inheritance in a litter of Irish Terriers. *Vet. Pathol.* **9**, 328.

Whitbread T.J., Gill J.J.B. & Lewis D.G. (1983) An inherited enchondrodystrophy in the English Pointer dog, a new disease. *J. Small Anim. Pract.* **24**, 399–411.

Wilkinson G.T. & Robins G.M. (1979) Polyarthritis in a young cat. *J. Small Anim. Pract.* **20**, 293–7.

Wolff J. (1892) *Das Gesetz der Transformation der Knochen.* A. Hirschwald, Berlin.

Chapter 2
The Treatment of Fractures

INITIAL EXAMINATION OF THE FRACTURE PATIENT

Orthopaedic injuries alone are seldom life-threatening unless they are associated with gross haemorrhage. (A soft tissue swelling the size of a clenched fist around a fracture site is equivalent to approximately 750 ml of blood.) Wounds, fractures and dislocations are usually obvious on clinical examination and there is a natural tendency to concentrate on these and miss the more serious internal injuries. Chest injuries particularly pneumothorax are common complications of fractures of the humerus and scapula. In all road traffic accidents, a careful clinical and radiological examination should be done to check for chest injuries, which should be treated before embarking on fracture fixation. Many chest injuries are missed on clinical examination but are picked up on radiographic examination. Cases with tension pneumothorax or intrapulmonary haemorrhage are obviously an anaesthetic risk and surgery should be delayed (usually a matter of days) until resolution occurs. Nitrous oxide will rapidly increase the volume of any existing pneumothorax and should not be used in the anaesthesia of such cases.

A serious potential risk of pelvic fracture is rupture of the bladder or urethra. Fortunately, this type of injury is uncommon. In a review of 123 pelvic fracture cases (Denny 1978), only one had bladder rupture and two had rupture of the urethra. Nevertheless, if there is any doubt about the integrity of the bladder or urethra, then cystography and/or urethrography should be undertaken.

The protocol for the initial assessment and management of acute trauma cases is well documented. For further information, see Houlton & Taylor (1987).

The priorities in the assessment and management of accident cases can be divided into 'general priorities' and 'local priorities'. These are listed below; orthopaedic injuries are at the bottom of the list and it is important to attend to the other problems first before undertaking fracture fixation or reduction of dislocations.

[66]

General priorities
1 Maintain an airway.
2 Maintain blood volume.
3 Relieve pain.

Local priorities
1 Head injuries — see p. 117.
2 Chest injuries.
3 Abdominal injury.
4 Spinal injury — see p. 169.
5 Orthopaedic injury — see below and Chapters 4 and 5.

Dislocations and ligamentous ruptures tend to be seen in mature dogs and cats over 1 year of age. The same trauma in immature animals is more likely to cause a fracture or separation of an epiphysis.

BASIC MANAGEMENT OF DISLOCATIONS

In all dislocations, reduction should be undertaken as soon as possible after the accident, preferably within 24 hours. After reduction of a hip dislocation, the leg should be strapped in flexion using an Ehmer sling for 5 days.

In cases of shoulder luxation, a body cast is applied for 3 weeks to prevent redislocation. The elbow, by contrast, requires little external support as good stability is restored immediately following reduction in most cases.

FIRST AID PROCEDURES FOR TEMPORARY IMMOBILIZATION OF FRACTURES OR INJURED JOINTS

Robert Jones bandage (Fig. 2.1a–c)
The Robert Jones bandage is a thick cotton wool bandage which acts as a splint and controls oedema. For these reasons, it is useful not only as a first aid measure for the temporary immobilization of fractures but also as a post-operative bandage for fractures which have been treated surgically. The bandage is comfortable to wear and is generally well tolerated despite its bulk.

Thomas extension splint (Fig. 2.1d)
Although this splint can be used as the sole method of fixation for stable fractures below the elbow or stifle, it is generally used only as a temporary splint for limb bone

fractures. The splint is usually constructed from an aluminium rod, but coat hanger wire can be used in small dogs. A ring is made in the rod to fit around the base of the leg. The base of the ring is bent in at an angle to avoid pressure on the femoral blood vessels and the ring is padded with cotton wool. The splint is pushed firmly into the inguinal region and the cranial bar of the splint is bent to conform to the leg's normal angulation in the standing position. Elastoplast strips are used to fix the foot to the end of the bar. The upper part of the leg is also attached to the cranial bar with Elastoplast, while a thick band of Elastoplast is placed round both bars and the hock.

Velpeau sling bandage (Fig. 2.1e (i), (ii), (iii))
This bandage is used to immobilize shoulder and scapular injuries and to prevent weight bearing. A conforming gauze bandage is wrapped around the paw, the leg is flexed and the bandage is brought up over the lateral aspect of the shoulder and around the chest. Several layers are applied and then covered with elastoplast.

Ehmer sling (Fig. 2.1f)
The Ehmer sling prevents weight bearing on the hind leg

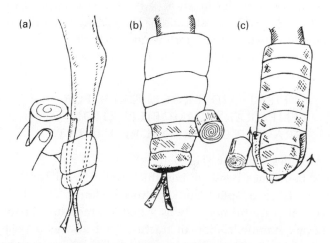

Fig. 2.1a–c (a) Robert Jones bandage. Elastoplast strips are placed down the anterior and posterior aspect of the foot (these will prevent the bandage slipping off the leg) and can be used for traction during application of the cotton wool layers. (b) A 1 lb roll of cotton wool is split into two narrower ½ lb rolls and these are used to pad the leg. The total amount of cotton wool required ranges from ½–2 lb depending on the size of the dog. (c) The ends of the Elastoplast are flapped back to reveal the pads of the foot and then attached to the end of the bandage using Elastoplast. The cotton wool is tightly compressed with a Vetwrap elasticated bandage.

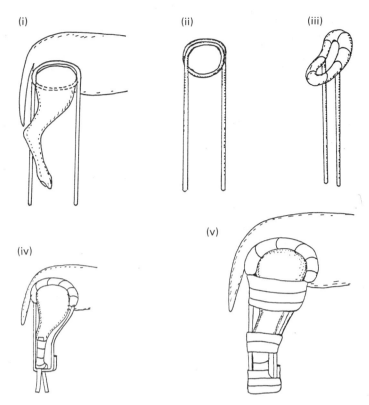

(i) (ii) (iii)

(iv) (v)

Fig. 2.1d Application of the Thomas extension splint. (i & ii) a ring is made in the aluminium rod to fit round the base of the leg; (iii) the base of the ring is bent at an angle and padded with cotton wool; (iv) the splint is positioned and bent to conform with the animal's normal standing position; (v) fixed to the limb with Elastoplast.

and its main use is to provide partial immobilization of the hip following reduction of a dislocation. An Elastoplast bandage is used for the Ehmer sling. The bandage is taken round the foot first, the leg is flexed and the bandage is

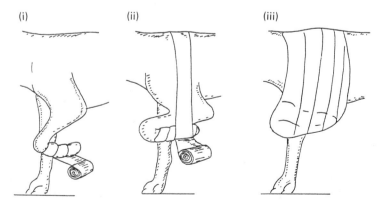

(i) (ii) (iii)

Fig. 2.1e Velpeau sling bandage.

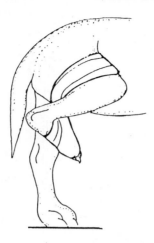

Fig. 2.1f Ehmer sling.

then passed around the medial aspect of the stifle, brought over the cranial aspect of the distal femur then taken down the *medial* side of the tibia to the hock and so on until several layers have been applied as shown in Fig. 2.1f. If the bandage is applied in this way it rotates the femoral head firmly into the acetabulum minimizing the risk of dislocation. The bandage is removed after 5 days.

FRACTURE HEALING

Once a fracture has been reduced, and provided the blood supply to the fragments is intact, the main requirement for successful healing is the provision of adequate immobilization. The degree of stability achieved affects the size of callus formation — the more unstable the fracture the greater the size of the callus (Hutzschemreuter *et al.* 1969). Conversely a completely stable fracture should heal without callus formation (Muller 1963). Rigid immobilization of a fracture can be achieved by internal fixation and compression of the fracture site. The aim of compression treatment of fractures is to achieve primary bone union in which direct longitudinal reconstruction of the bone occurs without any radiologically visible periosteal or endosteal callus (Muller *et al.* 1970). Primary bone should be strived for in the management of articular fractures but is not so essential in the management of diaphyseal fractures. Is complete immobilization essential for healing? Fracture healing will proceed in the presence of a certain amount of tension. A considerable amount of bending will also be tolerated, but torsion or rotation impedes healing because it causes tearing of the fibroblastic network of the callus and this may lead to non-union. Currently the external fixator is the fashionable method of fracture fixation. The device can be used to vary the amount of movement at the fracture site, i.e. rigid fixation during the early stages with an increase in micromovement or stress during the latter stages of healing. Studies have shown that controlled stress across the fracture both speeds the rate and improves the quality of bone healing (McKibbin 1978).

SELECTION OF APPROPRIATE METHOD OF FIXATION (Fig. 2.2)

Diaphyseal fracture
Fractures involving the diaphysis can be broadly divided into stable and unstable fractures (Figs 2.3a, b).

Stable fractures are the transverse, blunt oblique or

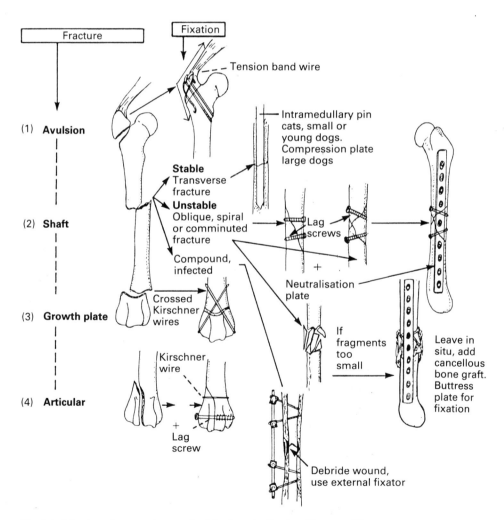

Fig. 2.2 Selection of appropriate method for fracture fixation (Denny 1986).

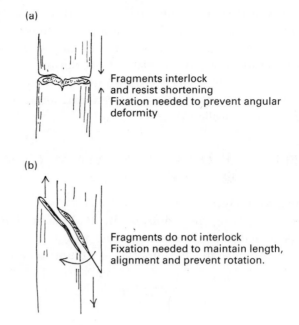

Fig. 2.3 (a) Stable fractures — transverse or greenstick; (b) unstable fractures — oblique, spiral or comminuted.

greenstick fractures in which the fragments interlock and resist shortening. The only fixation necessary is to prevent angular deformity and, depending on site, this may be done with either a cast, intramedullary pin, plate or external fixator.

The *unstable fractures* are oblique, spiral or comminuted. The fragments do not interlock. The method of fixation should maintain length of bone and prevent angulation and rotation. The ideal way of doing this is to reconstruct the bone with lag screws and apply a neutralization plate. If the fragments are too small for lag screw fixation, they are left *in situ* and a plate is applied to maintain bone length. In this situation, the plate acts as a buttress plate. The external fixator provides a useful alternative; this device is extremely versatile and can be used in the management of any diaphyseal fracture. It is the method of choice for fixation of open or infected fractures.

Avulsion fractures
In an avulsion fracture, for example fracture of the tibial tuberosity, the fragment is distracted by the tensile force of the muscle tendon or ligament which inserts on the fragment. The fragment should be stabilized with Kirschner wires used in combination with a tension band wire to counteract the tensile force acting on the fragment.

Articular fractures

In articular fractures, for example fracture of the lateral condyle of the humerus, early open reduction is essential to allow accurate reconstruction of the joint surfaces. Fixation is achieved with a transcondylar lag screw and a Kirschner wire to prevent rotation.

Growth plate fractures and separations

Early open reduction should be carried out. Kirschner wires are used for fixation; see below.

TIMING OF SURGERY

It is important to consider the soft tissue response to injury when considering the optimal time to carry out internal fixation of a fracture. The local circulation will be disturbed causing hypoxia, acidosis and oedema of the tissues, an ideal situation for infection to become established. Surgery should either be undertaken before the circulation becomes compromised, ideally within 6 h (maximum 24 h), or it should be delayed for between 4 and 6 days to allow the circulation to the soft tissues to become re-established. Urgent surgical treatment is needed for articular fractures, growth plate fractures and compound fractures.

Early surgery is also preferable for pelvic fractures and severely comminuted shaft fractures before muscle contracture makes reduction difficult.

If antibiotic prophylaxis is to be provided, high blood concentrations are established by intravenous injection 1 h before surgery. A 5-day course of treatment is given. Ampicillin is used most frequently. Poor asepsis, prolonged operating time and disruption of blood supply to the bone by rough handling of tissues and stripping periosteum or soft tissue attachments all predispose to infection. Antibiotic prophylaxis is no substitute for poor standards of asepsis and surgical technique.

CLOSED REDUCTION AND CONSERVATIVE TREATMENT OF FRACTURES

Conservative methods of fracture treatment include:
1 Cage rest.
2 Robert Jones bandage.
3 Thomas extension splint.
4 Casts and splints.

Cage rest

Pelvic fractures which involve non-weight-bearing areas of the pelvis, i.e. the pubis and the ischium, can be simply managed by confining the animal to a cage for 4−6 weeks. Cats with orthopaedic injuries seem to get better despite treatment; they respond well to cage rest and if there is doubt about the correct management of a pelvic or limb bone fracture in a cat then cage rest often gives satisfactory results.

Robert Jones bandage, Thomas extension splint
(Fig. 2.1a−d)

These methods of fracture immobilization tend to be used as a first aid measure for temporary immobilization of fractures until internal fixation is carried out. The Robert Jones bandage is also often used for 5−10 days post-operatively to provide additional support and to control oedema.

Casts and splints

Casts or splints can be used as a definitive form of fracture treatment under the following criteria. The method should be reserved for stable fractures (greenstick, transverse, or blunt oblique). At least 50% of the fracture surfaces should be in contact following reduction for satisfactory healing to occur. It is essential to immobilize the joint above and below the fracture, consequently the method is limited to fractures distal to the elbow and stifle. As a general rule avulsion fractures and articular fractures should not be treated by closed reduction and external coaptation. Plaster of Paris is still a popular casting material but is tending to be superseded by fibre-glass casting materials such as Vetcast (3M UK plc) and Zimflex (Zimmer UK) which are extremely strong and light.

APPLICATION OF A PLASTER OF PARIS CAST TO IMMOBILIZE AN UNDISPLACED TRANSVERSE FRACTURE OF THE RADIUS AND ULNA

1 The dog should be anaesthetized for application of the cast.

2 Strips of Elastoplast are applied down the anterior and posterior aspects of the leg and these can be used to exert traction on the limb during application of the cast (Fig. 2.4 (i)).

3 A stockinet is applied to the limb; this should extend from below the toes to well above the elbow (Fig. 2.4 (ii)).

4 Two or three layers of cast padding (Soffban, Smith and Nephew) are applied next starting from the toes and working up to the elbow (Fig. 2.4 (iii)).

5 An assistant holds the leg in extension; one hand is used to steady the leg above the elbow while the other exerts traction on the Elastoplast foot tapes (Fig. 2.4 (iv)). Two slabs of plaster of Paris are prepared; they should be four

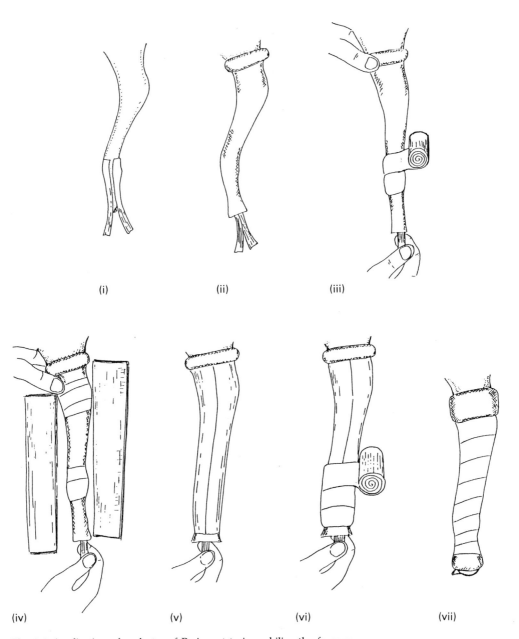

(i) (ii) (iii)

(iv) (v) (vi) (vii)

Fig. 2.4 Application of a plaster of Paris cast to immobilize the forearm.

layers thick and of sufficient length to extend from above the elbow to the foot (Fig. 2.4 (iv)). The slabs are soaked in lukewarm water and then applied to the anterior and posterior aspect of the leg. Next, run your hands up and down the cast to ensure the slabs are evenly applied and conform to the shape of the leg (Fig. 2.4 (v)). Take a roll of plaster of Paris, hold on to the free end and dunk the roll into water till it is thoroughly saturated, i.e. until all the air bubbles have stopped coming out of it. Squeeze excess water from the plaster and apply it over the slabs in a wrapround fashion starting from the foot and working up the leg (Fig. 2.4 (vi)). Finally, fold back the stockinet at the top and bottom of the cast together with the foot tags and stick these down with a little more plaster of Paris (Fig. 2.4 (vii)). It is important that the stockinet at the distal end of the cast is folded back sufficiently for the pads to be exposed so that they can be checked regularly to ensure that the circulation to the foot has not been compromised. Although plaster of Paris sets rapidly the cast will take at least 8 h to dry out. Once it has dried out several layers of Elastoplast are used to protect it. The cast is changed at 2 weeks when soft tissue swelling will have subsided. The second cast is left on for 4 weeks or longer till sufficient callus has developed to immobilize the fracture.

The cast should be inspected by a veterinary surgeon at least once a week. The owner should feel the cast each day to check that it feels warm and is not rubbing. The pads should also be checked daily to ensure the circulation to the foot is not being compromised. Warn the owner that if the cast begins to smell or the dog starts to chew frantically at the cast, stops putting weight on the leg or goes off his food, veterinary attention must be sought immediately and the cast changed.

EXTERNAL SKELETAL FIXATION

The external fixator is an extremely versatile method of fixation which can be used to stabilize a great variety of fractures and osteotomies. The Kirschner splint (Benkat UK) and the AO/ASIF External Skeletal Fixator (Straumann Great Britain Ltd) are used most often in small animal orthopaedics. The Kirschner splint is available in three sizes, the small set to be used in cats and small dogs weighing less than 8 kg, the medium set for animals weighing between 8 and 20 kg, and the large set for dogs weighing more than 20 kg.

The external fixator is particularly suitable for open fractures with gross soft tissue damage, infected fractures or severely comminuted fractures. The pins are placed at some distance away from the fracture site and are therefore less likely to encourage the spread of infection; the traumatized area is easily accessible for dressing; the device is relatively quick and easy to apply; and the pins can be driven transcutaneously.

In its simplest form the method involves the transcutaneous insertion of two half pins each in the proximal and distal bone segments which are then connected to an external bar by clamps (Fig. 2.5a). If no clamps are available the external bar can be secured to the half pins with wire and cylinders of bone cement or Technovit (Fig. 2.5b). A much cheaper alternative to bone cement is the use of car body fillers (Armstrong 1991). There are a variety available but the strongest is metal repair paste (Plastic Padding Chemical Metal). This material is very light and could prove useful for use in cats and small dogs.

The fixator should be applied to the:
1 Craniolateral surface of the humerus.
2 Craniomedial surface of the radius.
3 Lateral surface of the femur.
4 Medial surface of the tibia.

Various configurations of external fixator may be used. They can be unilateral (type 1), bilateral (type 2), or biplanar (type 3) — for further information see Egger (1983), Brinker *et al.* (1990) and Carmichael (1991). Fixator assemblies can be adapted depending on the type of fracture. Basic principles of fixation apply and the aim is to have the pins engage a minimum of four cortices above and below the fracture site. Generally unilateral frames cause less damage to soft tissues or neurovascular structures and if proper configurations are used the unilateral frame can be as strong as the bilateral frame. The stability provided by the unilateral frame can be improved by moving the connecting rod closer to the skin (clamps 0.5 cm from skin surface), adding a second rod unilaterally, or using pins of larger diameter.

Application of a four pin unilateral (type 1) fixator to the tibia (Fig. 2.5a)

The leg is prepared for surgery in the usual way and the dog positioned to allow a medial approach to the tibia.

Open reduction of the fracture is carried out using a standard medial approach to the tibia. Pins 1 and 4 are

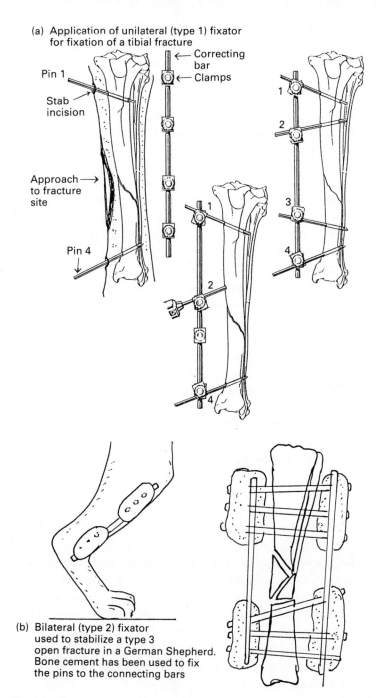

(a) Application of unilateral (type 1) fixator for fixation of a tibial fracture

(b) Bilateral (type 2) fixator used to stabilize a type 3 open fracture in a German Shepherd. Bone cement has been used to fix the pins to the connecting bars

Fig. 2.5a–b

inserted at the proximal and distal ends of the tibia. The pins are inserted through small separate stab incisions. It is easier to insert the pin if the pin hole is first pre-drilled with a small drill bit directed at approximately 65° to the long axis of the bone. Each pin is then inserted with a hand chuck until the tip just exits the far cortex. Once pins 1 and 2 have been inserted, four clamps are placed on a connecting bar. Final reduction of the fracture is carried out and the outer clamps on the connecting bar are attached to pins 1 and 4 and tightened. The central two clamps can then be used as drill guides to direct pins 2 and 3 into the bone above and below the fracture site. These pins should be placed so that they form a converging angle of approximately 45° with pins 1 and 4 respectively. Final adjustments can now be made and then all four clamps are tightened and the main surgical wound closed. The clamps, connecting bar and pin ends should be covered with Elastoplast leaving the limb exposed.

There will be some discharge from the pin holes for a few days but this is usually only a transient problem. Excess discharge should be carefully removed but the pin/skin interface should not be touched as this may interfere with granulation which is necessary to seal the area. External fixators are well tolerated by cats and dogs and are often worn for 2 or 3 months. Healing is by second intention with production of callus at the fracture site. The fixator is removed once there is radiographic evidence of healing.

One of the advantages of an external fixator is that by removing one or more of the pins during the later stages of healing, loading of the bone can be increased and it is thought that this increases the rate of fracture healing (De Bastiano *et al.* 1984).

INTRAMEDULLARY FIXATION

Intramedullary fixation is a simple method of fracture repair which is widely used in veterinary orthopaedics. The intramedullary devices include:

1 The Steinmann pin.
2 The Rush pin.
3 The Kirschner wire.
4 The Kuntscher nail.

The Steinmann pin is the most commonly used, the main indication being the treatment of stable fractures, i.e. transverse or blunt oblique fractures of the middle third of long bones. As the pin lies within the medullary cavity it resists bending in all directions. Fracture stability is related to the tightness of the pin fit within the medullary cavity, interlocking of the fragments and muscle pull giving functional compression. The medullary cavity of long bones in

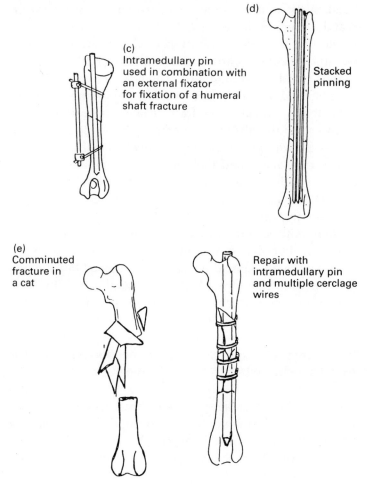

(d)

(c)
Intramedullary pin
used in combination with
an external fixator
for fixation of a humeral
shaft fracture

Stacked
pinning

(e)
Comminuted
fracture in
a cat

Repair with
intramedullary pin
and multiple cerclage
wires

Fig. 2.5c—e

the cat tends to be a uniform diameter so a tight pin fit can be achieved. In the dog, however, the medullary cavity varies in diameter so it is usually only possible to achieve three point fixation: one, at the point of insertion, two, at the fracture site or narrowest point of the medullary canal and three, by impacting the distal end of the pin into the cancellous bone of the metaphysis and epiphysis. A round intramedullary pin resists bending in all directions but has little resistance to shortening or rotation at the fracture site. Rotation or torsion is most likely to occur when a loose fitting pin is used for fixation and this may lead to non-union. Stability and resistance to rotation can be improved in several ways:

1 The intramedullary pin can be used in combination with an external fixator (Fig. 2.5c).

2 In oblique fractures stability can be improved with cerclage or hemicerclage wiring (Figs 2.16 and 2.17).
3 Instead of a single intramedullary pin, several smaller pins can be stacked within the medullary cavity (Fig. 2.5d).
4 A Kuntscher nail which is V-shaped or clover leaf in cross section can be used instead of the intramedullary pin (Fig. 2.10). This technique has largely been superseded by stacked pinning in small animal orthopaedics.

Although an intramedullary pin disturbs endosteal callus formation it causes little interference with the healing of the cortex and periosteum. Size of callus varies with stability achieved; if stability is good there will be minimal callus formation but if it is poor due to a loose fitting pin there will be extensive periosteal callus formation.

Intramedullary fixation should be avoided in comminuted fractures in dogs. The pin provides no longitudinal support or resistance to shortening forces and collapse, rotation and non-union are to be expected. Cats are an exception. Most shaft fractures in the cat even if they are severely comminuted can be successfully managed using a Steinmann pin in combination with cerclage wire (Fig. 2.5e). In the dog the intramedullary pin should be reserved for stable fractures of the middle third of the femoral or humeral shaft.

Steinmann pin
The Steinmann pin is the pin most frequently used in veterinary orthopaedics and little specialist equipment is needed for its insertion (Figs 2.6–2.9).

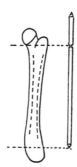

Fig. 2.6 Pain measured against a radiograph of the normal femur and pre-cut.

EQUIPMENT (Arnolds Ltd)
1 Intramedullary pin insertor with Jacobs chuck.
2 Selection of Steinmann pins (1/16 to ¼ inch diameter, 7–12 inch in length).
3 Stainless steel wire (18, 20 and 24 gauge).

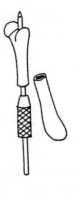

Fig. 2.7 Pin introduced into proximal shaft of femur in a retrograde manner using a chuck, pin emerges in trochanteric fossa.

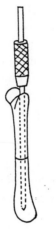

Fig. 2.8 Position of chuck reversed, fracture reduced, pin driven down into distal shaft of femur.

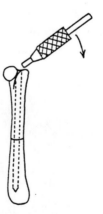

Fig. 2.9 Pin broken off flush in trochanteric fossa.

4 Hacksaw, wire cutters, wire twisters, pin cutters.
5 Two pairs of bone holding forceps.
The use of a Steinmann pin for fixation of a fractured femur is illustrated in Figs 2.6–2.9.

In large dogs it may be necessary to insert two or three Steinmann pins to fill the medullary cavity. Provided the pin has been broken off below the tip of the greater trochanter and remains in this position it can be left *in situ* after healing is complete. In immature dogs rapid longi-tudinal growth of the bone often seals the pin within the diaphysis. However in mature dogs there is a tendency for the pin to migrate dorsally ('ride up') and cause soft tissue damage. In this event the pin is removed provided that fracture healing is complete. Some surgeons prefer to remove all intramedullary pins and use a longer pin which is cut off just below the skin surface to allow for easy removal.

The main disadvantage of the intramedullary pin is that rotational stability is poor. However this is outweighed by advantages such as:

1 Ease and speed of insertion and removal of the pin.
2 Low cost.
3 The intramedullary pin is a stronger method of fixation than the plate, and bone is also stronger following fracture healing when this method is used (Braden *et al.* 1973).
4 A pin which crosses an epiphyseal plate causes minimal disturbance in bone growth when compared with other methods of internal fixation.

The Kuntscher nail

The Kuntscher nail (Kuntscher 1965) is a clover leaf or V-shaped hollow nail (Fig. 2.10). It is available in diameters ranging from 2 to 20 mm and in any length required. One end of the nail is sharpened for impaction and at the other end there is a hole to engage an extractor hook.

Equipment for insertion of the nail is relatively expensive when compared with that for Steinmann pins. The use of nails has been limited in canine orthopaedics to transverse

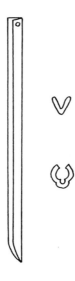

Fig. 2.10 Kuntscher nail.

shaft fractures of the femur and to a lesser extent humeral fractures. The nail is inserted at the extremity of the bone and then driven down the medullary cavity. The shape of the Kuntscher nail ensures a good grip in cancellous bone and provided a nail is selected which tightly impacts the medullary cavity, rotation at the fracture site is kept to a minimum.

The Rush pin
The design of the Rush pin is illustrated in Fig. 2.12. The pin has a pointed 'sledge runner' tip for ease of insertion while the other end is hooked to ensure good fixation and simplify removal. The pins are available in various sizes with diameters ranging from 5/32−¼ inch and lengths from 1−7 inch.

The Rush pin immobilizes the fracture by its spring-like action which results in three-point pressure within the medullary cavity (Fig. 2.14). This method of fixation is most commonly used for supracondylar fractures of the femur and humerus. Two pins are used and the mode of insertion is illustrated in Figs 2.11−2.14.

THE USE OF TWO RUSH PINS FOR FIXATION OF A SUPRACONDYLAR FRACTURE OF THE FEMUR
The fracture is reduced and an awl-reamer or Steinmann pin is used to penetrate the cortex of the distal fragment to allow insertion of the Rush pin. The angle of insertion should be 30−40° to the long axis of the bone (Fig. 2.11). The first Rush pin is introduced and used to maintain reduction of the fracture (Fig. 2.12); the second Rush pin is introduced (Fig. 2.13).

Once the fracture is correctly held in alignment the pins are hammered alternately until each is seated and the hook head grips the cortex.

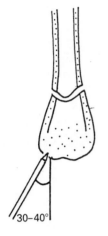

Fig. 2.11

Figs 2.11−2.14 Rush pin fixation of a supracondylar fracture of the femur.

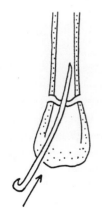

Fig. 2.12

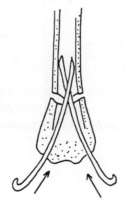

Fig. 2.13

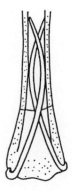

Fig. 2.14

Orthopaedic wire is made of monofilament stainless steel and is available in sizes ranging from 18 to 28 gauge. Eighteen gauge wire is the thickest and has a diameter of 1.2 mm.

Wire sutures may be used as the sole method of fixation particularly in fractures of the mandible and skull. Simple interrupted sutures are used to retain the fragments in place. A straight traumatic needle serves as a cheap substitute for a small diameter drill bit to drill holes through the fragments through which the wire is threaded.

Wire is frequently used in combination with intramedullary pins for fracture fixation, either to retain fragments in alignment or to provide rotational stability. If an intramedullary pin is used as the sole method of fixation for an oblique midshaft fracture of the femur, the fragments tend to override and there may be rotation at the fracture site. A simple way to overcome this problem is to supplement the pin with a 360° cerclage wire (Fig. 2.16). The 360° cerclage

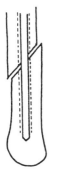

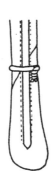

Fig. 2.15   Fig. 2.16

wire however is a controversial method of fixation. It has been condemned by some (Newton & Hohn 1974; Vaughan 1975) as it is said to cause non-union by interference with the periosteal blood supply. Others (Withrow & Holmberg 1977) favour cerclage and attribute failures of the method to poor case selection and poor technical application rather than interference with blood supply. Normal bone receives blood from a variety of sources; these include: the nutrient artery, the metaphyseal vessels and fascial attachments to the periosteum. If the blood supply in cortical bone was longitudinal to the long axis, then this could be 'strangled' by a cerclage wire, however this is not the case. Vascular supply within the cortical bone is perpendicular rather than longitudinal to the long axis and it has been shown

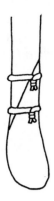

Fig. 2.17

(Cohen & Harris 1958) that the longitudinal vascular supply is limited to 1 or 2 mm. Consequently when two cerclage wires are used to stabilize an oblique fracture (Fig. 2.17) the segment of bone between them does not become necrotic. It is vascularized initially and in a centripedal fashion by vessels arising from the surrounding soft tissues and the periosteum. As healing progresses the normal centrifugal blood flow within the Haversian systems will be restored.

The proper application of cerclage wires should result in compression of the fracture and primary bone union will often occur. Conversely, a loose cerclage wire results in resorption of bone or lysis under the wire and leads to non-union of the fracture. The potential for bone necrosis may be exacerbated by excessive periosteal stripping and poor standards of asepsis.

Three hundred and sixty degree cerclage wire should be reserved for oblique or spiral shaft fractures. Eighteen gauge (1.2 mm diameter) wire is used for animals over 20 kg while at least 20 gauge (1 mm diameter) wire is used for animals under 20 kg. The wire should be applied tightly and specific wire tighteners are available for this purpose (Fig. 2.18). The wire is tied either by twisting (Fig. 2.19) or by use of an ASIF loop (Fig. 2.20).

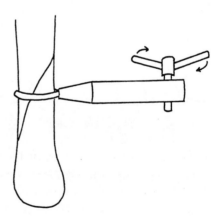

Fig. 2.18

If a twist knot is used, it is important to ensure that the first few twists are equally distributed on each wire (Fig. 2.19). Uneven twisting may cause the wire to break before it is fully tightened or the formation of a slip knot (Fig. 2.21) which may loosen.

Movement of a cerclage wire can cause lysis of the underlying bone. This complication can be minimized by

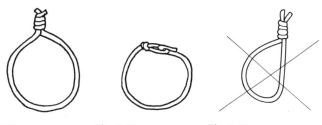

Fig. 2.19   Fig. 2.20   Fig. 2.21

Figs 2.19–2.21 The use of full cerclage wires in fixation of 18 consecutive long bone fractures in small animals. Redrawn with permission from Withrow S.J. and Holmberg D.C. (1972). (*J. Am. Anim. Hosp. Ass.* **13**, 735.)

ensuring that the wire is applied tightly and if necessary the cortex of the bone is notched to prevent the wire slipping. However, if absolute stability is to be ensured, the wire should penetrate the cortex of the bone (Fig. 2.22a and b) before it is passed round the fragments.

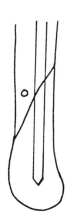   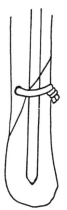

Fig. 2.22a   **Fig. 2.22b** Hemicerclage wire.

Wire may also be used in combination with pins or alone as a wire tension band to compress a fracture site. The application of this method of fixation is described on p. 95.

BONE PLATES

The correct application of a bone plate and screws should result in optimal stability at the fracture site and allow early pain-free limb function.

There has been considerable interest in the use of compression plates during the past 20 years. Although there is a definite role for this type of plate in veterinary orthopaedics, especially large animal work, the equipment is expensive. In the dog good results can be obtained using the cheaper traditional plates and self-tapping screws for fracture fixation. These plates are applied without compression and include:

1 The Sherman plate (Fig. 2.23). This is a weak plate and its use is mainly limited to small dogs.

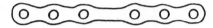

Fig. 2.23 Sherman plate.

2 The Lane bone plate (Fig. 2.24). This is similar to the Sherman plate but far weaker.

3 The Venables bone plate (Fig. 2.25). There are no constrictions between the screw holes and consequently the plate is strong and ideal for general veterinary orthopaedics. A heavy duty Venables plate is also available, and can be used in very large dogs.

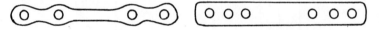

Fig. 2.24 Lane plate.   **Fig. 2.25** Venables plate.

4 The Burns bone plate (Fig. 2.26). This is a modification of both the Sherman and Venables type plates. It combines the attributes of both, i.e. strength and reduction in the size of the implant.

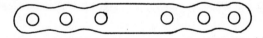

Fig. 2.26 Burns bone plate.

5 Finger plates are also available for fracture fixation in miniature dogs.

The Sherman screw is the standard orthopaedic screw and is self-tapping; a 9/64 inch diameter screw is suitable for most dogs.

Applications of a bone plate
Insertion of a bone plate using 9/64 inch diameter Sherman screws is illustrated in Figs 2.27–2.30.

The fracture is reduced and the longest plate that can be

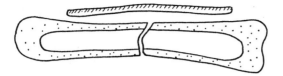

Fig. 2.27

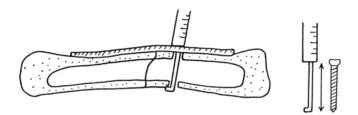

Fig. 2.28

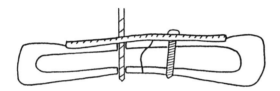

Fig. 2.29

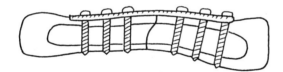

Fig. 2.30

easily inserted is chosen. This should allow at least two screws to be placed on either side of the fracture to provide satisfactory immobilization. The plate is accurately contoured to the shape of the bone using plate benders.

A 7/64 inch bit is used to drill the first screw hole about 1 cm from the fracture site. The hole should penetrate both cortices. A depth gauge is used to measure the length of the hole and a screw chosen of that length. The screw thread should grip in both cortices.

After insertion of the first screw, the next screw hole is drilled on the other side of the fracture site. The appropriate screw is inserted.

The rest of the screws are inserted working away from the fracture site.

The weakest point on any plate is the screw hole and

care should be taken in the application of a plate to avoid leaving an empty screw hole directly over the fracture site, otherwise the plate may break at this point before healing is complete. If it is only possible to insert one screw in the distal fragment then external support must be provided. Occasionally the screw thread that has been cut in the bone is stripped and under these circumstances the screw cannot be tightened. The screw should be removed and replaced by one of a larger diameter (5/32 inch). The indications for plate removal are given on p. 102.

AO/ASIF PRINCIPLES OF FRACTURE REPAIR

The AO group (The Association for the Study of Osteosynthesis) was formed by a group of Swiss Surgeons in 1958. Later, the group became known as ASIF, the Association for the Study of Internal Fixation. The AO/ASIF group defined biomechanical principles for the successful treatment of fractures by internal fixation. The basic research was done at the Laboratory for Experimental Surgery in Davos, Switzerland. Metallurgical expertise was gained from the watch industry and an entire system of implants and instruments was developed for fracture treatment.

The aim of the AO/ASIF method is to restore full function to the injured limb as quickly as possible. This is achieved by:

1 Atraumatic surgical technique.

2 Accurate anatomical reduction, especially in intra-articular fractures.

3 Rigid internal fixation.

4 The avoidance of soft tissue damage and fracture disease, i.e. joint stiffness, muscle wasting and osteoporosis, by early mobilization.

Rigid fixation is achieved by compression techniques; this may take the form of:

1 Functional compression as in tension band wiring.

2 Interfragmental compression which is achieved with lag screws.

3 Axial compression, which is achieved with a plate or a wire using the tension band principle, in which the fixation device is placed on the tension side of the bone (see Figs 2.42–2.45b).

4 Interfragmental compression used in combination with a neutralization plate or external fixator.

INTERFRAGMENTAL COMPRESSION

Interfragmental compression is a method of compressing two fragments of bone together and is achieved by the lag screw principle. This is illustrated in Figs 2.31 and 2.32. The method of drilling holes depends on the type of screw used but basically if fragment A is to be lagged to fragment B using a screw (Fig. 2.31), then the hole in fragment A must be large enough for the screw to pass through it without the thread getting a grip (gliding hole). The screw thread must only grip in the far cortex of fragment B (Fig. 2.32).

As the screw is tightened interfragmentary compression results (Fig. 2.33). If the screw thread gripped in both cortices it would be impossible to compress the fracture.

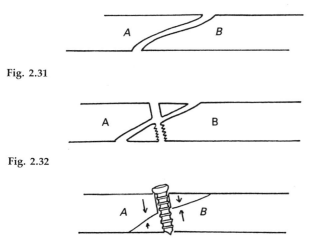

Fig. 2.31

Fig. 2.32

Fig. 2.33

ASIF bone screws are made with a much larger area of thread contact surface at more nearly right angles to the long axis of the screw than is present in most conventional bone screws, and this ensures a full grip in the bone. In addition a tap is used to cut a thread in the bone. This ensures a good fit for the screw thread without damage to the bone. If an ASIF bone screw of incorrect length is inserted it can be removed and replaced with another without risk of damage to the thread in the bone. Self-tapping screws on the other hand give rise to multiple microfractures as they are inserted. The result is fibrous tissue formation around the thread which offers the screw a poor hold in the bone.

Two types of ASIF bone screws have been developed, the cortex screw (Fig. 2.34) for use in the hard cortical bone

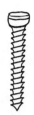

Fig. 2.34 Cortex screws are available in the following diameters:*
1.5 mm (drill bit 1.1 mm)
2.0 mm (drill bit 1.5 mm)
2.7 mm (drill bit 2.0 mm)
3.5 mm (drill bit 2.5 mm)
4.5 mm (drill bit 3.2 mm)
* Synthes, Straumann (Great Britain) Ltd.

of the diaphysis, and the cancellous screw (Fig. 2.35) for use in the soft cancellous bone of the metaphysis and epiphysis; this screw has a coarser thread for this purpose.

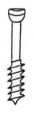

Fig. 2.35 Cancellous screws are available in the following diameters:*
4.0 mm (drill bit 2.0 mm)
6.5 mm (drill bit 3.2 mm).
* Synthes, Straumann (Great Britain) Ltd.

When cancellous screws are used for the fixation of condylar fractures it is not necessary to enlarge the hole in the proximal fragment provided the thread grips in the far fragment only (Figs 2.36 and 2.37).

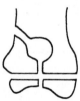

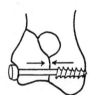

Fig. 2.36

Fig. 2.37

Interfragmental compression using screws alone can be employed for oblique or spiral fractures of the diaphysis when the length of the fracture is four times the diameter of the shaft (Fig. 2.38). The angle of insertion of lag screws is of some importance.

In an oblique fracture a screw at right angles to the fracture line will give maximum interfragmental compression (Fig. 2.38), while a screw placed at right angles to the shaft would offer maximum resistance to shortening but not complete interfragmental compression (Fig. 2.39). Maximum use of the good qualities shown in Figs 2.38 and 2.39 can be made by insertion of the screw along an im-

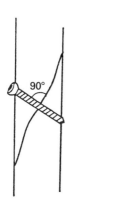

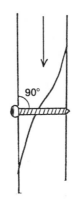

Fig. 2.38   Fig. 2.39

aginary line that bisects the angle between a perpendicular to the long axis of the shaft and a perpendicular to the fracture plane (Fig. 2.40). In practice several screws are inserted at different angles to each other to counteract shearing and torsional forces and at least one of the screws is placed at right angles to the long axis of the bone (Fig. 2.41).

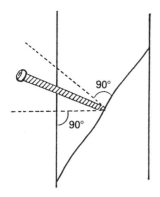

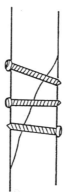

Fig. 2.40

Fig. 2.41

When screws are used as the sole method of internal fixation for a shaft fracture then external support should also be provided.

AXIAL COMPRESSION

Whenever possible axial compression is achieved by employing the tension band principle (Pauwels 1965) and this is illustrated in Figs 2.42–2.45a.

If a bone is thought of as a column, and a load is placed

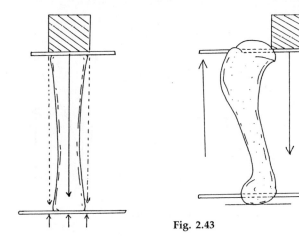

Fig. 2.42

Fig. 2.43

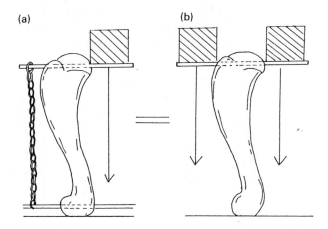

(a)

(b)

Fig. 2.44

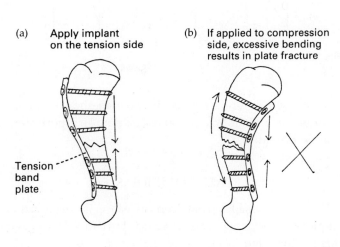

(a) Apply implant on the tension side

(b) If applied to compression side, excessive bending results in plate fracture

Tension band plate

Fig. 2.45

over its centre (Fig. 2.42) then within the column there are only compressive forces. However, if the load is placed on one side of the column (Fig. 2.43) then there are extra bending or compressive forces exerted on this side of the column with equal and opposite tensile forces on the other side of the column. These tensile forces can be neutralized with a tension band which is shown as a chain in Fig. 2.44a. It acts as if a load had been placed on this side of the column giving compression as in Fig. 2.44b.

Normally bones are unevenly loaded so that one side of the bone is under compression and another side under tension. Implants should be placed on the tension side of the bone otherwise they will be subjected to repeated bending and compressive forces and may break before fracture healing is complete (Fig. 2.45a, b). Unfortunately the loading of bone is not as simple as shown in Figs 2.42–2.45b. The stresses in bone are continually changing depending on:
1 Weight bearing.
2 Locomotion.
3 Muscle pull.
A fracture causes a total disruption in the normal stresses. Nevertheless the tension side of certain long bones has been established, i.e.
1 The proximal anterior humerus.
2 The caudal aspect of the olecranon.
3 The proximal lateral femur.
4 The antero-medial aspect of the distal tibia.
Although a plate should be placed on the tensile side of a bone whenever possible, this consideration takes third priority in the list shown below:

Plate position
1 On aspect of bone which is easiest to expose.
2 Consider position of lag screws in relation to the plate and choice of exposure.
3 Place on tensile side of bone if possible.

AXIAL COMPRESSION USING A WIRE TENSION BAND

This method is used for treatment of avulsion fractures of the olecranon, greater trochanter, patella, tibial crest, malleoli and os calcis. In all these fractures the fragment is distracted by the muscle, tendon or ligament which inserts on it. The tension band is placed so that it counteracts the tensile force on the fragments and redirects it to compress the fragment against the adjacent bone (Pauwels 1965).

Avulsion of the tibial crest is used as an example. This is a fairly common injury in the immature Greyhound and the fracture occurs through the growth plate. The tibial crest is distracted by the tensile force of the quadriceps muscles exerted through the straight patellar ligament (Fig. 2.46). The fracture is reduced and initial fixation is achieved with two Kirschner wires driven through the crest into the metaphysis (Fig. 2.47). A hole is drilled transversely through the tibia distal to the fracture site (Fig. 2.47). A length of stainless steel wire (20 gauge) is passed through the hole, the ends of the wire are brought across the anterior aspect of the tibia in a figure of 8 pattern and then passed through the straight patellar ligament before being twisted tight (Fig. 2.48a, b, c). As the wire is tightened (Fig. 2.48a) its proximal loop engages on the protruding ends of the Kirschner wires (Fig. 2.48a). Each Kirschner wire is then bent (Fig. 2.48a) and cut leaving a hook about ½ cm long which is rotated up to fit snugly with the tibial crest and insertion of the straight patellar ligament (Fig. 2.48b).

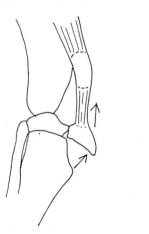

Fig. 2.46

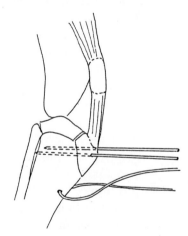

Fig. 2.47

The wire tension band counteracts the pull of the straight patellar ligament and the resultant vector (v) compresses the fracture site (Fig. 2.48b). The tension band is acting in exactly the same way as a guy rope holding up a tent pole (Fig. 2.48d). Imagine the tent pole is the tibial crest, the straight patellar ligament is one guy rope and the tension band wire is the other. The opposing pull of the two guy ropes will cause compression between the tent pole and

(a)

(b)

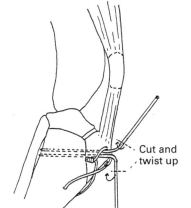

Cut and
twist up

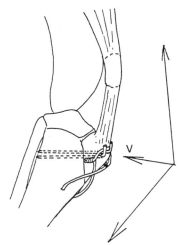

(c)

(d)

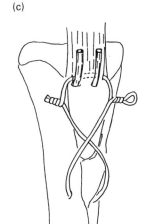

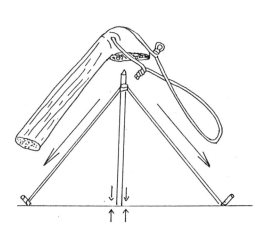

Fig. 2.48

the ground or, in this example, between the tibial crest
and the metaphysis.

Whenever a plate is used to compress a fracture it is in
fact acting as a tension band because the plate must be
placed under tension to give compression. Tension in the
plate is achieved either with a tension device (see Figs 2.49–
2.51) or by displacement of the plate through eccentrically
placed screws (see Figs 2.55–2.59).

AXIAL COMPRESSION USING PLATES

Axial compression using a plate and a tension device
This method is illustrated in Figs 2.49–2.51. It requires

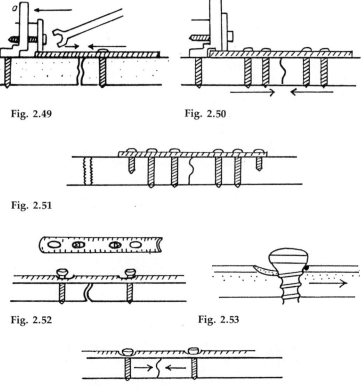

Fig. 2.49   Fig. 2.50

Fig. 2.51

Fig. 2.52   Fig. 2.53

Fig. 2.54

Figs 2.52−2.54 Redrawn with permission from Muller M.E., Allgower M. and Willenegger H. (1970) *Manual of Internal Fixation*. Springer Verlag, Berlin.

large exposure and its use is basically confined to fractures of the proximal or distal third of long bones.

The fracture is reduced (Fig. 2.49), a plate is applied and a screw inserted approximately 1 cm from the fracture site. The tension device *a* is then attached to the plate and screwed to the bone.

The tension device is tightened to compress the fracture (Fig. 2.50), the remaining screws are inserted and the device is removed. When possible to ensure that there is a gradual gradient between rigid bone under the plate and normal elastic bone the end screw is placed through one cortex only; this helps avoid the risk of refracture at the end of the plate (Fig. 2.51).

Axial compression using a semi-tubular plate
(Figs 2.52−2.54)

In many circumstances it is not possible to use a tension device to compress fractures and this led to the development of plates with screw holes that permitted a self-

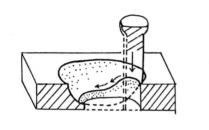

Fig. 2.55

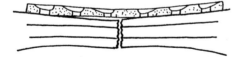

Fig. 2.56

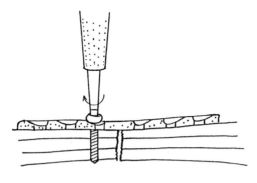

Fig. 2.57

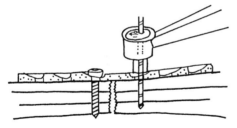

Fig. 2.58

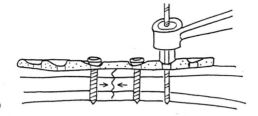

Fig. 2.59

Fig. 2.55–2.59 Redrawn by permission of Allgower M., Matter P., Perren
S.M. and Reudi T. (1973). *The Dynamic Compression Plate (DCP).* Springer
Verlag, Berlin.

compressing action. The two types of plate with this feature
are the semi-tubular plate and the dynamic compression
plate (DCP).

The screw is placed eccentrically (i.e. at one end of the
oval screw hole, Figs 2.52 and 2.53). The conical geometry
of the screw shoulder against the oval screw hole of the

plate (Fig. 2.53) ensures that as the screw is tightened the plate is placed under tension and the fracture is compressed.

The semi-tubular plate is light and its shape ensures a good fit on the underlying bone. It should only be used on the tension side of a bone as it has poor resistance to bending.

The dynamic compression plate (Allgower *et al.* 1973)

The main feature of the DCP is the design of the screw hole which is based on the spherical gliding principle. This enables the DCP to be used as a self-compressing plate. Insertion of the screw will displace the plate resulting in compression of the fracture as the screw head is tightened against the hemicylindrical slope of the screw hole (Fig. 2.55).

The spherical geometry of the screw hole also ensures that there is a congruent fit between the screw and the plate in any position along the screw hole, while permitting a certain degree of tilt between the screw and the plate.

The DCP is ideal for treating multiple fractures of a long bone in that individual fragments can be compressed together by the introduction of successive screws in the plate.

The application of the DCP as a self-compressing plate is illustrated in Figs 2.56–2.59. The fracture is reduced and the plate carefully contoured to fit the bone (Fig. 2.56). The plate is then secured to one of the main fragments by means of a screw inserted about 1 cm from the fracture site. A neutral guide is used for positioning the screw (Fig. 2.57). The second screw is placed in the opposite fragment but with the aid of the loaded drill guide; as this screw is tightened the fracture is compressed (Fig. 2.58). The remaining screws are inserted with the aid of the neutral drill guide (Fig. 2.59).

The loaded drill guide is generally used once on either side of the fracture. However, if further compression is needed, another screw may be inserted in the load position on either side of the fracture. The remaining screws are placed using a neutral drill guide.

The greatest fracture gap that can be compressed is 3.2 mm with a 2.7 DCP, 4.0 mm with a 3.5 DCP and 4.0 mm with a 4.5 DCP.

A prime indication for compression plate fixation is a simple transverse diaphyseal fracture, e.g. radius and ulna. The method provides optimal stability at the fracture site and primary bone union should result.

The ASIF range of plates and screws provides the possibility of successful treatment of fractures in animals of any size. ASIF plates are classified either by their type or function.

Plate type

DYNAMIC COMPRESSION PLATE

Figures below, e.g. 4.5, apply to plate size and diameter of cortical screw used with plate (Brinker *et al.* 1977).
1 4.5 DCP narrow or broad (used in large or giant breeds of dog).
2 3.5 DCP narrow or broad (medium to large breeds of dog).
3 2.7 DCP (small dogs or cats).
4 Mini DCP used with 2 mm cortex screws (toy and miniature breeds of dog, and cats).

SEMITUBULAR PLATE (½, ⅓ OR ¼ SEGMENTS)

The quarter tubular plate is the most useful. It takes 2.7 mm screws, is used in cats and small breeds of dog, and also in mandibular fractures and acetabular fractures in dogs.

SMALL FRAGMENT PLATES

These come in a variety of shapes, 'T' plates, angled plates, etc. used with 2.7 mm cortex screws. They are useful for pelvic fractures and mandibular fractures.

MINI PLATES

These can be used with 2 mm or 1.5 mm cortex screws. Useful for radius and ulna fractures in toy and miniature breeds of dog.

SPECIAL PLATES (Fig. 2.60)

The *reconstruction plate* can be cut to length and contoured in any direction. It is especially useful in pelvic fractures.

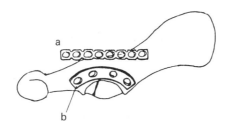

Fig. 2.60 Special AO/ASIF plates: (a) the reconstruction plate; this plate can be bent in any direction and cut if necessary, useful for pelvic fractures; (b) the curved acetabular plate designed to fit round the dorsal acetabular pin.

The *acetabular plate* is designed to curve around the dorsal acetabular rim.

Double hook plates are designed to stabilize fractures and osteotomies near the ends of long bones.

There are other ASIF plates but the ones listed above are used most often in small animal orthopaedics.

Plate function

Although DCP means dynamic compression plate the DCP is not always used as a compression plate; it may also function as a neutralization plate or as a buttress plate.

THE NEUTRALIZATION PLATE

This means the use of any plate without compression (especially for comminuted fractures) to transmit all torsional and bending forces from the proximal to the distal fragment of a bone and thus prevent these forces acting on fracture surfaces which have been stabilized by interfragmental compression using lag screws (Fig. 2.61a).

BUTTRESS PLATE

If a plate is used to shore up a fragment of bone or to span an area of comminution where fragments are too small for lag screw fixation then the plate is said to function as a buttress plate (Fig. 2.61b).

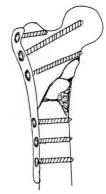

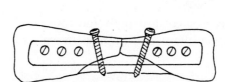

Fig. 2.61a Neutralization plate.

Fig. 2.61b Buttress plate.

The indications for plate removal

Normally there is no need to remove plates which have been used to stabilize fractures in middle-aged dogs. Plates that have been used for fixation of the jaw and pelvis in dogs of any age are also left *in situ* after healing is complete.

When plates are used in the treatment of long bone

fractures in dogs under 3 years of age, particularly working dogs, it is usual to remove the plate after 3–4 months to avoid the phenomenon of 'stress protection'. Normal bone is constantly subjected to mechanical stresses that result in some bone deformation or strain every time weight is put on it or when isotonic contraction of muscle occurs. These constantly changing stresses seem to be essential for the maintenance of the functional architecture of bone. When a rigid plate is used for fracture fixation the underlying bone is protected from stress (Allgower *et al.* 1973). According to Wolff's law of adaptation to functional demand this stress protection will cause bone destruction to prevail over osteogenesis in the course of remodelling leading to osteoporosis and a risk of refracture at one or other end of the plate. Stress protection depends on the rigidity of the plate inserted and fortunately this phenomenon is rare in dogs provided implants of the correct size are used by (Brinker *et al.* 1977).

Although it is desirable to remove the plates after healing of long bone fractures in young dogs, in the case of the humerus it is often safer to leave the plate *in situ* to avoid iatrogenic damage to the radial nerve. (It is often difficult to identify the nerve during exposure of the plate through the development of scar tissue from the initial open reduction.)

Other indications for plate removal are when fracture healing is complicated by infection and osteomyelitis or when a plate crosses a growth plate in an immature animal. Rejection of plates and screws due to corrosion or foreign body reaction has now become a rare occurrence as materials used in the manufacture of these implants are of high quality.

When a plate is used for fixation of fractures of the radius or tibia there is little soft tissue cover. This sometimes leads to skin reactions over the plate or lameness due to temperature changes between the plate and bone and under these circumstances the implant should be removed.

Growth plate injuries

Local disorders of bone growth form an important group of orthopaedic problems that occur in dogs and cats. A typical long bone is developed from three primary centres of ossification, one for the diaphysis and one for each epiphysis. In many bones secondary centres are also present and it is from these that various processes such as the tuberosities develop. Longitudinal growth of bone occurs from the growth plate, a zone of cartilage interposed between the diaphysis and the epiphysis. The cells of the growth plate are shown in diagrammatic form in Fig. 2.62a. Closest to the epiphysis are the germinal or resting cartilage cells; these give rise to a zone of proliferating young cartilage cells. Then there is a zone of hypertrophic cartilage cells; the matrix between the cells is scanty. This zone is the weak link in the growth plate. In a traumatic epiphyseal separation (epiphysiolysis) cleavage occurs through the zone of hypertrophic cartilage cells. This is of clinical importance because the germinal cells remain with the epiphysis so there is still potential for longitudinal growth of bone after reduction of the separation. Proceeding into the metaphysis from the growth plate the cartilage calcifies and undergoes enchondral ossification.

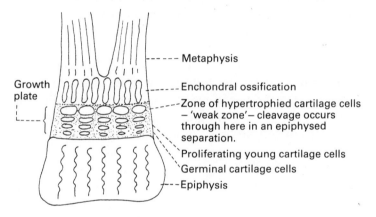

Fig. 2.62a

Growth plate disorders can result from:
1 Trauma—a fracture or crush injury or a disruption of blood supply to the germinal cells.
2 Bridging of the growth plate with a metal implant will eventually cause premature closure of the growth plate. Implants should be removed within 4 weeks if growth is to continue.

The blood supply to the epiphysis influences the prognosis following epiphyseal separation. Fortunately most epiphyses have the type of blood supply shown in Fig. 2.62b and this remains intact despite displacement. However, if the epiphysis is covered by articular cartilage (Fig. 2.62c) as for example the capital femoral epiphysis, then blood vessels can only enter at the perichondrium and these will be disrupted when separation occurs, leading to avascular necrosis of the epiphysis.

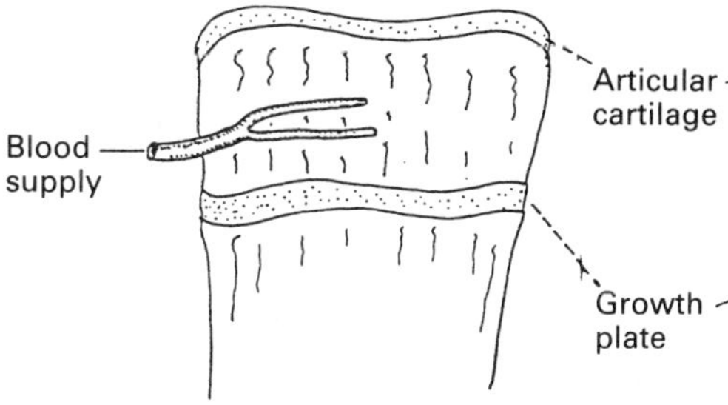

Fig. 2.62b

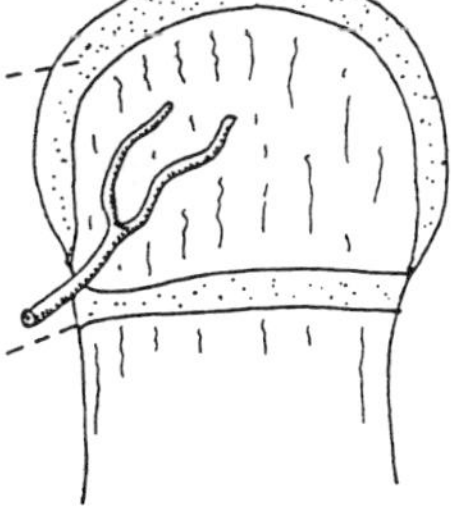

Fig. 2.62c

Salter & Harris (1963) have classified growth plate injuries into six types (Fig. 2.62d):

Type 1 Separation without fracture. After realignment healing is rapid and the prognosis is good. The exception is separation of the capital femoral epiphysis (see above).

Type 2 This is the most common. Separation of the epiphysis occurs associated with fracture of a triangular piece of the metaphysis. Provided accurate reduction is carried out the prognosis is good.

Type 3 This type is uncommon. It is seen near the end of growth. Accurate reduction is important to reconstruct the joint surface.

Type 4 Transepiphyseal fracture. Unless precisely re-aligned, union will occur between the epiphysis of one fragment and the metaphysis of the other causing premature fusion which results in angulation and deformity.

Type 5 This type is probably more common than is thought but it is not usually recognized until deformity occurs. There is a crush injury of the growth plate and diagnosis is difficult because there is rarely displacement. Premature fusion with deformity and shortening are inevitable.

Type 6 A blow to the periosteum results in a bridge of bone being formed across the growth plate leading to angulation.

General principles for the treatment of fractures involving the growth plate
This section concerns the management of Salter type 1 and 2 injuries where there is separation of the epiphysis, sometimes called epiphysiolysis.

1 Reduction of the epiphyseal separation should be carried out as early as possible—closed reduction is ideal but it is often difficult to achieve owing to the small size of the epiphysis. If reduction is managed and the leg is immobil-

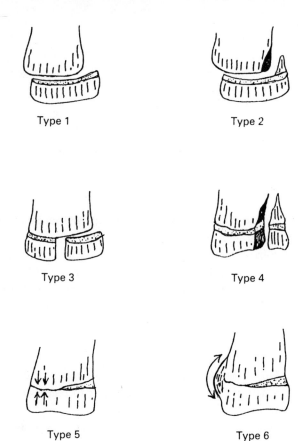

Type 1

Type 2

Type 3

Type 4

Type 5

Type 6

Fig. 2.62d For classification of the six types of growth plate injuries *see* text.

ized in a cast, then minimal disturbance to longitudinal bone growth is likely.

2 In the majority of cases open reduction is necessary. This must be done with a minimum of trauma and great care should be taken to avoid leverage on the epiphyseal side of the growth plate, otherwise the germinal cells will be damaged and premature closure caused.

3 If internal fixation is used, the ideal method is Kirschner wires or small Steinmann pins placed across the growth plate with as little deviation from the long axis of the bone as possible (Figs 2.62e and 2.62h). Provided the pins do not occupy more than 20% of the surface area of the growth plate, then minimal disturbance in longitudinal growth will result. However, although the ideal method of fixation has been mentioned, the method will depend on the age of the animal and epiphysis involved. For example, when separation of the distal epiphysis of the femur has occurred

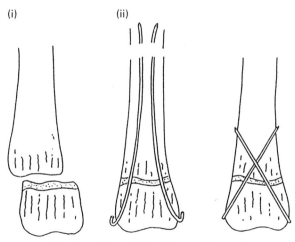

Fixation of the epiphysis in puppies under
6 months of age

Fig. 2.62e   **Fig. 2.62f**

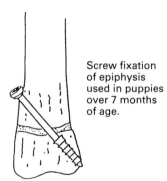

Screw fixation
of epiphysis
used in puppies
over 7 months
of age.

Fig. 2.62g This method should
not be used in younger animals.

in a puppy under 6 months of age, then crossed Kirschner
wires (Fig. 2.62f) are the preferred method of fixation
because they cause minimal interference with growth.
However, they do not provide the stability of a screw. A
screw (Fig. 2.62g) is used for fixation in larger dogs over 7
months of age because there is only limited growth potential left. The screw provides optimal stability and the fracture should heal with minimal callus formation, which is
important as far as joint function is concerned. When a
screw is used to stabilize an epiphysis in a puppy under 6
months of age (a procedure that should be avoided) then it
must be removed after 3–4 weeks to prevent premature
closure of the growth plate.

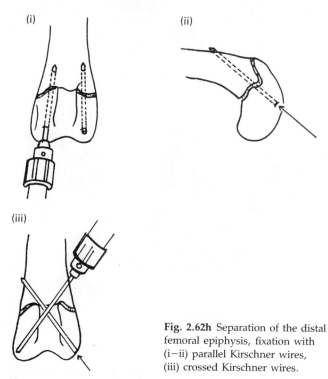

Fig. 2.62h Separation of the distal femoral epiphysis, fixation with (i—ii) parallel Kirschner wires, (iii) crossed Kirschner wires.

4 Epiphyseal separations and fractures heal very rapidly, often within 4 weeks.

5 A puppy that has been treated for an epiphyseal separation or fracture must be checked at regular intervals in case shortening or angular deformity results. Often no matter how careful the reduction has been, premature closure of the growth plate occurs. If this results in loss in length of a bone, it is often of minor significance as dogs accommodate well to limb shortening. A far more serious complication is angular deformity and this is most commonly seen as a result of growth plate injuries of the radius and ulna (see p. 250).

SHAFT FRACTURES IN PUPPIES AND KITTENS

The management of fractures in puppies and kittens under 5 months of age differs from methods described for adult animals. Fractures heal very rapidly in 2—4 weeks. Plenty of callus is produced which undergoes rapid and complete remodelling, leaving none or very little evidence of the original fracture. Closed reduction and external fixation should be used whenever possible in puppies. However,

Brinker *et al.* (1983) recommend that internal fixation is indicated for:

1 Fractures causing rotational deformity or excessive shortening.
2 Displaced fractures of articular surfaces.
3 Fractures affecting the growth plate.

A small diameter intramedullary pin can be used for fixation of a shaft fracture because there is much more cancellous bone for the pin to embed in compared with the adult. Bone plates should rarely be used and are removed early (1 month).

Kirschner wires are used to reconstruct fractures involving joint surfaces — but in some cases a cancellous screw may be needed to give better stability.

REFERENCES

Allgower M., Matter P., Perren S.M. & Reudi T. (1973) *The Dynamic Compression Plate (DCP)*. Springer Verlag, Berlin, Heidelberg, New York.

Armstrong G.H. (1991) Use of car body fillers in external fixation. *Vet. Rec.* **August**, 151.

Braden T.D., Brinker W.O., Little R.W., Jenkins, R.B. & Butler D. (1973) Comparative evaluations of bone healing in the dog. *J. Am. Vet. Med. Assoc.* **163**, 65.

Brinker W.O. (1978) *Small Animal Fractures*. East Lansing, Michigan, Department of Continuing Education Services, Michigan State University Press.

Brinker W.O., Flo G.L., Lammerdine J.J. *et al.* (1977) Guidelines for selecting proper implant size for treatment of fractures in the dog and cat. *J. Am. Anim. Hosp. Assoc.* **13**, 476.

Brinker W.O. Piermattei D.L. & Flo G.L. (1983) *Handbook of Small Animal Orthopaedics and Fracture Treatment*. W.B. Saunders Company, Philadelphia, London, p. 195.

Brinker W.O., Piermattei D.L. & Flo G.L. (1990) *Handbook of Small Animal Orthopaedics and Fracture Treatment*, 2nd edn. W.B. Saunders Company, Philadelphia, pp. 24–8.

Carmichael S. (1991) The external fixator in small animal orthopaedics, *J. Small Anim. Pract.* **32**, 486–94.

Cohen J. & Harris W.H. (1958) The three dimensional anatomy of haversian systems. *J. Bone Joint Surg.* **40A**, 419.

De Bastiano G., Aldegheri R. & Renzo Brivio L. (1984) The treatment of fractures with a dynamic external fixator. *J. Bone Joint Surg.* **66B**, 538–45.

Denny H.R. (1978) Pelvic fractures in the dog, a review of 123 cases. *J. Small Anim. Pract.* **19**, 151.

Denny H.R. (1986) Acute trauma in small animals 3: orthopaedic injuries. *In Practice* 168–75.

Egger E.L. (1983) Static strength evaluation of six external skeletal fixation configurations. *Vet. Surg.* **12**, 130–6.

Houlton J.E.F. & Taylor P.M. (1987) *Trauma Management in the Dog and Cat*. Wright, Bristol.

Hutzschemreuter P., Perren P., Steinmann S., Geret V. & Klebl M. (1969) Some effects of rigidity of internal fixation on the healing pattern of osteotomies. *Injury* **1**, 77–90.

Kuntscher G. (1965) Intramedullary surgical technique and its place in orthopaedic surgery. *J. Bone Joint Surg.* **47A**, 809.

McKibbin B. (1978) The biology of fracture healing in long bones. *J. Bone Joint Surg.* **60B**, 150–62.

Muller M.E. (1963) Internal fixation for fresh fractures and non-unions. *Proc. Roy. Soc. Med.* **56**, 455.

Muller M.E., Allgower M. & Willenegger H. (1970) *Manual of Internal Fixation.* Springer Verlag, Berlin, Heidelberg, New York.

Newton C.D. & Hohn R.B. (1974) Fracture non-union resulting from cerclage appliances. *J. Am. Vet. Med. Assoc.* **164**, 503.

Pauwels F. (1965) *Gesammelte Aghandlungen zur Funktionellen Anatomie des Bewegungs-apparates.* Springer Verlag, Berlin, Heidelberg, New York.

Salter R.B. & Harris W.R. (1963) Injuries involving the epiphyseal plate. *J. Bone Joint Surg.* **45A**, 587.

Vaughan L.C. (1975) Complications associated with the internal fixation of fractures in the dog. *J. Small Anim. Pract.* **16**, 415.

Withrow S.J. & Holmberg D.C. (1977) Use of full cerclage wires in the fixation of 18 consecutive long bone fractures in small animals. *J. Am. Anim. Hosp. Assoc.* **13**, 735.

Chapter 3
The Skull and Spine

THE SKULL

Fractures of the mandible

Upper airway obstruction can occur in the cat or dog with fractures of the mandible and/or maxilla, particularly if the animal is concussed, because blood and mucus tend to accumulate in the back of the pharynx. The first priority is to remove this material and, if necessary, pass an endotracheal tube to maintain an airway.

Fracture of the mandibular symphysis is the most common jaw fracture in the cat, 73.3% of cases (Umphlet & Johnson 1988), while in the dog the majority of fractures involve the premolar (31%) and the molar (18%) regions (Umphlet & Johnson 1990).

The common sites of mandibular fracture are:

1 The symphysis.
2 The horizontal ramus between the canine and first premolar teeth.
3 The horizontal ramus at the level of the carnassial tooth.
4 The junction of the horizontal and vertical ramus.

The vertical ramus is less prone to fracture because it is well protected by muscle and the zygomatic arch.

The majority of mandibular fractures are caused in road traffic accidents. Kicks, bites, gun shot wounds and dentistry account for the remaining cases. Paradontal disease predisposes to fracture and could account for the relatively high incidence of the injury in Poodles and Pekingese. Clinical signs of fracture include bleeding from the mouth, excessive salivation and malocclusion of the teeth. The jaw is displaced towards the side of fracture.

Although fractures of the mandible are usually compound, infection is seldom a serious problem due to the antibacterial and cleansing action of saliva (Weinmann & Sicher 1955). The aim of treatment is to immobilize the fracture and restore good occlusion of the teeth to allow an early return to normal feeding.

First aid immobilization of mandibular fractures is simply achieved by closing the mouth and applying a muzzle so that the upper jaw acts as a splint for the lower. A muzzle can be used as the sole method of treatment and is loosened at feeding times to allow the animal to drink liquids. The methods of fixation for mandibular fractures are listed below.

Fractures of the symphysis

CERCLAGE WIRE (Winstanley 1976)
Good fixation of the symphysis in cats and dogs can be achieved with a cerclage wire placed around the mandible just caudal to the canine teeth (Fig. 3.2). The wire is passed under the soft tissues so that it lies in close contact with the bone. A large hypodermic needle is bent into a half circle; it can be used as a guide to pass the wire around the symphysis (Fig. 3.1). The cerclage wire tends to become buried beneath the mucous membrane and can be left *in situ*. The symphysis should heal within 5 weeks; if the wire is still visible or causing soft tissue reaction it is removed after this period.

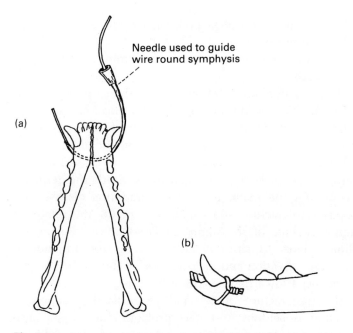

(a)

Needle used to guide
wire round symphysis

(b)

Fig. 3.1

THE LAG SCREW (Lawson 1963; Wolff 1974)
The mucous membrane is elevated and a lag screw inserted transversely just behind the canine teeth and anterior to the middle mental foramen (Fig. 3.2). This method provides optimal stability and avoids vital structures.

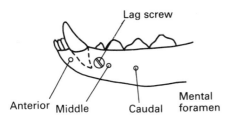

Fig. 3.2

TRANSVERSE PIN (Leonard 1971; Spellman 1972)
An alternative to the lag screw is to transfix the mandible
with a pin (site of entry is as in Fig. 3.2).

Fractures of the horizontal ramus of the mandible

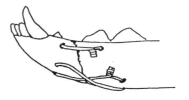

Fig. 3.3

ANTERIOR RAMUS (Fig. 3.3)
A wire suture is placed close to the buccal margin of the
fracture. Holes for the wire are drilled between the teeth
roots. Stability can be improved by placing a wire tension
band over the ventral aspect of the fracture. Exposure is
achieved through a ventral skin incision.

Fractures of the horizontal ramus caudal to the second premolar tooth

PLATE FIXATION (Sumner-Smith & Dingwall 1971, 1973)
Most fractures of the horizontal ramus in both dogs and
cats are best managed by plate fixation. It is important to
achieve accurate anatomical reduction of the fracture to
ensure normal dental occlusion. The best way of checking
dental occlusion is to close the mouth; unfortunately this
cannot be done with an endotracheal tube in the normal
position. This problem can be overcome after induction of
anaesthesia by making a pharyngostomy incision (through
the lateral pharyngeal wall of the piriform fossa, just caudal
to the articulation between the stylohyoid and epihyoid
bones), through which the endotracheal tube is passed and
then directed down the larynx. Anaesthesia is then maintained in the normal way and the endotracheal tube does
not interfere with normal jaw occlusion during surgery.
The plate is applied to the lateral surface of the mandible
close to the ventral border of the ramus. It is essential that
the plate is carefully contoured to the shape of the bone to
prevent malocclusion. Exposure of the fracture is through a
skin incision over the ventral aspect of the ramus. The

platysma muscle is incised and retracted dorsally to expose the bone (Fig. 3.4).

Application of the plate close to the ventral border of the ramus (Fig. 3.5) avoids the risk of penetration of tooth roots and the mandibular nerve by screws.

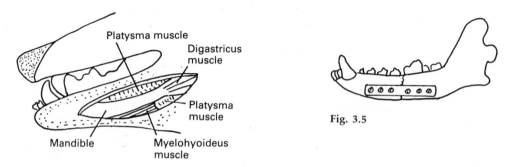

Fig. 3.4

Fig. 3.5

EXTERNAL FIXATOR

In comminuted fractures of the ramus or in dogs with poor bone stock as a result of paradontal disease then the use of an external fixator may be more readily applicable than a plate. The shape of the mandible in breeds like the Pekingese may make use of a conventional connecting bar on the fixator difficult and in this situation the pins or Kirschner wires are first driven into the bone fragments (at least two in each) and are then joined on the lateral aspect of the jaw with bone cement or dental acrylic (Figs 3.6a and b).

TRANSVERSE PINNING (Lawson 1957)

Transverse pinning is a simple and effective form of fixation.

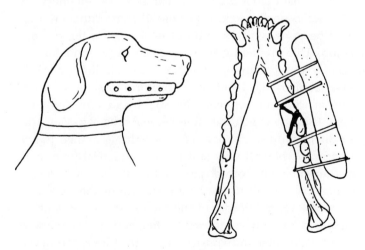

Fig. 3.6a External fixator for mandibular fractures.

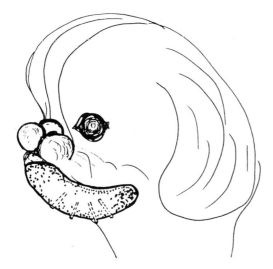

Fig. 3.6b Plate of bone cement moulded around the ventral aspect of the mandible for Pekingese with bilateral ramus fractures. Kirschner wires placed in the mandible are incorporated externally in cement.

The pin passes horizontally posterior to the fracture through the sublingual tissue and must be inserted at right angles to the median plane through all cortices (Fig. 3.7).

WIRE SUTURES

Wire sutures placed around the base of teeth or through holes drilled in the bone can be used for fixation in small dogs (Fig. 3.8). Whatever fixation is used for fractures of the horizontal ramus of the mandible an attempt should be made to repair torn gums and buccal mucous membrane to limit further contamination of the fracture site.

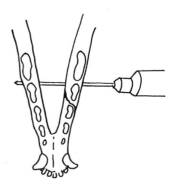

Fig. 3.7

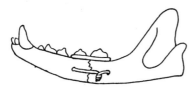

Fig. 3.8

Fractures of the vertical ramus

The vertical ramus is well protected by muscle and provided there is little displacement of the fragments fractures of this region can be treated conservatively (Lawson 1963). However plate fixation has been described (Sumner-Smith & Dingwall 1971). A skin incision is made over the angle of the jaw (Fig. 3.9). The periosteum is incised along the

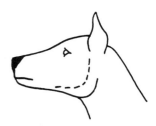

Fig. 3.9

caudal aspect of the ramus and elevated with the attached masseter muscle to expose the vertical ramus taking care to avoid the vital structures shown in Fig. 3.10. Small ASIF plates are ideal for fracture fixation using 2.0 mm or 2.7 mm cortex screws. Alternative wire sutures are used for fixation.

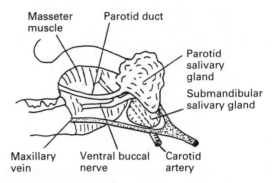

Fig. 3.10 Reproduced by permission of Sumner–Smith G. and Dingwall J.S. (1973) The plating of mandibular fractures in the dog. *Vet. Rec.* **92**, 39.

Fractures of the mandible — aftercare
Liquid or soft food should be fed for at least 3 weeks after fixation. Cats with severe trauma to the jaw may need feeding through a pharyngostomy tube for a few days after surgery. Systemic antibiotics are indicated in all cases where the fracture is compound. If malocclusion prevents eating then extraction of the offending teeth may be necessary.

Fractures of the nasal, premaxilla and maxillary bones
Although fractures of these bones are often initially associated with epistaxis and obstruction of the nasal passages this is usually a transient problem and the fractures will heal without surgical interference. Occasionally a dog will be encountered with gross instability of the nose resulting from multiple fractures. Under these circumstances fixation can be provided by half pin splintage. The fragments are transfixed with pins and the ends of the pins are incorporated in an acrylic resin 'bumper' moulded round the nose (Fig. 3.11a, b). Alternatively resin bars can be placed on either side of the nose.

Feline high-rise syndrome and hard palate fractures
The term 'high-rise syndrome' was first used by Robinson in 1976 to describe the injuries seen in cats which had fallen two or more storeys (24 or more feet). Injuries most commonly sustained include thoracic, facial and oral trauma

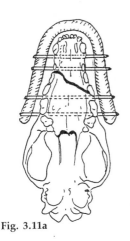

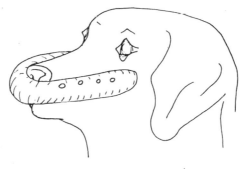

Fig. 3.11b

Fig. 3.11a

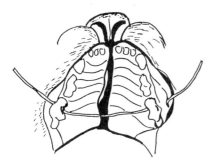

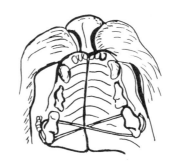

Fig. 3.11d

Fig. 3.11c Repair of a hard palate fracture in the cat using a tension band wire.

and limb injuries. The survival rate for treated cats was 90% (Whitney & Mehlhaff 1987). Because cats fall in a splay-legged position, they often land on all four limbs, which causes either direct trauma to the head or secondary injury through bouncing. Therefore facial injuries are frequently seen in cats, particularly split mandibular symphysis and split hard palate. Whitney & Mehlhaff recommend conservative treatment for hard palate fractures in cats (soft food for at least 1 month) and they report that all healed without surgery. At this clinic a tension band wiring technique is used to close the split in the hard palate, the wire is placed between the roots of the canine teeth (Fig. 3.11c and d) and is removed 4–6 weeks later. This provides rapid relief from pain and the cat is usually willing to take soft food within a day or two of surgery.

Fractures of the neurocranium (Hoerlein 1971; Oliver 1975)
Fractures of the neurocranium may be associated with brain damage, either directly or indirectly through haemorrhage

into the cranial vault. Few cases are presented for treatment presumably because the injury is often fatal. Associated signs will, of course, vary with the degree and location of the brain damage. Linear fractures may require no treatment except the administration of corticosteroids (betamethasone or dexamethasone, 2–4 mg/kg/day) to control oedema. Mannitol should not be used for the control of oedema except during or after surgery as it may potentiate further haemorrhage.

Intracranial haemorrhage and oedema may be associated with:

1 Loss of consciousness.

2 Dilatation of one or both pupils or other evidence of cranial nerve injury.

3 Motor dysfunction such as hemiparesis or decerebrate rigidity.

If any of these signs are present and progressive, then cranial decompression should be considered as an emergency procedure.

Pressure may be relieved by trephining the skull close to the fracture.

Depression fractures may impinge on or lacerate the cerebral cortex. Pressure should be relieved as quickly as possible by careful elevation of the fragments from the dura mater. Haemorrhage is controlled and the dura closed either by direct suture or by application of a temporal fascia graft if a defect is present. Closure of the dura mater is important because of its function as a barrier to infection of the central nervous system. The defect in the skull is covered with the temporal muscle. Alternatively if the fragment is large it may be retained in position with wire sutures.

Luxation of the temporomandibular joint
(Leonard 1971; Knecht & Schiller 1974)
Open 'jaw locking' as a result of temporomandibular luxation is a well-recognized but uncommon clinical entity in the dog. Traumatic over-extension of the temporomandibular joint results in forward and upward displacement of the mandibular condyle.

Under general anaesthesia manual reduction is achieved by placing a fulcrum (1–3 cm diameter wooden rod) transversely across the mouth. This procedure moves the mandibular condyle backwards and ventrally to re-engage the temporal joint surface. It may be necessary to tape the mouth closed (between meals) for 10–14 days to maintain reduction.

Temporomandibular ankylosis in the cat (Sullivan 1989)
Fractures or luxations involving the temporomandibular
joint particularly in the cat may result in temporomandibular
ankylosis. The range of jaw movement becomes increasingly
restricted so the cat has difficulty feeding and grooming
itself. Administration of corticosteroids does little to halt
the progression of the ankylosis or to prevent recurrence if
the jaw has been forcibly stretched open under general
anaesthesia. The best option in these cases is excision
arthroplasty of the affected joint with removal of the mandibular condyle, adjacent osteophytes and scar tissue.
Sullivan (1989) reported good results in two cats treated in
this way both being able to eat and groom normally when
examined 18 months after surgery.

TECHNIQUE FOR EXCISION OF THE
TEMPOROMANDIBULAR JOINT
The first problem is of course intubation. Be prepared to
do a tracheotomy if the mouth cannot be quickly prised
open soon after induction of anaesthesia. To open the
mouth insert the tips of a pair of artery forceps between
the caudal molars of the upper and lower jaw nearest the
ankylosed joint; gradually open the artery forceps and this
should create enough force to gradually spread the jaw
open. Having opened the mouth the endotracheal tube is
passed and anaesthesia maintained in the usual way. The
temporomandibular joint is best approached by a horizontal
lateral incision directly over the joint which is located
immediately ventral to the caudal extremity of the zygomatic
arch. The masseter muscle attachments to the zygomatic
arch are freed and the muscle is reflected ventrally to expose
the joint taking care of the branches of the facial nerve.
The mandibular condyle is removed using small rongeurs
or a high speed dental burr. However in most cases, because
of the extensive periarticular new bone formation around
the joint, it is first necessary to remove the caudal third of

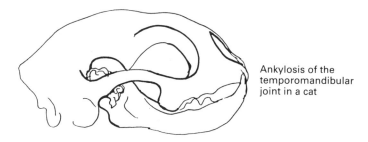

Ankylosis of the
temporomandibular
joint in a cat

Fig. 3.11e Ankylosis of the temporomandibular joint in a cat.

the zygomatic arch before advancing in a ventromedial direction removing proliferative bone, part of the vertical ramus and the mandibular condyle until the jaw can be readily opened (Figs 3.11e and f).

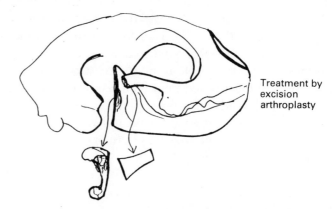

Treatment by excision arthroplasty

Fig. 3.11f Treatment by excision arthroplasty.

Subluxation of the temporomandibular joint
(Cameron *et al*. 1975; Robins & Grandage 1977)
Subluxation of the temporomandibular joint may result in repeated bouts of open mouth jaw locking. The condition is encountered in Basset Hounds and a single case has also been described in an Irish Setter. It has been suggested that the primary aetiological factor is temporomandibular dysplasia.

This allows the coronoid process to become displaced lateral to the rostral part of the zygomatic arch as the mouth is closed and prevents closure (Fig. 3.12). The condition can be relieved by resection of the ventral part of the zygomatic arch (Fig. 3.13).

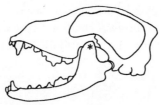

Fig. 3.12

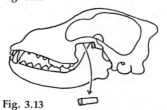

Fig. 3.13

Figs 3.12–3.13 Temporo-mandibular joint dysplasia and open mouth jaw locking in the dog. Reproduced by permission of Robins G.N. and Grandage J. (1977). (*J. Am. Med. Ass.* **171**, 1072). * Coronoid process.

Mandibular neurapraxia (Robins 1976)

Mandibular neurapraxia is the term used to describe a condition in the dog which is probably caused by bilateral, temporary paralysis of the mandibular branch of the trigeminal nerve as a result of wide opening of the mouth.

In affected cases the lower jaw hangs down passively but manipulation of the mandible is not resented and the mouth can be passively closed. However, the lower jaw drops as soon as it is released. The condition usually resolves within 3 weeks. The mouth is kept loosely muzzled during this period and the dog is fed a semi-liquid diet with the muzzle in place.

Mandibular neurapraxia should be differentiated from other conditions which result in inability to close the mouth such as:

1 Oral foreign body.
2 Fracture of the mandible.
3 Luxation or subluxation of the temporomandibular joint.

THE SPINE

Neurological examination (Palmer 1965; Griffiths 1972)

The basic layout of the central nervous system (CNS) is simply illustrated in Fig. 3.14. The system can be divided into two parts, the lower motor neurone and the upper motor neurone. The lower motor neurone is the effector unit of the CNS and consists of a ventral horn cell, its axon and termination in voluntary muscle. The upper motor neurone relays impulses from the cerebral cortex via the corticospinal tracts to the lower motor neurone (Fig. 3.14).

The lower motor neurone is not only activated by the upper motor neurone but also by local reflex arcs. The activity of these reflex arcs is influenced and modified by the upper motor neurone. Hence injury to the spinal cord at the thoracolumbar junction tends to disrupt upper motor neurone control over the hind legs. Although reflex activity in the legs remains, it is hyperactive because the inhibitory effect of the upper motor neurones has been lost.

Lower motor neurone injury in clinical cases is usually synonymous with peripheral nerve injury so that both motor and sensory components are lost; the result is:

1 Loss of voluntary motor activity.
2 Loss of reflex motor activity.
3 Loss of tone and flaccidity.
4 Fibrillation.
5 Muscle atrophy.

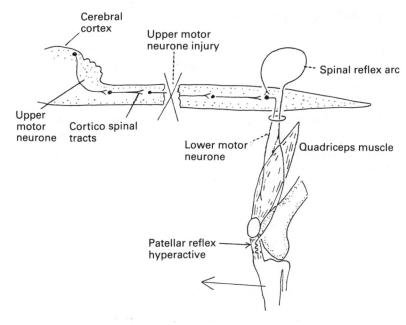

Fig. 3.14

Peripheral nerve injury—the forelimb

The brachial plexus is derived from the last three cervical and first two thoracic nerves. The nerves of the forelimb and the muscles they supply are given in Fig. 3.21. Worthman (1957) carried out experimental neurectomies in the dog and demonstrated that, with the exception of the radial nerve, nerves of the forelimb could be sectioned without producing an alteration in the dog's gait although the dependent muscles atrophied. Section of the radial nerve resulted in paralysis of the extensors of the elbow, carpus and digits. The limb was held in flexion and could bear no weight. There was desensitization of the dorsal and lateral parts of the forearm and dorsal aspect of the paw.

Worthman (1957) considers that the most common causes of radial nerve paralysis are fractures of the first rib and humerus. However, many dogs presented after road accidents with apparent radial nerve paralysis have an avulsion of the brachial plexus. In the most severely affected cases this injury results in paralysis of all forelimb muscle groups with accompanying sensory loss. Most cases of avulsion of the brachial plexus have a very poor prognosis for a useful recovery of limb function (Griffiths *et al.* 1974). Amputation of the limb is indicated if there is no evidence of recovery within 3 months, or earlier should the limb become severely excoriated by contact with the ground or by self-mutilation.

What are the alternatives to amputation?

SKIN FLAP

A 'web' of skin may be established in the angle of the elbow to keep the joint in flexion and prevent excoriation of the lower limb by contact with the ground (Figs 3.15 and 3.16).

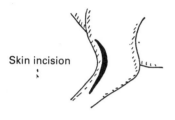

Skin incision

Fig. 3.15

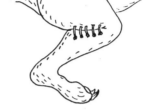

Fig. 3.16

CARPAL ARTHRODESIS

In dogs with low lesions of the radial nerve that are able to extend the elbow but still knuckle at the carpus, fusion of the carpus may help to restore limb function. However, in the author's experience dogs treated in this way may continue to have problems due to knuckling of the digits with excoriation of the skin. In the cat, arthrodesis of the carpus in a hyperextended position (45°) is said to be an effective form of treatment for low radial nerve injuries (crossed Kirschner wires are usually used for fixation in the cat).

MUSCLE RELOCATION TECHNIQUES
(Bennett & Vaughan 1976)

Limb function can be restored or improved in dogs with certain peripheral nerve injuries by means of muscle relocation techniques. Successful application of this method is dependent on the availability of a muscle from a different group to the paralysed muscles, which must have an intact nerve supply and must be in a position to allow physical transposition. It is often difficult to fulfil these criteria as more than one nerve is often injured as in brachial plexus avulsion.

After radial nerve paralysis elbow function can be restored by cutting the tendon of insertion of the biceps brachii muscle and relocating the point of insertion to the posterior medial aspect of the olecranon where the tendon is sutured to the periosteum. Ability to extend the carpus and digits is restored by side-to-side anastomosis between the tendon of the flexor carpi radialis or flexor carpi ulnaris muscle and the common digital extensor tendon. When treatment has been successful an improvement in limb function should occur within 6 weeks with recovery in 3 months.

Hindlimb peripheral nerve injury

The lumbosacral plexus is derived from the last three lumbar and the first three sacral nerves. The clinical signs associated with paralysis of specific nerves of the hindlimb have been described by Worthman (1957).

OBTURATOR NERVE

This innervates the external obturator, pectineus, adductor and gracilis muscle. Obturator paralysis therefore results in an inability to adduct the limb.

FEMORAL NERVE

This innervates the quadriceps muscle group and paralysis results in inability to protract or fix the stifle when weight bearing which in turn leads to collapse of the hock. Sensation is lost on the medial aspect of the leg.

SCIATIC NERVE

This innervates the hamstring muscle group and then terminates in the peroneal and the tibial nerves which supply all the muscles below the stifle. The peroneal innervates the extensors of the digits and flexors of the hock. Paralysis results in hyperextension of the hock and knuckling of the digits. Muscle relocation techniques have been used to restore limb function following peroneal nerve paralysis (Bennett & Vaughan 1976). A side-to-side anastomosis is performed between the tendon of the functional long digital flexor and the tendon of the non-functional long digital extensor muscle.

Upper motor neurone lesions

Upper motor neurone lesions result in spastic paralysis in which there is:

1 Limited voluntary movement.
2 Intact reflex activity which is often hyperactive.
3 Increased tone.
4 Abnormal reflexes—uncontrolled tail wag when a hind limb is stimulated, involuntary urination (mass reflex) in response to stimulation of the hindquarters.

The commonest site of cord compression is in the thoraco-lumbar region most often as a result of a disc protrusion. Clinical signs can be divided into five groups according to the severity of cord compression:

Grade I Thoracolumbar pain.

Grade II Hindlimb paresis/ataxia with or without pain.

Grade III Paraplegia (an inability to stand unaided and no, or only limited, voluntary movement).

Grade IV Paraplegia with urinary retention and overflow.

Grade V Paraplegia with urinary retention and overflow and loss of conscious pain sensation.

Paralysis of the hindlimbs associated with disc protrusion in the thoracolumbar region is usually spastic in nature unless there has been irreversible damage to the spinal cord with ascending and descending myelomalacia. In the neurological examination of the dog with hindlimb paresis or paraplegia the withdrawal (pedal) reflex is assessed by pinching the interdigital skin of the foot. It is important to differentiate between a pedal reflex which can be present after complete cord transection and withdrawal of the limb due to pain; the latter is very important with regard to prognosis. When pinching the foot the dog's head end should be carefully observed for conscious reaction to pain.

The patellar reflex is tested by tapping the straight patellar ligament which should result in a reflex jerk of the limb. Muscle tone (resistance to passive movement) is best assessed by manipulation of the limb when the dog is lying on its side.

In the animal with hindleg ataxia conscious proprio-ception can be simply assessed by knuckling the foot. If the dog is aware that this has been done it will quickly return the foot to its normal position. An alternative is to stand the dog's foot on a piece of paper. The paper is moved away and if the dog is unaware of the position of its foot it will be moved passively on the paper.

The panniculus reflex is useful to assess the site of cord injury. Pricking or pinching the flank results in local con-traction of the panniculus muscle. The muscle has a seg-mental sensory nerve supply from the first thoracic to the third lumbar nerve while its motor supply is derived from the lateral thoracic nerve. Reflex contraction is usually absent caudal to the site of cord injury.

Other signs or tests to indicate the site of cord compression are as follows:

1 Lesions cranial to the third lumbar vertebra disrupt the sympathetic nerve supply to the hindlimbs resulting in hyperthermia through loss of vasomotor control.

2 Lesions between the third and fourth lumbar vertebrae result in a depressed patellar reflex.

3 Lesions between the fourth and sixth lumbar vertebrae result in hind leg weakness and urinary retention.

4 Lesions of the cauda equina are considered on p. 171.

If there is radiographic evidence of cord compression in the thoracolumbar region (i.e. disc protrusion, fracture or dislocation) and the dog has flaccid paralysis of the hindlegs, this usually indicates that there has been irreversible damage to the spinal cord with extensive haemorrhage and ascending myelomalacia. It is important to recognize the *ascending syndrome* because it carries a hopeless prognosis and affected animals should be destroyed on humane grounds. The clinical signs of the ascending syndrome are:

1 Generalized pain and dullness.

2 Flaccid paralysis of the hindlegs, tail and anal sphincter.

3 Penis hangs flaccidly from the prepuce.

4 As myelomalacia extends cranially, the Schiff Sherrington reflex becomes apparent in which there is rigid extension of both forelegs.

5 Later the forelegs become flaccid.

6 Death occurs 5 or 6 days after the onset of paraplegia when there is involvement of the phrenic outflow at C5, C6 and C7.

Flaccid paralysis of the hindlegs can also result from ischaemic myelopathy due to fibrocartilaginous embolism or spontaneous spinal haemorrhage. There is an acute onset of paralysis but no spinal pain. The condition tends to be seen in young dogs of the larger breeds. It can be differentiated from the ascending syndrome in that there is often pain sensation still present in the hind legs, despite the paralysis. Radiographs of the spine are normal and approximately 65% of dogs recover the use of their hindlegs within 6 weeks.

Conditions which should be considered in a differential diagnosis of hindleg paresis, ataxia or paraplegia are listed below.

Conditions causing a sudden onset of paraplegia include:

1 Thoracolumbar disc protrusion—commonest sites T12/13, T13/L1.

2 Spinal fractures and dislocations—commonest sites terminal thoracic and terminal lumbar regions.

3 Spontaneous spinal haemorrhage.

4 Cord infarction caused by fibrocartilaginous embolism (De Lahunta & Alexander 1976; Hayes *et al.* 1978).

Conditions causing a gradual onset of paresis include:

1 Chronic degenerative radiculomyelopathy (CDRM) (Griffiths & Duncan 1975).
2 Congenital deformities of the spine.
3 Peripheral neuropathies.
4 Demyelination of the cord due to distemper virus or toxoplasmosis.
5 Spinal tumours.

CHRONIC DEGENERATIVE RADICULOMYELOPATHY

This condition is seen in older dogs of the larger breeds, especially the German Shepherd. There is a slowly progressive ataxia and weakness of the hindlegs. The nails tend to be excessively worn and there are deficits in conscious proprioception. The patellar reflex is often depressed. There are degenerative lesions in the lumbar dorsal columns and the condition has been classified as a 'dying back' disease of the central nervous system. Affected animals are usually destroyed 6 months to 1 year from the time of diagnosis because of the increasing severity of hindleg ataxia. There is no effective treatment. Some owners have their dogs fitted with carts once the hindleg ataxia becomes so severe that the animal can no longer exercise. The cart will allow the dog to be reasonably active for a further 2 years or more before the spinal cord changes begin to affect the forelegs necessitating euthanasia. CDRM is sometimes confused with hip dysplasia. Admittedly, many older dogs presented with CDRM will have radiographic evidence of hip dysplasia and osteo-arthritis but this is often of no clinical significance unless there is obvious pain on manipulation of the hips. Hip dysplasia does not cause deficits in conscious proprioception and excessive wear of the nails!

CONGENITAL SPINAL DEFORMITIES

Many spinal deformities are asymptomatic. Morgan (1968) reported an incidence of 47% of such deformities in a series of 145 canine spines. These included:
1 Fusion of vertebral bodies.
2 Cervical ribs.
3 Change in location of anticlinal vertebra.
4 Hemivertebrae.
5 Lumbarization of T13.
6 Sacralization of L7.
7 Lumbarization of S1.
8 Fusion of S3 and Co1.
9 Incomplete fusion of S2 and S3.

Congenital spinal deformities which are likely to cause clinical signs include the following.

Spina bifida
This is a rare condition in dogs and cats. There is failure of fusion of the left and right sides of one or more vertebral segments. Radiographs show poor development or absence of neural arches and spines on lateral views and vertical fissures may be seen in the affected vertebrae on ventro-dorsal projections.

Hemivertebrae
This condition is seen most often in screw-tailed breeds of dog (Bulldog, French Bulldog and Boston Terrier). The defect involves a number of vertebral bodies which have a wedge-shaped deformity. This produces crowding of the ribs, scoliosis and kyphosis (Figs 3.17a−d). In severe cases the resulting deviation causes spinal cord compression and hindleg paresis/ataxia at 3−4 months of age. The prognosis is poor and the motor dysfunction is likely to become worse. Some pups do seem to compensate for the deformity and stabilize. In the early stages steroid therapy may help alleviate the signs. If decompressive laminectomy is to be undertaken it is important to carry out myelography to make certain that the hemivertebrae are the cause of cord compression and that there are no other spinal lesions present.

Atlanto-axial subluxation and cervical spondylopathy
See pp. 134−148.

PERIPHERAL NEUROPATHIES
These can be divided into inherited and acquired neuropathies. For a comprehensive review of these the reader is referred to Duncan (1989).

The inherited peripheral neuropathies in dogs are classed as autosomal recessive and include:

1 *Giant axonal neuropathy* (Duncan & Griffiths 1981). Affects German Shepherds 14−15 months of age. Clinical signs include hindleg weakness and ataxia. Megaloesophagus appears to be a cardinal feature of the disease.

2 *Progressive axonopathy* of Boxer dogs (Griffiths *et al.* 1980). The disease is inherited as an autosomal recessive trait. The age of onset is usually between 3 and 6 months. The main presenting sign is an ataxia of the hindlimbs, decreased muscle tone, absence of the patellar reflexes, preser-

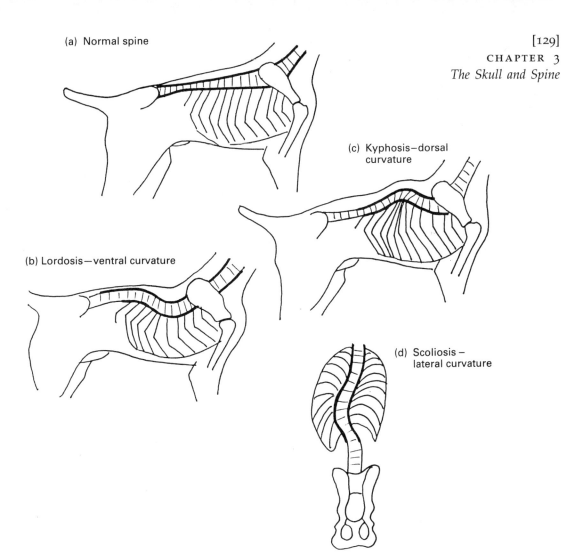

(a) Normal spine

(b) Lordosis—ventral curvature

(c) Kyphosis—dorsal curvature

(d) Scoliosis—lateral curvature

Fig. 3.17

vation of the pedal reflexes, good conscious pain sensation and virtual absence of muscle atrophy. The signs are symmetrical. Nerve roots and, to a lesser extent, peripheral nerves show demyelination/remyelination changes.

3 Sensory neuropathy in Dachshunds.

4 Sensory neuropathy in Pointers.

5 Hypertrophic neuropathy in Tibetan Mastiffs.

6 Globoid cell leucodystrophy in West Highland White Terriers.

Acquired canine neuropathies include *distal denervating disease* (Griffiths & Duncan 1979). This is a degenerative neuropathy of the distal motor axon in dogs. Affected animals present with quadriparesis, local reflex activity is depressed and there is muscle atrophy. Spontaneous recoveries have been recorded.

Feline inherited polyneuropathies include:

1 *Neuropathy of inherited hyperchylomicroanaemia.*

2 *Neuropathy of Niemann—Pick disease* (lysosomal storage disease).

The most important acquired feline neuropathy is *ischaemic neuropathy* due to thromboembolism. Occlusion of the aortic trifurcation with emboli produced as a sequel to cardiomyopathy causes an acute onset of paresis or paraplegia with pain, loss of femoral pulse, cold limbs and pale foot pads. It is the release of serotonin (5-HT) from platelets, not just loss of blood supply, which is the main cause of muscle and nerve ischaemia. Treatment is aimed at the underlying cardiac disease; analgesics are used as necessary and aspirin therapy is recommended for the rest of the cat's life to inhibit platelet function (25 mg/kg every 3 days) (Flanders 1986). A very guarded prognosis is given in all cases as although the cat may recover from the neuropathy further relapses are likely if the cardiomyopathy is not cured.

SPINAL NEOPLASIA IN CATS

The commonest cause of spinal cord dysfunction in cats is neoplasia, especially lymphosarcoma (Northington & Juliana 1978).

CLINICAL SIGNS ASSOCIATED WITH LESIONS OF THE CERVICAL SPINAL CORD

1 Pain.

2 Pain and foreleg paresis.

3 Hemiparesis.

4 Quadriparesis.

5 Quadriplegia.

However in the condition cervical spondylopathy (canine wobbler syndrome), although the site of cord compression is in the cervical region, hind leg ataxia is the main presenting sign.

Differential diagnosis of neck pain

Conditions with positive findings on plain radiographs of the cervical spine include:

1 Intervertebral disc protrusion.

2 Atlanto-axial subluxation.

3 Cervical spondylopathy; pain is a feature in some 30% of cases.

4 Discospondylitis (p. 163).

5 Fractures.

6 Vertebral tumours.

7 Extradural spinal cord tumours may involve vertebrae.

Conditions with negative findings on plain radiographs include:

1 Spinal cord tumours. Myelography is needed to confirm the presence of the lesion; the tumour can be intradural but extramedullary or it can be intramedullary.

2 *Polyarteritis/spinal haemorrhage syndrome*, seen in Beagles and Foxhounds (Joshua & Ishmael 1968; Kelly *et al.* 1973). Myelogram is usually negative in these cases.

3 *Granulomatous meningoencephalomyelitis* (Thomas & Eger 1989). There are no specific diagnostic tests for this condition; myelogram is usually negative. Remissions occur with steroid therapy.

Radiographic diagnosis of spinal lesions

This is dependent upon good positioning and a demonstration of fine detail. General anaesthesia is essential to allow correct positioning of the dog. Lateral views of the spine are usually the most helpful but should be supplemented by ventrodorsal views as necessary. The long axis of the spine does not normally lie parallel to the table top when the dog is lying on its side, so soft pads must usually be placed under the nose, neck and lumbar spine (Fig. 3.18).

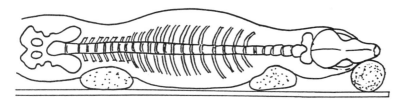

Fig. 3.18

The sagittal plane through the vertebrae should also be parallel to the film. This is achieved by keeping the upper legs parallel to the top of the table with pads (Fig. 3.19).

The neurological examination of the spine peripheral nerves is summarized in Fig. 3.21.

Myelography (Wheeler & Davies 1985)

Myelography is a technique used to outline the spinal cord with a positive contrast medium, Iohexol (Omnipaque, Nycomed UK), which is injected into the subarachnoid space. Injection of contrast into the cysterna magna is the most useful although lumbar puncture is indicated on

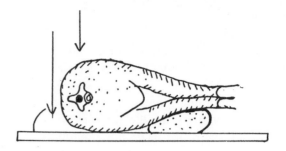

Fig. 3.19

occasions. Suggested doses of Omnipaque 300 (300 mg I/ml) are:

Large dogs 4–10 ml Omnipaque 300.

Medium dogs 3–6 ml Omnipaque 300.

Small dogs 1–3 ml Omnipaque 300.

Indications for myelography in dogs and cats are:

1 To confirm the presence of a suspected spinal lesion when plain radiographs are negative.

2 To determine the significance of multiple lesions, e.g. disc lesions seen on plain radiographs.

3 To assess cord compression.

4 To assist in decisions about appropriate methods of surgery, e.g. the choice between a ventral slot procedure or a spinal fusion operation in the management of a Doberman with cervical spondylopathy.

Myelography is carried out with the dog under general anaesthesia; diazepam (Valium, Roche) is used as premedication. A spinal needle or hypodermic needle is used; 20 gauge, 1.5 inch is suitable for the majority of dogs. The dorsal aspect of the upper neck and back of the skull are clipped and prepared aseptically. The dog is placed in right lateral recumbency with the head flexed at 90° to the spine and the nose parallel to the table top, and held in this position by an assistant. The site for cysternal puncture is midway along a line drawn from the occipital protuberance to meet a transverse line joining the wings of the atlas (Fig. 3.20). The spinal needle is advanced perpendicular to the skin and advanced directly in the midline. Resistance is felt as the tip of the needle penetrates the ligamentum flavum at the atlanto-occipital space (the needle is now almost at the right depth); a 'pop' or sudden loss of resistance will be felt as the needle enters the subarachnoid space and cerebrospinal fluid should flow as soon as the stylette is removed. If venous blood appears it generally means the needle is not in the midline and it should be redirected in

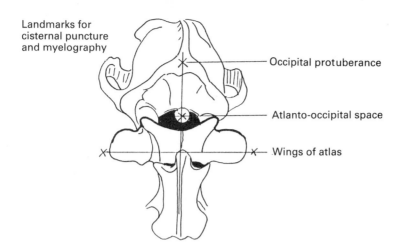

Landmarks for cisternal puncture and myelography

— Occipital protuberance

— Atlanto-occipital space

— Wings of atlas

Fig. 3.20 Landmarks for cisternal puncture and myelography.

the proper position. The appropriate amount of Omnipaque is slowly injected and the needle removed. After injection the head is elevated and the table is tilted at 30° with the head up, a radiograph is taken immediately and subsequent radiographs taken depending on the flow of the contrast column. The angle of tilt can be increased to 45° if necessary. In normal dogs the contrast column will reach the lumbosacral joint in about 10 min. Occasionally the flow of contrast will stop at the low cervical region; this is not necessarily significant unless the obstruction persists after further time has elapsed and the table has been tilted to a steeper angle. During recovery from anaesthesia the dog should be placed in a kennel with its head raised until consciousness has been regained.

Lumbar puncture
This is not an easy technique. The injection is made dorsally between L4/L5 or L5/L6; needles used are 2−3 inches, 21−23 gauge spinal. The dog is positioned in right lateral recumbency. The hindlegs are pulled cranially arching the lumbar region and increasing the space between the neural arches. The needle is inserted in the midline, cranial to the spinous process of L5 and directed ventrally and cranially at a 45° angle to pass through the interarcuate ligament and the spinal cord until it is stopped by the floor of the spinal canal. The needle is withdrawn approximately 1 mm and contrast is injected into the subarachnoid space. A check radiograph can be taken after injection of a small quantity of contrast to ensure the needle is in the correct position.

Atlanto-axial subluxation (Geary *et al.* 1967; Gage & Smallwood 1970; Ladds *et al.* 1970; Gage 1975; Cook & Oliver 1981)

Atlanto-axial subluxation is occasionally encountered in toy breeds of dogs, particularly Pomeranians and Yorkshire Terriers. The condition is characterized by compression of the cervical spinal cord with pain and motor dysfunction. Clinical signs usually become apparent before the dog reaches a year of age. Four specific anatomical abnormalities may result in atlanto-axial subluxation. These include:

1 Congenital absence of the dens which is said to be the most common.

2 Congenital odontoid process separation.

3 Tearing or stretching of the ligaments between the atlas and axis.

4 Fracture of the odontoid process with concurrent rupture of the atlanto-axial ligament.

Onset of clinical signs may be sudden or gradual, the former being the most common. The signs include cervical pain and motor dysfunction ranging from paresis of the fore or hind legs to total quadriplegia.

A lateral radiograph of the cervical spine with the head in a flexed position will confirm the presence of atlanto-axial subluxation (Figs 3.22 and 3.23).

The luxation can be reduced and the vertebrae stabilized by two wire sutures (24 gauge) passed under the dorsal arch of the atlas and through the dorsal spine of the axis (Figs 3.24, 3.25 and 3.26). A dorsal midline approach is used to expose the vertebrae.

In addition a cancellous bone graft may be packed around the wire sutures to promote bony union between the vertebrae as the wires alone may break with time with a recurrence of symptoms.

Manipulation during surgery may result in respiratory arrest. Respiratory failure may also occur post-operatively due to oedema of the cord. Consequently the animal should be carefully monitored during anaesthesia and for 24 h post-operatively. Steroids are given to control oedema. Antibiotic cover is also provided.

Cervical pain should abate within a few days of surgery and motor dysfunction resolve within 4–8 weeks. This is dependent on the time lapse between onset of signs and treatment and also the degree of damage to the cord.

Atlanto-axial subluxation was diagnosed in 30 dogs

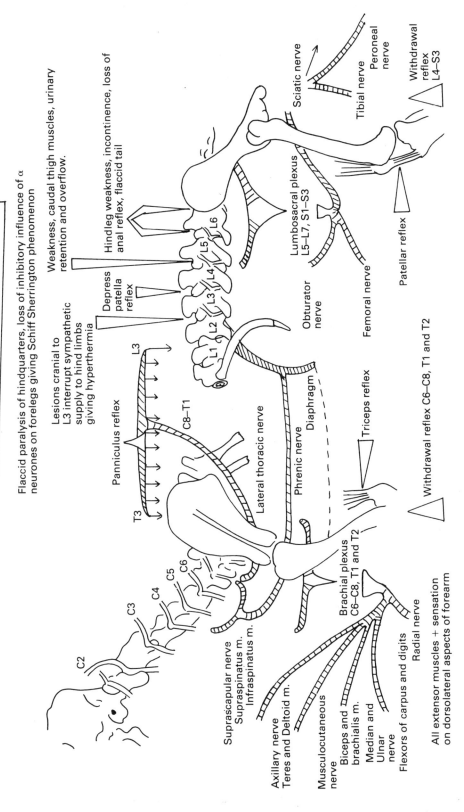

Ascending myelomalacia

Flaccid paralysis of hindquarters, loss of inhibitory influence of α neurones on forelegs giving Schiff Sherrington phenomenon

Lesions cranial to L3 interrupt sympathetic supply to hind limbs giving hyperthermia

Weakness, caudal thigh muscles, urinary retention and overflow.

Hindleg weakness, incontinence, loss of anal reflex, flaccid tail

Depress patella reflex

Panniculus reflex

L3

T3

C8–T1

Lateral thoracic nerve

Phrenic nerve

Diaphragm

Triceps reflex

Withdrawal reflex C6–C8, T1 and T2

Brachial plexus C6–C8, T1 and T2

Radial nerve

Flexors of carpus and digits

Median and Ulnar nerve

Biceps and brachialis m.

Musculocutaneous nerve

Axillary nerve
Teres and Deltoid m.

Suprascapular nerve
Supraspinatus m.
Infraspinatus m.

C2
C3
C4
C5
C6

L1 L2 L3 L4 L5 L6

Obturator nerve

Lumbosacral plexus
L5–L7, S1–S3

Femoral nerve

Patellar reflex

Withdrawal reflex
L4–S3

Sciatic nerve

Tibial nerve

Peroneal nerve

All extensor muscles + sensation on dorsolateral aspects of forearm

Fig. 3.21 Neurological examination — summary.

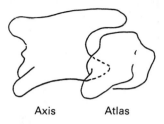

Axis   Atlas

Fig. 3.22 Normal alignment of the atlas and axis.

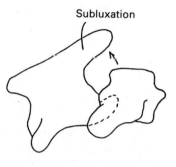

Subluxation

Fig. 3.23 Dorsal tilting of the spine of the axis is seen in subluxation.

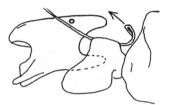

Fig. 3.24   **Fig. 3.25**

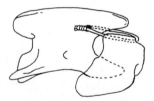

Fig. 3.26

referred to the Department of Veterinary Surgery, University of Bristol between 1977 and 1986 (Denny *et al.* 1988) and in six others seen at a private orthopaedic referral clinic in Bristol between 1987 and 1990. The condition was encountered in six small breeds of dog and was seen most frequently in the Yorkshire Terrier.

Sixty per cent of cases were under 1 year of age when presented to the clinic, with a peak incidence at 8 months. The age incidence in the mature dogs ranged from 2 to 6 years.

The most common presenting sign was cervical pain (76% of cases) and in most dogs this was accompanied by varying degrees of motor dysfunction. The duration of clinical signs ranged from 2 days to 21 months — average 3 months. Lateral radiographs of the neck both in the extended and the flexed position were used to confirm the diagnosis.

Six dogs with no evidence of neck pain and only mild neurological deficits were managed conservatively; one of these, a 5-month-old Cavalier King Charles Spaniel, made a good recovery with 1 month's cage rest only.

A 6-month-old Terrier X which had been quadriparetic for 2 months was euthanased. This animal had hydrocephalus and gross deformity of the atlas and axis.

Twenty-seven dogs were treated surgically. In 13, the atlas and axis were exposed using a dorsal approach; the vertebrae were stabilized using a wire suture (24 gauge) passed under the dorsal arch of the atlas and through the dorsal spine of the axis. This was supplemented by a cancellous bone graft in one case. Seven of the 13 dogs recovered within 4–8 weeks of surgery and one dog remained mildly quadriparetic. Respiratory problems with gasping-type medullary breathing followed by cardiac arrest occurred in five dogs at the end of surgery; only one of these animals was successfully resuscitated.

The dorsal approach to the atlas and axis makes it difficult to monitor anaesthesia in small breeds with atlanto-axial subluxation. There is a high risk of inducing respiratory arrest when the wire suture is placed and the vertebrae are reduced. A ventral procedure for stabilizing the atlanto-axial subluxation proved much safer in a series of 14 dogs. The procedure was based on a technique using threaded pins described by Sorjonen & Shires (1981).

The dog is placed in dorsal recumbency with the neck hyperextended over a sandbag. This reduces the atlanto-axial subluxation and avoids any manipulation of the vertebrae during surgery. A ventral midline skin incision is made over the cranial half of the neck. The sternohyoideus muscles are divided in the midline and the trachea and oesophagus are retracted towards the animal's left side. The larynx is also retracted towards the left, once the attachments of the right sternohyoideus muscle are severed close to the larynx. The thyroid gland, recurrent laryngeal nerve, right vagus and carotid are identified and protected throughout the surgery. The longus colli muscle is elevated from the ventral surface of the axis and atlas and retracted with self-retaining retractors. The joint capsule overlying the ventral articular facets between the atlas and axis is identified and sectioned with a number 15 scalpel blade. A lag screw (1.5 mm cortical screw, Straumann, Great Britain

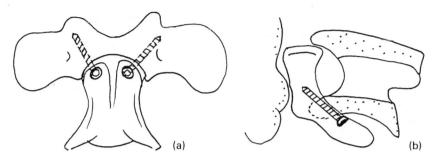

Fig. 3.27 Atlanto axial subluxation—ventral lag screw fixation of articular facets.

Ltd) is placed across each of the ventral articular facets between the axis and atlas (Fig. 3.27a and b). Care is taken to ensure that the screws are directed dorsolaterally across the articular facets away from the neural canal. The pilot hole for the screw is drilled through both ventral facets with a 1.1 mm drill bit and the hole in the ventral facet of the axis is over-drilled with a 1.5 mm bit. A 1.5 mm tap is used to cut a thread in the pilot hole. The soft tissues are protected during drilling and tapping by the use of metal foil; for example, an empty catgut packet moulded to the wound margins. After wound closure, the neck is supported with a cotton wool collar for 10 days and the animal is kept strictly confined for 4 weeks.

There were no complications during surgery and 11 of the dogs made uneventful recoveries within 2 months. This was maintained during follow-up periods ranging from 3 to 23 months. One dog died suddenly 10 days after surgery (cause unknown) and another dog was destroyed 3 weeks after surgery because of fits. This animal had granulomatous encephalitis as well as an atlanto-axial subluxation.

Based on the results presented here, lag screw fixation appears to be the treatment of choice for atlanto-axial subluxations. These clinical observations support the results of experimental work by Sorjonen & Shires (1981) using the ventral procedure. The method provides good stability and there is no need to manipulate the vertebrae during surgery as positioning the neck in hyperextension beforehand reduces the luxation. The neural canal is not entered and it is relatively easy to monitor the dog during surgery.

Atlanto-axial subluxation in the cat

Atlanto-axial subluxation, secondary to hypoplasia of the odontoid process, was reported in an 11-month-old Siamese cat (Shelton *et al.* 1991). Stabilization was achieved through the ventral approach using Kirschner wires placed across the ventral articular facets (Sorjonen & Shires 1981). Cancellous bone was collected from the vertebral body of the third cervical vertebra and packed around the articular facets to promote fusion. The cat made an uneventful recovery.

Cervical spondylopathy (canine wobbler syndrome)
Cervical spondylopathy is well documented and for further information the reader should refer to Denny *et al.* (1977), Read *et al.* (1983), Lewis (1989, 1991) and Mckee *et al.* (1989, 1990).

Cervical spondylopathy is a syndrome characterized by a hind leg ataxia which is now recognized in certain breeds of dogs, notably the Great Dane and the Dobermann Pinscher. The pathogenesis of the syndrome is not completely understood but is currently ascribed to compression of the cervical spinal cord, either as a result of instability of one or more of the vertebrae C5, C6, and C7 in the Dobermann (Fig. 3.28) or as a result of deformity of a vertebra, usually C6 or C7, causing stenosis of the canal (Fig. 3.29). Alternatively, both instability and deformity may coexist. Vertebral deformity with stenosis of the neural canal is seen more often in Great Danes.

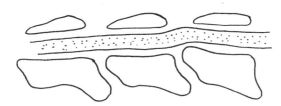

Fig. 3.28

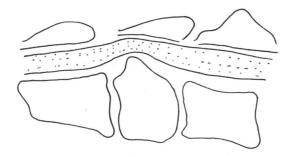

Fig. 3.29

The condition appears to be most prevalent in the Great Dane and the Dobermann Pinscher but it also has been recognized in the following breeds: Basset Hound, St Bernard, Rhodesian Ridgeback, Old English Sheepdog, Boxer, German Pointer, Rough Collie, Weimaraner, Chow, Pyrenean Mountain Dog, Retriever, Irish Setter, English Mastiff, Borzoi, and English Pointer.

In Great Danes male animals are usually affected while the sex distribution in other breeds is equal. Seventy per cent of Danes are under 1 year of age at the onset of clinical signs. Only 30% of Dobermanns are under a year of age; the rest present between 1 and 12 with a peak at 4 years.

Animals are presented with variable histories which include clumsiness, difficulty in rising from a prone position, hind leg weakness, falling or collapse at exercise, cervical pain and, in the case of male dogs, inability to cock the leg or serve bitches.

Affected animals have hind leg ataxia and there is also forelimb involvement in some. Ataxia is most obvious at the walk and can be exacerbated by making the animal turn sharply. In extreme cases this manoeuvre results in loss of balance and collapse, while in others it induces crossing or wide abduction of the hind limbs. Some dogs resume an almost normal action when made to run a straight course. The main finding on neurological examination is a deficit in conscious proprioception. Knuckling of the digits, with excessive wear of the nails, is a common finding. Cervical pain may be present and passive flexion of the neck can result in transient collapse.

Radiographic examination is necessary to confirm the clinical diagnosis of cervical spondylopathy. The examination is carried out under general anaesthesia with the animal in lateral recumbency. Radiographs of severely affected cases show evidence of gross misalignment of adjacent vertebrae or deformity, with the neck positioned conventionally in extension (Figs 3.28 and 3.29). More commonly, however, particularly in younger animals, flexed radiographs are required to demonstrate conclusively the characteristic upward tilting of the anterior borders of affected vertebral bodies.

In order to obtain full flexion of each cervical vertebral segment it is necessary to flex the entire spinal column so that the animal lies in a curled up position. Careful padding of the lower neck is required in order to avoid sagging which causes overlapping of the interspaces by obliquely projected vertebral end-plates. The muzzle is also raised, so that the sagittal plane of the skull is parallel to the table top. This position should be maintained for as short a time as possible since it tends to produce respiratory airway obstruction. A survey at this clinic suggests that cervical spondylopathy is a widespread problem in the Dobermann Pinscher. Forty clinically normal dogs belonging to breeders were screened radiographically and vertebral instability was confirmed in every case. Approximately 30% of Dobermanns have evidence of cervical disc protrusion. This has probably occurred secondary to vertebral instability and accounts for the onset of clinical signs in some older dogs. Other causes include hypertrophy and elevation of the dorsal annulus fibrosus. These changes result from abnormal forces exerted on the disc material, and are secondary to vertebral instability or deformity. Vertebral instability can also cause hypertrophy of the ligamentum flavum which will cause dorsal impingement into the spinal canal.

Because of the variety of pathological changes that can be present it is important, especially if surgery is contemplated, to carry out myelography so that the exact site and the nature of cord compression can be determined.

CURRENT VIEWS ON THE MANAGEMENT OF CERVICAL SPONDYLOPATHY IN THE DOBERMANN
(Denny & Ibrahim 1989)
The management of cervical spondylopathy in the Dobermann Pinscher is described with reference to 122 cases. One hundred and seventeen were seen at the Department of Veterinary Surgery, University of Bristol between 1974 and 1988, and the other five were seen at the author's clinic during 1987–1988.

Fifty were managed conservatively (steroids and rest). On follow-up only 39.1% recovered or improved following treatment. In 39.1% the condition remained static, while in 21.8% there was deterioration despite treatment.

Seventy-two dogs were managed surgically by screw fixation of the vertebral bodies (Denny et al. 1977). In the majority of dogs fusion of the cervical vertebrae C4–C7 was carried out. Cancellous bone grafts were used to promote early fusion and the results of different grafting techniques will be presented. A successful outcome was achieved in 73.7% of cases, i.e. the dogs made full recoveries or improved sufficiently to lead a normal life. The condition of 2.6% of surgically treated cases remained static while 23.7% continued to deteriorate despite treatment.

Cervical fusion is achieved by screw fixation of the vertebral bodies using the technique described by Gage & Hoerlein (1975). A ventral midline approach is used (see cervical disc fenestration, p. 149). The vertebrae to be stabilized are exposed by cutting the attachments of the longus colli muscle to the ventral process; the muscle is then elevated from the vertebral body and retained laterally with retractors. A large window is cut in the ventral surface of the intervertebral disc and the nucleus pulposus removed with a dental tartar scraper (Fig. 3.30).

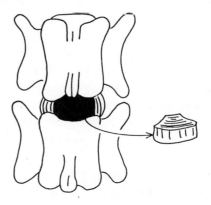

Fig. 3.30

The drill hole for each screw is started in the ventral midline at approximately the caudal third of the cranial vertebra. The drill bit is carefully advanced in a caudodorsal direction across the intervertebral space to end in the middle of the caudal vertebral body (Fig. 3.31).

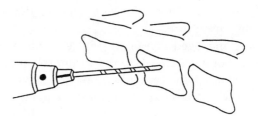

Fig. 3.31

A large bit is used to overdrill the hole in the cranial vertebral body so that when the screw is inserted the two vertebrae will be lagged together. A depth gauge is inserted into the hole and advanced until its tip meets the cortex forming the roof of the caudal vertebral body. A screw is selected which is about 4 mm shorter than the length indicated by the gauge in order to avoid the risk of the screw point entering the spinal canal as it is tightened. A single screw is placed through the cranial and caudal part of the body of each unstable vertebra to ensure optimal stability (Fig. 3.32). As many as five consecutive vertebrae have been fused without apparent interference with the range of neck movement.

A graft of cancellous bone is obtained from the proximal humerus (Fig. 3.33) and packed around the invertebral disc spaces to promote early bony function. Routine wound closure is then undertaken. Radiographs are taken post-operatively to check the position of the screw. It is not always possible to restore normal alignment of the vertebrae but this does not seem to interfere with recovery provided complete stability is restored. Exercise should be severely restricted for 4 weeks after surgery and a normal action should be resumed within 2 months.

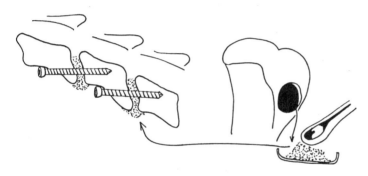

Fig. 3.32   Fig. 3.33

VERTEBRAL DISTRACTION FOR CERVICAL SPONDYLOPATHY USING A SCREW AND WASHER TECHNIQUE (Mckee *et al.* 1989, 1990)

In dogs with cervical spondylopathy, cord compression is not only due to vertebral abnormalities but also due to soft tissue structures impinging on the cord, e.g. hypertrophied dorsal annulus fibrosus. Myelographic studies have shown that traction on the neck will generally alleviate cord compression caused by soft tissue because traction stretches and flattens the hypertrophied dorsal annulus fibrosus and ligamentous structures. This finding leads to the development of vertebral distraction–fusion techniques. The simplest way of distracting the vertebrae is to place a large stainless steel washer (Veterinary Instrumentation) in the intervertebral disc space. The washer is held in place with a screw (Figs 3.34a and b). The surgical approach is almost

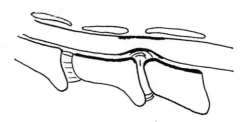

Fig. 3.34a Hypertrophied dorsal annulus fibrosus causing cord compression.

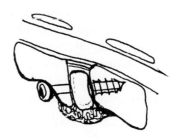

Fig. 3.34b Vertebral bodies distracted using washer and a lag screw. The dorsal annulus is flattened relieving compression. A cancellous bone graft is placed ventral to the bone disc space to promote bone fusion.

exactly the same as with the conventional cervical fusion operation, the only difference being the washer. Mckee *et al.* in their first series of cases described in 1989 had a long-term success rate of only 50% in a series of 30 Dobermann Pinschers. This was attributed to insufficient distraction of the vertebrae. They reported the results of a second series of dogs (Mckee *et al.* 1990) in which double washers were used to provide greater distraction of the vertebrae. The results were much better with 85% of cases improved following surgery. They also observed that dogs operated on within 2 weeks of the onset of signs were more likely to make a complete recovery compared to those receiving surgery after 2 weeks.

VENTRAL SLOT TECHNIQUE
Some cases of cervical spondylopathy are good candidates for ventral spinal decompression by the ventral slot technique, particularly when myelographic studies demonstrate large amounts of extruded disc material in the neural canal or there is a large disc protrusion. The procedure allows this disc material to be removed from the neural canal. For further details of the operation see the management of cervical disc protrusions (p. 151).

Cervical spondylopathy in Great Danes is usually diagnosed in puppies between 4 and 11 months of age. Affected animals may also show evidence of genu valgum, carpal valgus or osteochondritis dissecans. The main cause of cord compression is anterior stenosis of the spinal canal complicated by varying degrees of hyperplasia of the dorsal annulus fibrosus (Lewis 1989). C5/C6 is a common site of stenosis. Gross deformities of the vertebral body of C7 may also be seen.

Danes which are treated conservatively (restricted exercise and steroid therapy) generally become progressively more ataxic and for this reason most owners request euthanasia within 6 months of diagnosis (Denny *et al.* 1977). When stenosis exists it is possible to relieve this by dorsal laminectomy; however it should be remembered that the stenosis is often asymmetrical and may be present at more than one site in the cervical spinal canal. Careful lateral and ventrodorsal myelographic studies are necessary to confirm the site(s) and extent of stenosis. Dorsal laminectomy is not without hazard (Read *et al.* 1983) and many dogs show a deterioration in the early post-operative period and some may even be rendered quadriparetic for several weeks following surgery. Even though the dog's action may eventually improve following laminectomy, constrictive fibrosis at the site of surgery ('laminectomy membranes') may cause a recurrence of ataxia. Immature Danes with cervical spondylopathy also tend to develop growth disturbances like genu valgum or carpal valgus and for these reasons surgical treatment must carry a very guarded prognosis. A technique which avoids the risk of laminectomy membranes forming is to elevate the dorsal laminae as two flaps at the site of stenosis. The flaps are held open with wire sutures anchored around a screw placed across the adjacent articular facets. Mckee (1988) described the successful application of this method in a 5-month-old Great Dane with cervical vertebral canal stenosis.

BASSET HOUND

The condition is seen in animals under 8 months of age and cord compression arises directly as a result of anterior stenosis of the spinal canal at the C2/C3 junction and occasionally at C3/C4 (Lewis 1989). Dogs which reach maturity without neck pain or ataxia becoming too severe usually compensate reasonably well for the stenosis.

Surgical access for treatment by dorsal laminectomy is relatively easy because the stenosis involves the anterior cervical spine. The results have been encouraging and surgery is recommended if the dog does not appear to be responding to steroid therapy.

POSSIBLE CAUSES OF CERVICAL SPONDYLOPATHY

Diet
The nutritional status of affected animals is invariably normal.

Mechanical factors
It has been suggested that a large head on a long neck may impose abnormal stress on growing vertebrae. This might apply to the Great Dane but not the Dobermann Pinscher.

Trauma
An injury can precipitate clinical signs, particularly in the older dog.

Genetic factors
Evidence that cervical spondylopathy is an inherited defect is provided by:
1 The disproportionate breed incidence in Dobermanns and Great Danes.
2 The occurrence of the disorder in littermates.
3 The sex incidence in the Great Dane, the majority of animals being male.

As cervical spondylopathy appears to be so widespread in the Dobermann, eradication by planned breeding seems impracticable. However, it is obviously unwise to continue to breed from animals which are known to have produced offspring with clinical signs of cervical spondylopathy.

Cervical disc protrusion
The normal intervertebral disc consists of the outer annulus fibrosus and the inner nucleus pulposus (Fig. 3.35).

The nucleus pulposus is a gel-like structure which develops from the notochord. The annulus fibrosus has an inner zone consisting of fibro-cartilage and an outer zone of collagen lamellae. The nucleus pulposus is situated eccentrically within the annulus, the ventral annulus being one and a half times thicker than the dorsal. Consequently, most disc protrusions occur dorsally.

Hansen (1952) described disc degeneration and pro-

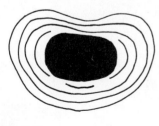

Fig. 3.35

trusion. He divided dogs into two groups, chondrodys-trophoid and non-chondrodystrophoid breeds.

In the chondrodystrophoid breeds such as the Dachshund and the Pekingese, the nucleus pulposus undergoes chondroid metamorphosis so that the nucleus is gradually replaced by hyaline cartilage. The process occurs between 8 months and 2 years of age.

In non-chondrodystrophoid dogs fibroid metamorphosis occurs with gradual replacement of the nucleus pulposus by collagenous tissue. This process occurs later in life, usually between 8 and 10 years.

These changes in the character of the nucleus pulposus precede degeneration. The chondroid nucleus undergoes calcification and similar changes can occur in the fibroid nucleus although far less commonly. Concurrent changes occur in the annulus fibrosus with fragmentation of the collagen lamellae.

Disc protrusion can consist of total rupture of the dorsal annulus fibrosus with extrusion of varying amounts of degenerative nucleus pulposus into the neural canal (Hansen Type I disc lesion). Alternatively, there may be only partial rupture of the annulus fibrosus with dorsal bulging of the disc (Hansen Type II lesion).

The clinical, radiological and pathological findings associated with cervical disc protrusion were described by Olsson & Hansen (1952). The same authors also described the technique of ventral fenestration of the affected disc. Since then several reports have been published on the management of dogs with cervical disc protrusion; these have been reviewed and the results of surgical treatment of a further 40 cases described (Denny 1978a). The results of this paper are published here.

The condition is most commonly encountered in the Beagle, Jack Russell Terrier, Dachshund and Cocker Spaniel. Age at the onset of clinical signs ranges from 1 to 12 years, with a peak incidence at 5 and 8 years. The most common presenting sign is cervical pain. The pain is often intense and the animal will scream if touched or moved (there is a saying that a cervical protrusion can be diagnosed without seeing the dog because of the cries of pain as the animal is brought into the waiting room). In less marked cases, the only evidence of pain is tautness of the cervical muscles as the dog guards its neck against passive manipulation. Affected animals are miserable and apprehensive. A hunched up attitude is adopted, usually with the head held down. One of the first presenting signs noticed is difficulty or unwillingness to lower the head to eat or drink. In addition there may be neurological deficits ranging from unilateral foreleg paresis, which is the most common, to hemiparesis, quadriparesis or quadriplegia.

Diagnosis of a cervical disc protrusion is confirmed by lateral radiograph of the cervical spine (Fig. 3.36). A narrow intervertebral disc space is taken as evidence of protrusion. Calcification of the disc is not necessarily of any clinical significance unless there is dorsal extrusion of calcified material into the neural canal.

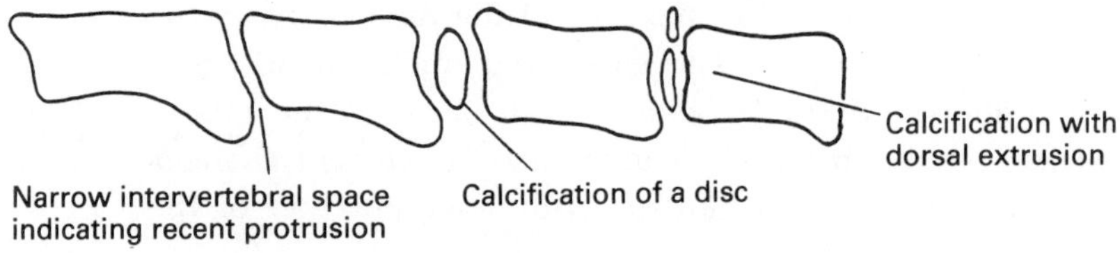

Narrow intervertebral space
indicating recent protrusion

Calcification of a disc

Calcification with
dorsal extrusion

Fig. 3.36 Radiographic changes in intervertebral disc disease.

The most common site of disc protrusion is between C2 and C3 and dogs presented with cervical pain alone often have protrusions of one of the first three cervical discs. Dogs presented with cervical pain associated with foreleg paresis, hemiparesis or quadriplegia are more likely to have protrusion of one of the last three cervical discs. The management of cases with cervical disc protrusion can be conservative or surgical. However, recurrence is more likely when conservative methods are used. This was demonstrated by Russell & Griffiths (1968) in an analysis of 110 cases. They found that recurrence in conservatively treated dogs over a 3-year period was 36.3%, whereas it was only 5.6% in dogs treated by ventral fenestration. Conservative treatment involves cage rest for 3 weeks and analgesics are given to control pain. If cervical pain persists, or neurological deficits become apparent, then fenestration should be recommended. In the majority of cases, fenestration is the treatment of choice. The operation simply involves cutting a window in the ventral surface of the annulus fibrosus of the disc to allow the nucleus pulposus to be removed and the protrusion to subside (Fig. 3.42).

If there has been complete rupture of the dorsal annulus fibrosus, then further extrusion of nucleus into the neural canal is prevented. The nucleus pulposus is replaced by scar tissue and therefore with regard to prophylaxis there is nothing further to be protruded or extruded into the neural canal.

Cervical disc fenestration

The dog is placed in dorsal recumbency with the head extended over a sandbag and the forelimbs pulled back lateral to the chest (Fig. 3.37). A ventral midline skin incision is made extending from the level of the atlas to the manubrium sternum (Fig. 3.37). The paired bellies of the sternohyoideus muscles are divided along the midline and retracted to expose the trachea (Figs 3.38 and 3.39).

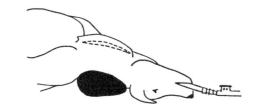

Fig. 3.37

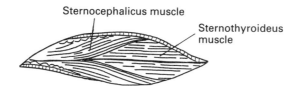

Fig. 3.38

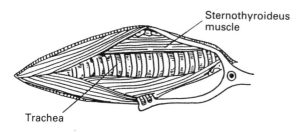

Fig. 3.39

The trachea and oesophagus are retracted towards the left side of the neck and the right vagus and carotid artery displaced to the right to expose the longus colli muscle (Fig. 3.40). The position of a specific disc can be determined by first palpating the caudal border of the wings of the atlas and the ventral process of each vertebra caudal to this point. The intervertebral disc lies immediately caudal to the ventral process.

The attachment of the longus colli muscle on each ventral process is cut. Self-retaining retractors are then used to displace the muscle laterally and expose the disc. A window

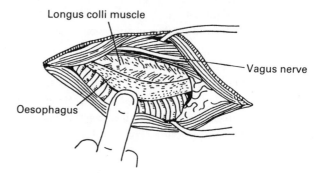

Longus colli muscle

Vagus nerve

Oesophagus

Fig. 3.40

is cut in the ventral surface of the intervertebral disc using a No. 15 scalpel blade and the nucleus pulposus removed with a dental tartar scraper (Figs 3.41 and 3.42). The first five cervical discs are routinely fenestrated.

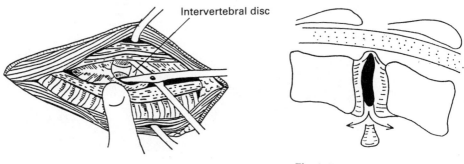

Intervertebral disc

Fig. 3.41

Fig. 3.42

The defects in the longus colli muscle are sutured to prevent haemorrhage. The remaining muscle layers are coapted with a continuous suture and the skin with interrupted sutures.

Although fenestration provides effective relief from recurrence of cervical pain, 30% of dogs continue to have intermittent periods of pain for an average period of 2 weeks after surgery (range 1—4 weeks). Severe neurological deficits as a result of disc protrusion are usually more commonly encountered in the thoracolumbar region as there is relatively little room for anything but the spinal cord within the neural canal. By comparison, the cervical neural canal is much larger than the cord, consequently disc protrusion in this region usually results in impingement on the nerve roots, causing pain and sometimes paresis of one limb rather than severe cord compression.

It might be argued that because the cervical neural canal

is relatively large compared with its contents, decompressive surgery is rarely necessary in dogs with cervical disc protrusions. The results of treatment by fenestration alone are encouraging in this respect. In dogs with cervical pain and foreleg paresis, paresis resolves within an average time of 3 weeks. In dogs with quadriparesis, the recovery period varies from 3 to 6 weeks. Fifty per cent of dogs with quadriplegia will recover provided fenestration is performed within 48 hours of the onset of signs. However, following fenestration some cases continue to have neck pain for many weeks following surgery while others with more severe signs of cord compression, i.e. foreleg paresis or quadriparesis may have a protracted recovery because of extruded disc material impinging on the nerve roots and/or spinal cord. The disc fenestration technique does not permit removal of this extruded disc material from the spinal cord and for this reason ventral decompression by the ventral slot technique (Seim & Prata 1982; Robins 1984) has become the treatment of choice in recent years, particularly in cases where disc material has been extruded into the neural canal (Hansen Type I lesion).

VENTRAL SLOT PROCEDURE

The site of cervical disc protrusion and cord compression should be confirmed by myelography. The surgical approach to the affected disc is identical to the disc fenestration procedure.

First the ventral spinous process adjacent to the disc is removed with rongeurs. Next a wide disc fenestration is performed using a No. 15 scalpel blade. As much of the ventral annulus as possible should be removed and any residual nucleus pulposus removed with a dental tartar scraper. A ventral slot is now cut into the adjacent vertebral bodies using a high speed bur (use the bur with an air drill, or a small electric hobby drill if amprolene gas sterilization facilities are available). The slot (Fig. 3.43) should not exceed more than half of the width of the disc and no more than a quarter of the length of each vertebral body. The slot penetrates the full depth of the vertebral body to the floor of the neural canal. The depth of the slot is gauged by observing change in the colour and consistency of the bone as it is removed with the bur. The outer cortical bone is hard and white, the medullary cancellous bone is soft and tends to bleed as it is removed, and then the inner medullary bone is reached which is white and dense again. It is essential to keep the slot in the midline

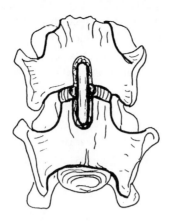

Fig. 3.43 Ventral slot procedure.

to avoid rupture of the laterally placed venous sinuses
once the neural canal has been entered. The slot should be
irrigated with saline during the burring process and the
debris removed with suction. Once the inner cortical bone
is reached, proceed with caution to avoid sudden penetration of the neural canal. Ideally the bone is burred
away until an almost transparent thin shell of bone remains.
This thin shell of bone can then be 'picked away' together
with remnants of the dorsal annulus using a fine bone
curette or dental tartar scraper. If the dorsal longitudinal
ligament can be identified it is carefully removed with a
No. 11 scalpel blade. Usually calcified disc material is clearly
visible in the bottom of the slot and this is carefully removed
with a fine angled curette or dental tartar scraper.

The two main potential complications of the surgery are
haemorrhage and spinal cord trauma. Bleeding from cancellous bone is usually controlled with suction, pressure
with a sponge or cautery, and occasionally bone wax
(Ethicon Ltd) is pressed into the bone. If the vertebral
sinus is ruptured, haemorrhage will be profuse. The slot
should be immediately packed with a saline-soaked swab
and suction used to remove blood. The swab is removed
after a couple of minutes and surgery continued. Continuous
suction may be necessary to allow visualization and removal
of the disc material and then further pressure or perhaps
the introduction of Gelfoam (Upjohn Ltd) is used to finally
arrest haemorrhage.

The ventral slot procedure can be combined with
prophylactic fenestration of the other cervical discs if
deemed necessary.

Wound closure is the same as in a routine disc fenestration
(see above).

In most cases the results of ventral decompression are

dramatic with an almost immediate relief from neck pain and improvement in motor function often within 24 h. A recent comparison of 111 dogs that had undergone ventral decompression or fenestration for solitary cervical disc protrusions was reported by Fry *et al.* (1991). Ventral decompression appeared to be significantly superior in all aspects to cervical disc fenestration except that the rates of intra-operative and post-operative complications were higher with the ventral decompression technique, which is not surprising as this is technically more difficult than disc fenestration.

THORACOLUMBAR SPINE

Thoracolumbar disc protrusions

Virtually all disc protrusions in the thoracolumbar region occur between T11 and L4, the commonest site of protrusion being between T12/T13 and T13/L1.

The condition is most frequently encountered in the Dachshund and Pekingese. The clinical and radiological findings associated with protrusion have already been described (pp. 125−6).

Clinical signs associated with thoracolumbar disc protrusion can be divided into five groups according to the severity of cord compression:

Grade I Thoracolumbar pain.

Grade II Hindlimb paresis/ataxia with or without pain.

Grade III Paraplegia (an inability to stand unaided and no, or only limited, voluntary movement).

Grade IV Paraplegia with urinary retention and overflow.

Grade V Paraplegia with urinary retention and overflow and loss of conscious pain sensation.

The dog with pain in the thoracolumbar region caused by a disc protrusion may be reluctant to exercise or unwilling to go up stairs. The animal tends to stand with the back arched and may cry out if touched in this region or if lifted off the ground. If the disc lesion causes paraplegia the dog usually presents with the history that it has 'gone off' its hind legs. It is important to know the speed of onset and duration of signs because this influences the prognosis. Usually the more rapid the onset the worse the prognosis. It is important to know if the dog has control over urination and defecation. Urinary retention is a poor prognostic sign. Has the dog had previous spinal problems? If so this will influence the decision to operate or not.

In the clinical examination, place the dog on grass or

other non-slippery surface and then assess whether the animal is paraplegic, paretic, or ataxic. Next palpate the spine looking for a focus of pain; a dog with pain caused by a thoracolumbar disc will tense the abdominal muscles when the back is palpated. The panniculus reflex is very useful to assess the level of cord damage; the panniculus muscle has a segmental sensory supply and there is usually cut off of the muscle twitch caudal to the site of injury (p. 125).

The most important part of the examination is to assess whether the dog still has pain sensation present in the hind legs. On stimulation of the toes there should be a central response, i.e. the dog should turn round, or cry out, that the painful stimuli are reaching the brain, confirming that at least some of the corticospinal tracts are intact. If there is no sensation present in the hind legs this indicates that there has been very extensive damage to the spinal cord. It is important to differentiate withdrawal of the foot due to pain from a pedal reflex which can be present or exaggerated even when there is complete cord transection. In this situation although the foot is withdrawn there is no central response.

The crossed extensor reflex is another useful test. This reflex stops a person falling over when one foot is lifted off the ground. To check this reflex the dog is placed on its side, one hind foot is pinched, and the normal dog will withdraw this foot only. If the crossed extensor reflex is present the contralateral hind leg will be extended as the pinched leg is withdrawn. This reflex, if present, indicates severe damage to the spinal cord and carries a poor prognosis.

Other tests are listed here: palpate the bladder, checking for retention and overflow, check the anal sphincter for tone, and check the tail for movement and sensation.

Seven per cent of cases with thoracolumbar protrusions develop flaccid paralysis due to ascending myelomalacia and it is impossible to predict which cases are going to do this although they tend to be animals which present with a very sudden onset of paraplegia (see p. 126).

Treatment of thoracolumbar disc protrusions may be conservative or surgical and Bojrab (1971) reported that the overall recovery rate was 85% based on the various methods of treatment reported in the literature. Conservative treatment involves enforced rest, preferably in a cage for 3–4 weeks. This type of treatment is recommended for the dog which has suffered its first attack of thoracolumbar pain or pain with hind leg paresis. Such dogs usually have dorsal protrusion of the disc without complete rupture of the annulus. Administration of corticosteroids or analgesics should be avoided in these cases. Otherwise pain relief with increased activity may result in a progression of the protrusion to rupture of the annulus with extrusion of the nucleus pulposus and severe cord compression.

If pain is severe and cannot be controlled by rest or with non-steroidal anti-inflammatory drugs then prednisolone is given, 0.5 mg/kg orally twice a day for 72 h to reduce inflammation of the nerve roots.

The paraplegic dog whether treated surgically or conservatively requires careful nursing. If urinary retention and overflow are present, the bladder should be expressed or drained by catheter at least twice daily. Antibiotic cover should be given to prevent urinary tract infection. Inability to move with urinary or faecal incontinence results in soiling of the coat and skin sores unless frequent bathing is carried out. The paraplegic dog must also be turned several times a day and bony prominences massaged to prevent the development of bed sores. Corticosteroids are given at high doses for 72 h after the onset of paraplegia to reduce cord oedema (dexamethasone, 2 mg/kg intravenously, repeated 4 h later, then 0.1 mg/kg intramuscularly twice daily for 2–3 days).

A treatment protocol for the different categories of dogs with thoracolumbar disc protrusions has been suggested by Wheeler (1988) and is presented here with a few additional suggestions based on results of fenestration (Butterworth & Denny 1991).

GRADE I (THORACOLUMBAR PAIN)
Conservative treatment is recommended for the first episode. Fenestration is recommended if the dog fails to respond within 3 weeks or has a recurrence of back pain. Fenestration usually provides rapid relief from pain, average 2.6 weeks, 92% success rate.

GRADE II (HIND LEG PARESIS/ATAXIA WITH OR WITHOUT PAIN)
Conservative treatment is recommended if this is the first episode, but if there is no response within 3 weeks or this is a recurrence of signs then fenestration is recommended unless the motor dysfunction is becoming worse in which

case decompression by hemilaminectomy should be used. The average recovery period after fenestration is 3.8 weeks, 93% success rate.

GRADE III (PARAPLEGIA)

Surgical treatment; although decompression hemilaminectomy is the best option, fenestration also gives good results and 85% of cases treated in this way recovered in an average of 5.5 weeks.

GRADE IV (PARAPLEGIA WITH URINARY RETENTION AND OVERFLOW)

Surgical treatment; decompression by hemilaminectomy is the best option but again good results have been obtained with fenestration particularly if the surgery is undertaken within 24 h of the onset. Average recovery period with fenestration is 8.3 weeks and 88% recovered.

GRADE V (PARAPLEGIA WITH URINARY RETENTION AND OVERFLOW AND LOSS OF CONSCIOUS PAIN SENSATION)

If signs have been present for less than 48 h then decompressive surgery is undertaken. If paraplegia has been present for more than 48 h then conservative management is recommended. Only 33% of dogs in this category treated by fenestration recovered and the recovery period was 2–3 months.

Carts are available for paraplegic dogs which have irreversible damage to the spinal cord. The cart consists of a frame on wheels which supports the hindquarters off the ground ('K-9 Cart', UK agent: Mrs D. Barrow, Poplar Farm, Oakley, Aylesbury, Bucks). These carts are well tolerated and enable the paraplegic dogs of all sizes to enjoy walks again. The cart is not so well tolerated by cats.

Generally the recovery rates for dogs in grades I–IV are similar if conservative treatment or fenestration is used, however fenestration carries a much better prophylactic result in that the risk of recurrence is reduced to virtually nil. Thirty per cent of dogs which are managed conservatively will have recurrences. Decompression carries a significant benefit for dogs in groups III and IV where the recovery period is shorter. In group V recovery rates with conservative treatment or fenestration have been put as low as 2–5% (Wheeler 1988), however if decompression is carried out within 48 h approximately 50% of these dogs regain hindlimb function.

SURGICAL TECHNIQUE, THORACOLUMBAR DISC FENESTRATION

A lateral approach for fenestration of thoracolumbar disc protrusions has been described by several authors (Seemann 1968, 1980; Flo & Brinker 1975; Denny 1978b, 1982).

Surgical technique

Thoracolumbar disc fenestration is not an easy operation and initial practice on cadavers is recommended. Specialist instruments for the operation include two pairs of self-retaining retractors, dental tartar scrapers and a periosteal elevator. Suction is useful but not essential.

The dog is placed on its right side with the thoracolumbar region arched over a wooden pole (Fig. 3.44). (This widens the disc space laterally and makes fenestration easier; the pole is moved as necessary to improve exposure of individual discs.) A lateral skin incision is made at the level of the transverse processes of the lumbar vertebrae from the ninth or tenth rib to the fifth lumbar vertebra (Fig. 3.44).

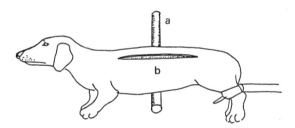

Fig. 3.44 The dog is placed on its right side with the thoracolumbar spine arched over a wooden pole (a). A lateral skin incision (b) is made from the ninth rib to the fifth lumbar vertebra.

The subcutaneous fat is retracted to reveal the lumbodorsal fascia which merges with the latissimus dorsi muscle in the costal region. The fascia, muscle and underlying layer of fat are incised and retracted (Figs 3.45a and b). The longissimus dorsi and the iliocostalis lumborum muscles can then be identified (Fig. 3.45c). Although the two muscles are fused in the lumbar region they can be distinguished as the longissimus dorsi muscle, which lies dorsally, has a glistening silvery appearance, while the iliocostalis lumborum muscle presents fleshy serrations which insert on the transverse processes of the lumbar vertebrae and last

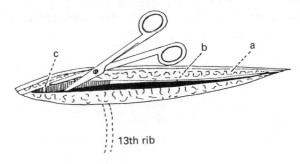

Fig. 3.45a The subcutaneous fat (a), lumbodorsal fascia (b) and the latissimus dorsi muscle (c) are incised.

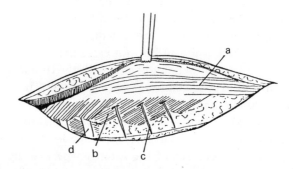

Fig. 3.45b The lumbodorsal fascia and the latissimus dorsi muscle are retracted to reveal the longissimus dorsi (a) and the iliocostalis lumborum (b) muscles. The dorsal branches of the lumbar nerves (c) and the last two ribs (d) can also be seen.

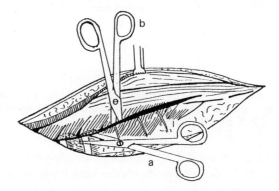

Fig. 3.45c The iliocostalis lumborum muscle is detached and elevated from the last three ribs (a). The iliocostalis lumborum muscle is then split longitudinally over the first four lumbar transverse processes (b).

four ribs. The iliocostalis lumborum muscle is detached and elevated from the last three ribs, and this area is packed with a swab to control haemorrhage (Fig. 3.45d) while the lumbar discs are being fenestrated.

Exposure of each of the first three lumbar discs is achieved by splitting the iliocostalis lumborum muscle in the direc-

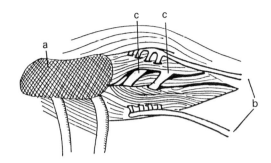

Fig 3.45d Haemorrhage from the severed costal attachments of the iliocostalis lumborum muscle is controlled by packing the area with a swab (a). Self-retaining retractors (b) are used to retract the iliocostalis lumborum muscle in the lumbar region while the transverse processes (c) are being exposed.

tion of its fibres in a caudal direction from the transverse process of the second lumbar vertebra (Fig. 3.45c). The muscle is elevated from the transverse process of the second lumbar vertebra and exposure of the process maintained with self-retaining retractors (Fig. 3.45d). The first lumbar disc, covered by a layer of fascia, lies just cranial to the transverse process. Exposure is completed by elevation of fascia and muscle from the edge of the transverse process in a cranial direction. This is done initially with a periosteal elevator and the lateral surface of the disc is then cleaned with the corner of a dry swab held with artery forceps. Care is taken to avoid the ventral branch of the first lumbar nerve and its associated blood vessels which cross the craniolateral surface of the disc (Fig. 3.46a and b). The vein is sometimes accidentally ruptured during exposure of the disc, but haemorrhage can be controlled by applying pressure with an elevator on the cranioventral corner of the disc (Fig. 3.46b). A 'window' is cut through the annulus fibrosus on the lateral side of the disc using a No. 15 scalpel blade and the nucleus pulposus is removed with a dental tartar scraper (Fig. 3.46c). The second and third lumbar and the thirteenth thoracic disc are exposed and fenestrated in the same way.

The swab covering the heads of the last three ribs is removed and exposure of the eleventh and twelfth thoracic discs carried out. These discs are covered by the levatores costorum muscles. Each muscle originates on the transverse process of a thoracic vertebra and inserts on the rib caudal to the process (Fig. 3.47). The origin of each muscle is partially severed with scissors (Fig. 3.47) and a periosteal elevator is used to retract the muscle in a ventral direction

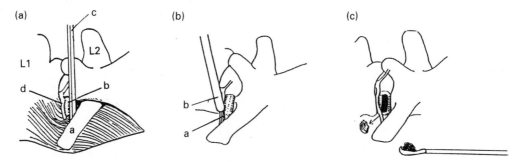

Fig. 3.46 (a) The transverse process (a) of the second lumbar vertebra is cleared of muscle. The first lumbar disc (b) lies immediately cranial to the transverse process. Fascia covering the lateral aspect of the disc is cleared in a cranial direction using a periosteal elevator (c) initially. The ventral branch of the first lumbar nerve (d) crosses the cranial edge of the disc.
(b) A vein (a) which runs with the spinal nerve is sometimes accidentally ruptured. Haemorrhage can be controlled by applying pressure with an elevator (b) on the cranioventral corner of the disc.
(c) A window is cut through the lateral side of the annulus fibrosus and the nucleus pulposus is removed with a dental tartar scraper.

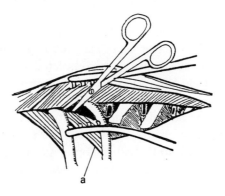

Fig. 3.47 Exposure of the twelfth thoracic disc. The origin of the levatores costorum muscle (a) is partially severed.

to complete exposure of the disc (Fig. 3.48). (Care is taken to avoid penetration of the pleural cavity during this procedure.) Lateral fenestration of the twelfth thoracic disc is then performed. Exposure and fenestration of the eleventh

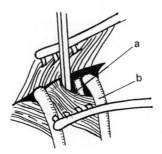

Fig. 3.48 Exposure of the twelfth thoracic disc. The levatores costorum muscle is retracted in a ventral direction to reveal the disc (a) lying just cranial to the head of the rib (b).

thoracic disc is achieved in the same way. Wound closure consists of separate layers of continuous sutures (vicryl) in the iliocostalis lumborum muscle, the latissimus dorsi fascia and the subcutaneous fat. The skin is coated with simple interrupted or vertical mattress sutures of oo monofilament nylon. A bandage is applied around the chest and abdomen.

Post-operatively, antibiotic cover is given for 5 days and most dogs can be discharged within this period. Bandage and skin sutures are removed at 10 days and owners are given general advice on nursing the dog.

Dogs presented within 24 h of a sudden onset of paraplegia are given hydrocortisone for 72 hours to control cord oedema. Dogs with urinary retention and overflow have their bladders emptied at least twice daily by catheter or manual expression until reflex emptying occurs (usually within 5 days). A frequent minor post-operative complication is flaccidity and bulging of the left abdominal wall. This is due to bruising of the ventral lumbar nerve roots during surgery. The flaccidity is a transient problem and normal muscle tone is regained within 2 weeks.

DECOMPRESSION BY HEMILAMINECTOMY
(Funkquist 1962; Schulman & Lippincott 1987; Black 1988; Wheeler 1988)
If a decompressive procedure is to be used it is important to determine the exact site of disc protrusion by myelography, and also to determine from ventrodorsal views of the spine the side of the neural canal to which the disc material has been extruded because this will influence the choice of approach from either the left or right side of the spine.

The dog is positioned in sternal recumbency but is rotated slightly, so that the side of the spine to be approached is uppermost. The skin incision is made just lateral to the dorsal midline starting in the caudal thoracic region and extended caudally over the lumbar spine. The subcutaneous tissues are divided to expose the lumbodorsal fascia (Fig. 3.45b). The fascia is incised close to the dorsal spinous processes and the muscles are elevated away from the spines on the side of the proposed hemilaminectomy. Next the dorsal articular facets are palpated and the vertebrae cranial and caudal to the proposed site of laminectomy identified (the last rib and transverse processes are useful landmarks). Muscle attachments are freed from the articular facets of these vertebrae; Gelpi retractors are used to maintain exposure. The articular facets directly over the site of disc protrusion are removed with rongeurs. The dorsal spinous process of the vertebra just cranial to the disc is grasped with a Backhaus towel clamp and elevated by an assistant. This increases the space at the articulation between the vertebrae. Compound spinal rongeurs with a 2 or 3 mm jaw width (Veterinary Instrumentation) are used to enlarge this space and expose the lateral side of the spinal cord. The hemilaminectomy is extended half the length of each vertebra adjacent to the disc lesion (Fig. 3.53). The procedure is simplified by the use of a high speed burr to remove the outer layer of cortical bone and the underlying cancellous bone leaving a thin sheet of inner cortical bone which is gently prised away with small rongeurs or a curette.

Once the hemilaminectomy is completed extruded disc material is removed from the floor of the spinal canal with a dental tartar scraper. Gentle flushing with saline from a syringe with catheter is also useful to remove final traces of disc material. Finally the soft tissues are retracted ventro-laterally to expose the affected disc which is fenestrated in routine fashion. The hemilaminectomy is covered with an autogenous fat graft. Prophylactic fenestration of adjacent discs is usually carried out before wound closure. Post-operative care is as described for disc fenestration (p. 161).

DECOMPRESSION BY MINI HEMILAMINECTOMY
(Jeffery 1988)
Mini hemilaminectomy for the removal of disc material from the neural canal is readily combined with the lateral fenestration of thoracolumbar discs. The same approach is used for both procedures. The relevant disc space is identified by counting the transverse processes caudal to the last rib. The transverse process immediately caudal to the affected disc is identified (Fig. 3.49a, b). The disc is cleared of fascia and muscle and the spinal nerve traced over the cranial margin of the disc into the intervertebral foramen. The overlying accessory process is removed with rongeurs and the radicular artery coagulated with diathermy. Bone around the relevant intervertebral foramen is thinned using a high speed burr and then the thin inner layer of bone is removed with fine rongeurs or hooked away with a fine dental tartar scraper. The mini hemilaminectomy is immediately dorsolateral to the affected disc but does not extend any further dorsal than the accessory process so the articular facets are left intact. Disc material is removed from the floor of the neural canal (see hemilaminectomy

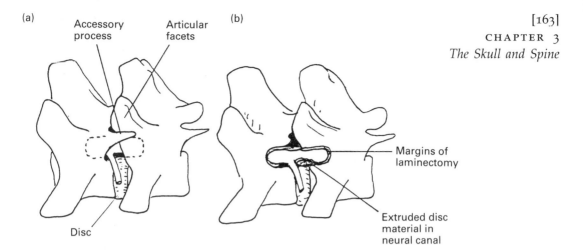

(a)

Accessory process

Articular facets

(b)

Disc

Margins of laminectomy

Extruded disc material in neural canal

Fig. 3.49 Mini hemilaminectomy technique (Jeffrey 1988).

above). The hemilaminectomy site is covered with an autogenous fat graft before wound closure.

This approach allows decompression of the cord with a minimum of trauma; there is no interference with the articular facets, and the hemilaminectomy is readily combined with prophylactic fenestration of the adjacent discs.

Intervertebral disc protrusions in the cat

Disc protrusions are a fairly common radiographic and post-mortem finding in the cat. Lesions are found most often in the cervical and lumbar regions, however neurological signs associated with disc disease are extremely uncommon in the cat (Heavner 1971). If pain or motor dysfunction are shown to be the result of a disc lesion then the principles of treatment are the same as in the dog.

Discospondylitis in the dog

Discospondylitis is an inflammatory disease of the intervertebral discs and vertebral bodies. The condition is caused by bacterial infection and *Staphyloccus aureus* is isolated most frequently (Bennett *et al.* 1981). The most common clinical features are spinal pain and stiffness with intermittent pyrexia. Lesions can affect any part of the spine but have been recorded most often in the cervical region and at the lumbosacral junction. Radiographs show destructive changes in the vertebral end plates and later reactive bone formation (Fig. 3.61a). Most cases respond well to prolonged antibiotic therapy (cephalosporin, ampicillin, clindamycin) given for 3–12 weeks. Occasionally surgical treatment is necessary in unresponsive cases. Curettage of the lesion has the advantage that material can be obtained directly for culture and sensitivity examination.

Discospondylitis in the cat

There are only occasional reports of discospondylitis in the cat (Norsworthy 1979; Malik *et al.* 1990), however Evans (1989) suggests that the condition is more common than generally thought. He recommends long-term treatment with ampicillin or amoxycillin. Codeine (0.25–1.00 mg/kg) can be given to provide analgesia when necessary.

Canine spinal 'arachnoid cysts' in the dog
(Dyce *et al.* 1991)

The 'arachnoid cyst' is an uncommon cause of neurological dysfunction. The lesion is invariably focal and comprises a dorsal subarachnoid dilatation which gives compression of the spinal cord. Myelographic studies reveal a characteristic dilatation in the subarachnoid space (Fig. 3.49c). Treatment by dorsal laminectomy and durectomy over the cystic area carries a good prognosis for recovery.

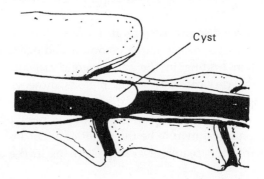

Fig. 3.49c Demonstration of a subarachnoid cyst of C2/C3 by myelography.

Spinal fractures and acute trauma to the spinal cord

Acute trauma to the spinal cord results from fractures, dislocations, disc protrusions or concussion. Fractures and/or dislocations of the spine most frequently occur in the terminal thoracic region (Hoerlein 1971). The injury generally causes paraplegia and the prognosis for recovery is poor unless there is still deep pain sensation present in the hindlimbs. Plain radiography is the most useful way of differentiating traumatic lesions of the cord. There will be negative findings if trauma to the cord is due to concussion (spinal haemorrhage).

When there has been acute trauma to the spinal cord treatment should be initiated within a few hours to be of benefit. Initial management is aimed at preventing further damage to the spinal cord, i.e. strict cage confinement, application of external spinal splint, and administration of corticosteroids. Various regimes for steroid therapy have been recommended in spinal trauma cases. Mckee (1990) advocates the following:

Day 1   Dexamethasone at 2 mg/kg by intravenous injection (can repeat).
Day 2   Same dose of dexamethasone given.
Day 3   Dose of dexamethasone reduced to 1 mg/kg, given intravenously.
Days 4–6   Prednisolone 0.5 mg/kg by mouth.
Days 7–9   Prednisolone 0.25 mg/kg by mouth.
Days 10–14   Prednisolone 0.25 mg/kg by mouth on alternate days.

The doses are reduced if cord damage is not severe or the animal is recovering rapidly. Treatment should be stopped if gastrointestinal haemorrhage occurs. This complication is even more likely to occur if corticosteroids are used in combination with non-steroidal anti-inflammatories and consequently this combination should be avoided.

Methylprednisolone (Solumedrone V, Upjohn) has a very rapid onset and may well prove to be the drug of choice for spinal cord trauma. The following dosage has been recommended (Rucker 1990); 30 mg/kg body weight initially, followed by 15 mg/kg at 2 and 6 h post-trauma, with continuous intravenous infusion of 2.5 mg/kg/h for the next 42 h.

The dose rate of methylprednisolone should not exceed 30 mg/kg.

If surgical treatment is to be undertaken, ideally this should be carried out within 6 h of the accident.

Fractures in the cervical region most frequently involve the atlas and axis. Although there may be considerable displacement of fractures of the cranial cervical vertebrae, the resultant neurological deficits are often remarkably mild. The main presenting sign is cervical pain. The prognosis is good and the majority of cases will recover with conservative treatment. Dogs with undisplaced fractures are given strict rest for 4 weeks while those with displaced or unstable fractures have the neck immobilized in a cast for 4 weeks.

Fractures of the caudal three lumbar vertebrae may compress the cauda equina causing intense pain, paresis or paraplegia, with urinary retention in some cases. There is plenty of room for the cauda equina within the neural canal and considerable vertebral displacement can be tolerated without necessarily causing permanent neurological dysfunction. Decompressive laminectomy is generally unnecessary but reduction and fixation of the fracture/dislocation should be undertaken to relieve pain. The prognosis is reasonably good except for cases with lumbosacral dislocation. Here the dog regains the use of its hindlegs but bladder paralysis persists.

FRACTURES OF THE CERVICAL VERTEBRAE

Fractures of the cervical vertebrae are uncommon in the dog (Stone *et al.* 1979; Denny 1983). Fractures most often involve the atlas and axis. The commonest site axial fracture is the dens and/or vertebral body.

Although there may be considerable displacement of fractures of the cranial cervical vertebrae, the resultant neurological deficits are often remarkably mild and the main presenting sign is cervical pain (De Lahunta 1977). However, deaths may occur from respiratory arrest when haemorrhage and oedema involve the brain stem following fracture (Gage 1968). Fractures of the caudal cervical vertebrae may cause quadriparesis or quadriplegia, and death may occur from respiratory failure if there is involvement of the phrenic outflow (De Lahunta 1977).

When fracture of a cervical vertebra is suspected, the dog must be handled with care to prevent further displacement of the fracture. Initial radiographic examination should ideally be carried out on the conscious animal. If the dog is anaesthetized for further radiographs or surgery then protective muscle tone is lost and the risk of fracture displacement is increased. This risk can be minimized by supporting the neck throughout the procedure and avoiding excessive flexion and extension. Diagnosis of cervical fracture can usually be confirmed from a lateral radiograph of the neck but in some cases ventrodorsal and oblique views may be necessary.

Most reported cases of cervical fracture have been treated surgically. Atlanto-axial subluxations with or without fractures of the dens have been stabilized by wiring the arch of the atlas to the dorsal spinous process of the axis (Figs 3.24−3.26) (Gage 1968; Oliver & Lewis 1973; Stone *et al.* 1979). When fractures have involved a cervical vertebral body, ventral plate fixation has been used (Stone *et al.* 1979) but experimental work by Swaim (1975) suggests that this technique is not always satisfactory as loosening of the screws and plate is a frequent complication. Another method of stabilizing cervical body fractures was described by Rouse (1979) with reference to three cases. Four pins were driven into the vertebral body, two cranial and two caudal to the fracture, and were left protruding about 1 cm below the ventral aspect of the vertebral body. The fracture was reduced and the free ends of the pins were incorporated in bone cement which acted as an internal splint (Fig. 3.50a). Rouse (1979) stresses the importance of reducing the fracture with the least possible trauma. Haemorrhage from the ventral vertebral sinus often occurs upon movement of the vertebral body fragments, and respiratory arrest is not uncommon, especially if extensive haemorrhage occurs within the neural canal. At the author's clinic nine dogs have been seen with fractures of the cervical vertebrae during a 10-year period. The fractures involved the atlas in four dogs, the axis in four and the fifth cervical vertebra in one. Clinical signs included neck pain, quadriparesis or quadriplegia.

One dog in the series was treated surgically; the remainder were managed conservatively. Dogs with undisplaced cervical fractures were given strict rest for 4 weeks and those with displaced or unstable fractures had the neck immobilized in a plaster of Paris collar for 4 weeks (Fig. 3.50b). The cast is applied with the dog conscious in a normal standing position with the neck extended. The dog may require hand feeding initially but should later manage to take food from a shallow, raised bowl. Fluids need to be given by hand while the cast is worn. Animals in this series made good recoveries with conservative treatment even though follow-up radiographs of some dogs showed quite marked displacement at the fracture site. The cervical neural canal is large relative to its contents and consequently affords

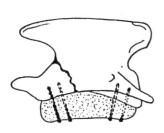

Fig. 3.50a

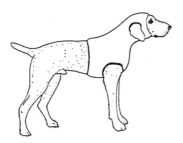

Fig. 3.50b

greater leeway for compression than other areas of the spine.

In conclusion, fractures of the cervical vertebrae are uncommon; the prognosis for recovery is good with conservative treatment even when there is an alarming degree of displacement of the fragments. Surgical treatment carries distinct risks but can be justified in dogs where atlanto-axial subluxation results from fractures of the dens.

FRACTURES OF THE THORACIC OR LUMBAR VERTEBRAE

Dogs presented with fractures of the thoracic or lumbar vertebrae immediately after road traffic accidents are usually paraplegic and have rigid extension of the forelimbs (Schiff Sherrington reflex). There is severe pain which can be localized to the area of the fracture and there may be obvious deformity in this region.

After a complete general and neurological examination radiographs should be taken of the spine in two planes. The types of fractures seen are:

1 Transverse fractures of the body of the vertebra.

2 Compression fractures in which the body of the vertebra is foreshortened and bony debris is displaced dorsally into the neural canal.

3 Fractures of the spinous and lateral processes: these do not involve the spinal cord directly and consequently there is no neurological deficit.

Subluxation and luxation of the vertebrae are also seen with or without concurrent fractures.

Prognosis for recovery following fractures or luxations of the thoracic or lumbar vertebrae is generally poor. If there is obvious displacement of the fragments or vertebrae then there is invariably cord transection or irreversible damage and the dog should be destroyed. Even when there is apparently little displacement of the vertebrae as in a subluxation, severe cord compression has often resulted because such injuries tend to occur in a 'whip lash' fashion, the vertebra being suddenly displaced dorsally in the accident and then sliding back into near normal alignment.

Surgical treatment should be reserved for the dog in which there is little displacement of the fragments or vertebrae. However, this is not quite so critical in the late lumbar region where there is relatively more room for the cord—cauda equina within the neural canal.

Treatment if it is to be of any value should be carried out within hours of the accident. A laminectomy is performed

over the site of cord compression to relieve pressure and
allow inspection of the cord (Figs 3.51–3.54). (If there is
evidence of gross tearing or contusion then the dog should
be destroyed.) The vertebrae can be stabilized in a number
of ways and these are illustrated in Figs 3.55–3.61.

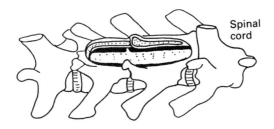

Fig. 3.51 Dorsal laminectomy of lumbar vertebrae: lateral view.
Reproduced by permission of Trotter E.J. (1975). *Current Techniques
in Small Animal Surgery*. Lea & Febiger, Philadelphia.

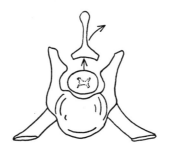

Fig. 3.52 Dorsal laminectomy of
lumbar vertebrae: anterior view.

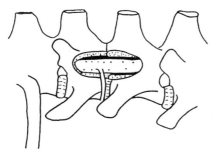

Fig. 3.53 Hemilaminectomy of lumbar vertebrae: lateral spinal cord.

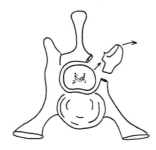

Fig. 3.54 Hemilaminectomy of
lumbar vertebrae: anterior view.

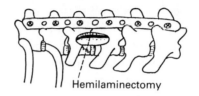

Hemilaminectomy

Fig. 3.55

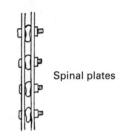

Spinal plates

Fig. 3.56

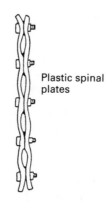

Plastic spinal plates

Fig. 3.57

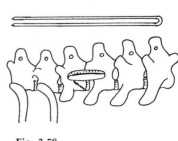

Fig. 3.58

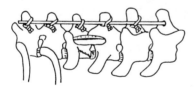

Fig. 3.59

Fig. 3.60a

Fig. 3.60b

Surgical approach

A dorsal midline skin incision is made over the fracture and the lumbodorsal fascia is incised. A periosteal elevator is used to separate the lumbar musculature from the spinous processes and the muscle attachments are severed from the articular and accessory processes of the involved vertebrae. Blunt dissection and lateral retraction of muscle is continued down to the transverse processes or the rib heads of the vertebrae.

An alternative is the lateral approach as described for thoracolumbar disc fenestration (p. 157) and this is indicated if plate fixation (Fig. 3.60a) or transfixion pinning (Fig. 3.60b) of the vertebral bodies is to be performed.

After laminectomy and spinal fixation the dog will require careful nursing. Care of the paraplegic dog has already been described on p. 155.

Methods of internal fixation for fractures of thoracic and lumbar vertebrae

Figures 3.55 and 3.56 show fixation using spinal plates applied to the dorsal spines of the vertebrae. Bolts are placed through the spine (Fig. 3.55, lateral view; Fig. 3.56, dorsal view) (Hoerlein 1971). Alternatively, plastic spinal plates can be used. Bolts are placed between the spinous processes and the plates grip the processes by friction (Fig. 3.57, dorsal view).

Fixation using a U-shaped pin and wire sutures is illustrated in Figs 3.58 and 3.59 (Gage 1971). Plate fixation of the vertebral bodies (Swaim 1971, 1972) is shown in Fig. 3.60a, and transfixion pinning of the vertebral bodies in Fig. 3.60b (Gage 1969).

Cauda equina lesions (Denny *et al*. 1982)

The cauda equina is described as the terminal portion of the spinal cord and adjacent nerve roots contained by the last three lumbar vertebrae, the sacrum and coccygeal vertebrae. It comprises nine nerve segments—one lumbar,

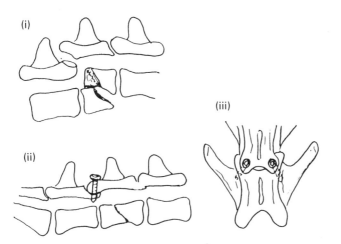

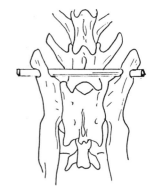

Fig. 3.60c (i) Tracing of a lateral radiograph showing fracture of the centrum of L6 with dislocation of the articular facets between L6/7, in a 6-month-old male German Shepherd dog. (ii) Radiograph taken after surgical reduction and immobilization with two screws through the articular facets. The dog recovered within 6 weeks of surgery and had no further problems during a 1-year follow up period. (iii) Dorsal view of L6/L7 position of lag screw.

Fig. 3.60d The use of a transiliac pin for fracture of the body of L7 with dislocation of articular facets at L7/S1. Can also be used to stabilize dislocation of the lumbosacral junction (technique by Slocum & Rudy 1975).

three sacral and five coccygeal. The peripheral nerves of clinical importance which are derived from these segments include the sciatic, pudendal, pelvic and caudal nerves. The cauda equina syndrome (CES) has been defined as a neurological condition caused by compression, displacement or destruction of the cauda equina.

Lawson (1971), in an assessment of canine paraplegia, described the characteristic features of lesions at various levels of the spinal column. A lesion at the sixth lumbar vertebra produces complete sciatic nerve paralysis with total dysfunction of the hind legs except for the muscles supplied by the femoral and obturator nerves. A seventh lumbar vertebral lesion produces partial sciatic nerve paralysis and paralysis of the tail and bladder with sensory loss in the tail and around the anus. A third sacral vertebral lesion has the same effect as a seventh lumbar lesion except that the sciatic nerve is unaffected. Coccygeal vertebral lesions cause paralysis and loss of sensation of the tail only.

CAUSES OF CAUDA EQUINA SYNDROME
Listed in order of decreasing frequency:
1 Lumbosacral spondylosis ± disc protrusion.
2 Lumbosacral discospondylitis. (Possible association with urinary tract infection, *Staph. aureus* isolated from the disc most frequently.)
3 Fractures and dislocations.
4 Tumour.

CLINICAL FEATURES
1 Traumatic lesions—intense local pain paresis or paraplegia. Urinary retention.
2 Discospondylitis—history of chronic urinary tract infection in some dogs. Stiffness or pain on rising. Hind leg lameness or weakness sometimes shifting from one leg to another. Urinary incontinence. A lateral radiograph of the lumbosacral junction shows destruction of end-plates of vertebral bodies and much new bone formation (Fig. 3.61a).
3 Lumbosacral spondylosis ± disc protrusion.

The larger breeds of dog are affected and the animals are presented with the same type of history as in the lumbosacral discospondylitis group. The most frequent clinical finding is lumbosacral pain, elicited by downward pressure. Although hind leg lameness is most often unilateral, bilateral and sometimes shifting, hind leg lameness is seen. A few dogs show evidence of pain on palpation of the hips

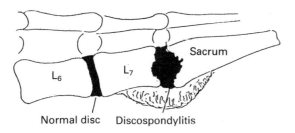

Fig. 3.61a

or stifle joints, but no other abnormalities except for muscle wasting are detected on clinical or radiological examination of the affected limb. Unilateral or bilateral hind leg paresis with a tendency to knuckle at the digits is occasionally seen. It is important to remember that lumbosacral spondylosis is a common incidental radiographic finding (Fig. 3.61b) in older dogs and is not necessarily of any clinical significance unless sufficient new bone is produced to impinge on the lumbar nerve roots.

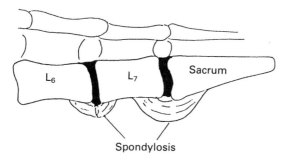

Fig. 3.61b

TREATMENT AND PROGNOSIS
Traumatic lesions of the last three lumbar vertebrae and the sacrum do not necessarily cause severe neurological deficits as the spinal canal in this region is large relative to its neural contents. Even with marked displacement good recoveries may follow reduction and internal fixation (Fig. 3.60c).

Dogs with discospondylitis generally respond well to prolonged antibiotic therapy (ampicillin or a cephalosporin). However, the response to conservative treatment in dogs with lumbosacral spondylosis or disc protrusion tends to be transient or incomplete. Surgical treatment by laminectomy (Fig. 3.61) and facetectomy gives better results in the long term.

SURGICAL TECHNIQUES

Lumbosacral laminectomy

The dog is placed in sternal recumbency with the lumbar spine arched over a sandbag and a midline skin incision is made over the lumbosacral junction (Fig. 3.61c(i)). The lumbodorsal fascia (Fig. 3.61c(ii)) is incised and retracted to reveal the longissimus dorsi and multifidus lumborum muscles (Fig. 3.61c(iii)) which are divided in the midline and retracted laterally, after section of the fascial attachments to the dorsal spines of the last lumbar vertebra and the sacrum. The dorsal surfaces of these vertebrae are cleared of muscle and the interarcuate ligament covering the lumbosacral intervertebral foramen is identified (Fig. 3.61c(iv)). The ligament is carefully removed to reveal the epidural fat covering the cauda equina. The dorsal spines of the last lumbar vertebra and the first sacral segment are removed with bone cutters (Fig. 3.61c(v)). Dorsal laminectomy is performed with rongeurs (Fig. 3.61c(vi)) and the caudal half of the neural arch of the last lumbar vertebra and the cranial half of the neural arch of the first sacral segment are removed. The cauda equina can be gently retracted to one side to allow inspection of the underlying disc and removal of prolapsed or infected disc material. When CES is thought to have resulted from lumbosacral

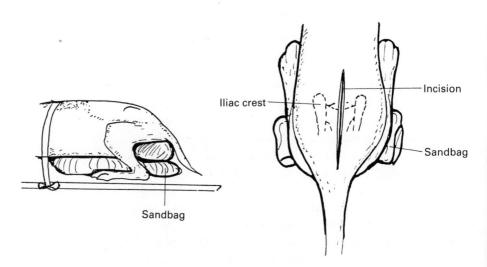

Fig. 3.61c(i) Positioning for lumbosacral laminectomy.

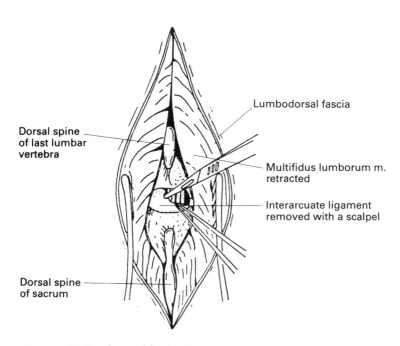

Lumbodorsal
fascia

Lumbodorsal
fascia

Dorsal spine of
7th lumbar vertebra

Multifidus
lumborum m.

Fig. 3.61c(ii) Lumbosacral
laminectomy.

Fig. 3.61c(iii) Lumbosacral
laminectomy.

Dorsal spine
of last lumbar
vertebra

Lumbodorsal fascia

Multifidus lumborum m.
retracted

Interarcuate ligament
removed with a scalpel

Dorsal spine
of sacrum

Fig. 3.61c(iv) Lumbosacral laminectomy.

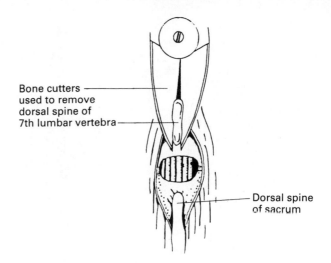

Bone cutters used to remove dorsal spine of 7th lumbar vertebra

Dorsal spine of sacrum

Fig. 3.61c(v) Lumbosacral laminectomy.

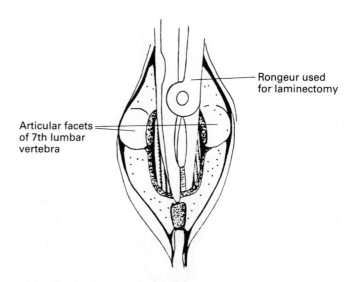

Rongeur used for laminectomy

Articular facets of 7th lumbar vertebra

Fig. 3.61c(vi) Lumbosacral laminectomy.

spondylosis with lateral occlusion of an intervertebral foramen, then facetectomy is carried out to allow decompression of the seventh lumbar nerve (Fig. 3.61c(vii)) and removal of osteophytes. Bilateral facetectomy is not recommended as this causes vertebral instability.

Before wound closure, a rectangular strip of subcutaneous fat is elevated, one end remaining attached while the other is used as a graft to cover the laminectomy site. The muscles

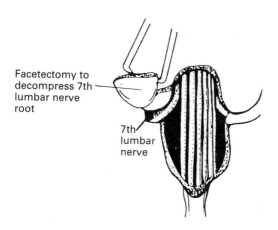

Facetectomy to decompress 7th lumbar nerve root

7th lumbar nerve

Fig. 3.61c(vii) Lumbosacral laminectomy.

and lumbodorsal fascia are closed in layers using vicryl and the skin with simple interrupted sutures of monofilament nylon. The surgical wound is protected with a bandage which is removed at 5 days. Owners are advised to restrict the dog's exercise severely for 6 weeks with no jumping or stairs during this period.

Lumbosacral disc fenestration — ventral approach
(Betts *et al.* 1976)
A midline laparotomy incision is made from the pubis to midway between the xiphoid and the umbilicus with lateral reflection of the prepuce in the male dog. The small intestines are packed off cranially and the bladder and colon retracted to identify the bifurcation of the abdominal aorta.

The seventh lumbar disc lies in the bifurcation between the internal iliac arteries; the median sacral artery and vein cross its ventral surface. The blood vessels are carefully retracted to allow ventral disc fenestration. In cases of vertebral instability, disc fenestration is followed by spinal fusion. A lag screw is driven through the caudal end-plate of the seventh lumbar vertebra across the intervertebral space and into the body of the sacrum. The laparotomy is closed in routine fashion.

Fracture/luxations of the sacrococcygeal area (Sharp 1989)
Sacrococcygeal fractures or luxations are common in cats. Hindlimb dysfunction occurs if there has been a traction injury to the more proximal nerve roots of the cauda equina. Limb function usually improves within a week of injury. The prognosis varies and the following guide to recovery

is given by Sharp (1989) based on a review of over 50 cats with sacrococcygeal injuries. All the cats with coccygeal deficits only (i.e. paralysed tail) recovered. Seventy-five per cent of cats which had urinary retention in addition to the coccygeal deficit recovered. Cats with both these deficits together with reduced anal tone or perineal sensation had only a 60% recovery rate, while those in which the situation was further complicated by lack of urethral sphincter tone (bladder readily expressed by pressure) had the worst prognosis with only 50% recovering. The series demonstrated that if the cats did not regain ability to urinate normally within 1 month of injury then incontinence was permanent. Tail amputation can always be carried out later if faecal and urinary soiling are a problem.

REFERENCES

Bennett D. & Vaughan L.C. (1976) The use of muscle relocation techniques in the treatment of peripheral nerve injuries in dogs and cats. *J. Small Anim. Pract.* **17**, 99.

Bennett D., Carmichael S. & Griffiths I.R. (1981) Discospondylitis in the dog. *J. Small Anim. Pract.* **22**, 539−47.

Betts C.W., Kneller S.K. & Skelton J.A. (1976) An unusual case of traumatic spondylolisthesis in a Red Bone Hound. Diagnosis and therapy. *J. Am. Anim. Hosp. Assoc.* **12**, 470.

Black A.P. (1988) Lateral spinal decompression in the dog: a review of 39 cases. *J. Small Anim. Pract.* **29**, 581−8.

Bojrab M.J. (1971) Disc disease. *Vet. Rec.* **89**, 37.

Butterworth S.J. & Denny H.R. (1991) Follow up of 100 cases with thoracolumbar disc protrusions treated by lateral fenestration. *J. Small Anim. Pract.* **32**, 443−7.

Cameron Stewart W., Baker G.J. & Lee R. (1975) Temporomandibular subluxation in the dog: a case report. *J. Small Anim. Pract.* **16**, 345.

Cook J.R. & Oliver J.E. (1981) Atlanto-axial luxation in the dog. *Compendium of Continuing Education Pract. Vet.* **3**, 242−50.

De Lahunta A. (1977) *Veterinary Neuroanatomy and Clinical Neurology*. Philadelphia, Saunders, pp. 191−338.

De Lahunta A. & Alexander J.W. (1976) Ischaemic myelopathy secondary to presumed fibrocartilaginous emboli in 9 dogs. *J. Am. Anim. Hosp. Assoc.* **12**, 37.

Denny H.R. (1978a) The surgical treatment of cervical disc protrusions in the dog: a review of 40 cases. *J. Small Anim. Pract.* **19**, 251.

Denny H.R. (1978b) The lateral fenestration of canine thoracolumbar disc protrusions: a review of 30 cases. *J. Small Anim. Pract.* **19**, 259.

Denny H.R. (1982) The lateral fenestration of thorocolumbar disc protrusion in the dog. *The Veterinary Annual*, 22nd edn. Scientechnic, Bristol, p. 169.

Denny H.R. (1983) Cervical fractures in the dog. *The Veterinary Annual*, 23rd edn. Scientechnic, Bristol, p. 236.

Denny H.R. & Ibrahim R. (1989) Management of cervical spondylopathy in the Dobermann Pinscher. *Proc. WSAVA/BSAVA 1989 Congress*, Cherry Print Ltd, Wakefield, p. 178.

Denny H.R., Gibbs C. & Gaskell C.J. (1977) Cervical spondylopathy in the dog: a review of 35 cases. *J. Small Anim. Pract.* **18**, 117.

Denny H.R., Gibbs C. & Holt P.E. (1982) The diagnosis and treatment of cauda equina lesions in the dog. *J. Small Anim. Pract.* **23**, 425.

Denny H.R., Gibbs C. & Waterman A. (1988) Atlanto-axial subluxation in the dog, a review of thirty cases and an evaluation of treatment by lag screw fixation. *J. Small Anim. Pract.* **29**, 37−47.

Duncan I. (1989) Canine and feline peripheral polyneuropathies. In: Wheeler S. (ed.), *Manual of Small Animal Neurology.* BSAVA.

Duncan I.D. & Griffiths I.R. (1981) Canine giant axonal neuropathy; some aspects of its clinical, pathological and cooperative features. *J. Small Anim. Pract.* **22**, 491.

Dyce J., Herrtage M.E., Houlton J.E.F. & Palmer A.C. (1991) Canine spinal 'arachnoid cysts'. *J. Small Anim. Pract.* **32**, 433−7.

Evans R. (1989) Special neurology of the cat. In: S. Wheeler (ed.) *Manual of Small Animal Neurology.* BSAVA.

Flanders A. (1986) Feline aortic thromboembolism. *Compendium of Continuing Education* **8**, 473.

Flo G.L. & Brinker W.O. (1975) Lateral fenestration of thoracolumbar discs. *J. Am. Anim. Hosp. Assoc.* **11**, 619.

Fry T.R., Johnson A.L., Hungerford L. & Toombs J. (1991) Surgical treatment of cervical disc herniations in ambulatory dogs. *Prog. Vet. Neurol.* **2**, 165−73.

Funkquist B. (1962) Thoracolumbar disc protrusions with severe cord compression in the dog. *Acta Vet. Scand.* **3**, parts I−III.

Gage E.D. (1968) Surgical repair of a fractured cervical spine in the dog. *J. Am. Vet. Med. Assoc.* **153**, 1407.

Gage E.D. (1969) A new method of spinal fixation in the dog. *Vet. Med. Small Anim. Clin.* **64**, 295.

Gage E.D. (1971) Surgical repair of spinal fractures in small breed dogs. *Vet. Med. Small Anim. Clin.* **66**, 295.

Gage E.D. (1975) Atlanto-axial subluxation. In: Bojrab M.J. (ed.) *Current Techniques in Small Animal Surgery.* Lea & Febiger, Philadelphia.

Gage E.D. & Smallwood J.E. (1970) Surgical repair of atlantoaxial subluxation in a dog. *Vet. Med. Small Anim. Clin.* **65**, 692.

Geary J.C., Oliver J.E. & Hoerlein B.F. (1967) Atlanto-axial subluxation in the canine. *J. Small Anim. Pract.* **8**, 577.

Griffiths I.R. (1972) Some aspects of the pathogenesis and diagnosis of lumbar disc protrusion in the dog. *J. Small Anim. Pract.* **13**, 439.

Griffiths I.R. & Duncan I.D. (1975) Chronic degenerative radiculomyelopathy in the dog. *J. Small Anim. Pract.* **16**, 461.

Griffiths I.R. & Duncan I.D. (1979) Distal denervating disease; a degenerative neuropathy of the distal motor axon in dogs. *J. Small Anim. Pract.* **20**, 579.

Griffiths I.R., Duncan I.D. & Lawson D.D. (1974) Avulsion of the brachial plexus−2 clinical aspects. *J. Small Anim. Pract.* **15**, 177.

Griffiths I.R., Duncan I.D. & Barker J. (1980) A progressive axonopathy of Boxer dogs affecting the central and peripheral nervous system. *J. Small Anim. Pract.* **21**, 29.

Hansen H.J. (1952) *Acta Orthop. Scand. Suppl.* **11**, 1−117.

Hayes M.A., Creighton S.R., Boysen B.G. & Holfield N. (1978) Acute necrotizing myelopathy from nucleus pulposus embolism of arteries and veins in large dogs with early disc degeneration. *J. Am. Anim. Hosp. Assoc.* **173**, 289.

Heavner J.E. (1971) Intervertebral disc syndrome in the cat. *J. Am. Vet. Med. Assoc.* **159**, 425.

Hoerlein B.F. (1971) *Canine Neurology—Diagnosis and Treatment*, 2nd edn. W.B. Saunders Co., Philadelphia.

Jeffery N.D. (1988) Treatment of acute and chronic thoracolumbar disc disease by mini hemilaminectomy. *J. Small Anim. Pract.* **29**, 611−16.

Joshua J.O. & Ishmael J. (1968) Pain syndrome associated with spinal haemorrhage in the dog. *Vet. Rec.* **83**, 165.

Kelly D.F., Grunsell C.S.E. & Kenyon C.J. (1973) Polyarteritis in the dog: a case report. *Vet. Rec.* **92**, 363.

Knecht C.D. & Schiller A.G. (1974) *Canine Surgery*, 2nd edn. American Vet. Publications, Wheaton, Illinois.

Ladds P., Guffy M., Blauch B. & Splitter G. (1970) Congenital odontoid separation in two dogs. *J. Small Anim. Pract.* **12**, 463.

Lawson D.D. (1957) Fixation of mandibular fractures in the dog and cat by transfixing pinning. *Vet. Rec.* **69**, 1029.

Lawson D.D. (1963) Mandibular fractures in the dog. *Br. Vet. J.* **119**, 492.

Lawson D.D. (1971) The diagnosis and prognosis of canine paraplegia. *Vet. Rec.* **89**, 654.

Leonard E.P. (1971) *Orthopaedic Surgery of the Dog and Cat*, 2nd edn. W.B. Saunders Co., Philadelphia.

Lewis D.G. (1989) Cervical spondylomyelopathy (wobbler syndrome) in the dog; A study based on 224 cases. *J. Small Anim. Pract.* **30**, 657–65.

Lewis D.G. (1991) Radiological assessment of the cervical spine of the dobermann with reference to cervical spondylomyelopathy. *J. Small Anim. Pract.* **32**, 75–82.

Mckee W.M. (1988) Dorsal laminar elevation as a treatment for cervical vertebral canal stenosis in the dog. *J. Small Anim. Pract.* **29**, 95–103.

Mckee M. (1990) Surgical management of spinal fractures and luxations. *In Practice* **November**, 227–32.

Mckee W.M., Lavelle R.B. & Mason T.A. (1989) Vertebral stabilisation for cervical spondylopathy using a screw and washer technique. *J. Small Anim. Pract.* **30**, 337–42.

Mckee W.M., Lavelle R.B., Richardson J.L. & Mason T.A. (1990) Vertebral distraction fusion for cervical spondylopathy using a screw and double washer technique. *J. Small Anim. Pract.* **31**, 22–7.

Malik R., Latter M. & Love D.N. (1990) Bacterial discospondylitis in a cat. *J. Small Anim. Pract.* **31**, 404–6.

Morgan J.P. (1968) Congenital spinal defects. *J. Am. Vet. Radiol. Soc.* **9**, 21.

Norsworthy G.D. (1979) Discospondylitis as a cause of posterior paralysis. *Fel. Pract.* **9**, 39–40.

Northington J.W. & Juliana M.M. (1978) Extradural lymphosarcoma in 6 cats. *J. Small Anim. Pract.* **19**, 409–16.

Oliver E. & Lewis E. (1973) Lesions of the atlas and axis in dogs. *J. Am. Anim. Hosp. Assoc.* **9**, 304.

Oliver J.E. (1975) Craniotomy, craniectomy and skull fractures. In Bojrab M.J. (ed.) *Current Techniques in Small Animal Surgery*. Lea & Febiger, Philadelphia, p. 359.

Olsson S.E. & Hansen H.J. (1952) Cervical disc protrusion in the dog. *J. Am. Vet. Med. Assoc.* **121**, 361.

Palmer A.C. (1965) *Introduction to Animal Neurology*, 1st edn. Blackwell Scientific Publications, Oxford.

Read R.A., Robins G.M. & Carlisle C.H. (1983) Caudal cervical spondylomyelopathy (wobbler syndrome) in the dog; a review of 30 cases. *J. Small Anim. Pract.* **24**, 605.

Robins G.N. (1976) Dropped jaw—mandibular neurapraxia in the dog. *J. Small Anim. Pract.* **17**, 753.

Robins G.N. (1984) The treatment of cervical disc disease in the dog by ventral decompression. *The Veterinary Annual*, 24 edn. John Wright & Sons, Bristol, pp. 293–304.

Robins G.N. & Grandage J. (1977) Temporomandibular joint dysplasia and open mouth jaw locking in the dog. *J. Am. Med. Assoc.* **171**, 1072.

Robinson G.W. (1976) The high-rise syndrome in cats. *Fel. Pract.* **6**, 40–3.

Rouse G.P. (1979) Cervical spine stabilization with methylmethacrylate. *Vet. Surg.* **8**, 1.

Rucker N.C. (1990) Management of spinal cord trauma. *Prog. Vet. Neurol.* **1**, 397–411.

Russell R.W. & Griffiths R.C. (1968) Recurrence of cervical disc syndrome in surgically and conservatively treated dogs. *J. Am. Vet. Med. Assoc.* **153**, 1412.

Schulman A. & Lippincott C.L. (1987) Dorsolateral hemilaminectomy in the treatment of thoracolumbar intervertebral disc disease in dogs. *Compendium of Continuing Education* **9**, 305−10.

Seemann C.W. (1968) A lateral approach for thoracolumbar disc fenestration. *Mod. Vet. Pract.* **49**, 73.

Seemann C.W. (1980) Anatomic orientation for lateral thoracolumbar disc fenestration. *Vet. Med. Small Anim. Clin.* **75**, 1865.

Seim H.B. & Prata R.G. (1982) Ventral decompression for the treatment of cervical disc disease in the dog, A review of 54 cases. *J. Am. Anim. Hosp. Assoc.* **18**, 233.

Sharp N.J.H. (1989) Neurological deficits in one limb. In: Wheeler S. (ed.) *Manual of Small Animal Practice.* BSAVA, p. 197.

Shelton S.B., Bellah J., Chrisman C. & McMullen H. (1991) Hypoplasia of the odontoid process and secondary atlanto-axial subluxation in a Siamese cat. *Prog. Vet. Neurol.* **2**, 209−11.

Slocum B. & Rudy R.L. (1975) Fractures of the 7th lumbar vertebra in the dog. *J. Am. Anim. Hosp. Assoc.* **11**, 167−74.

Sorjonen D.C. & Shires P.K. (1981) Atlanto-axial instability. A ventral surgical technique for decompression, fixation and fusion. *Vet. Surg.* **10**, 22−29.

Spellman G. (1972) *Vet. Med. SAC* **67**, 1213.

Stone E.A., Betts C.W. & Chambers J.N. (1979) Cervical fractures in the dog: a literature and case review. *J. Am. Anim. Hosp. Assoc.* **15**, 463.

Sullivan M. (1989) Temporomandibular ankylosis in the cat. *J. Small Anim. Pract.* **30**, 401−5.

Sumner-Smith G. & Dingwall J.S. (1971) The plating of mandibular fractures in the dog. *Vet. Rec.* **88**, 595.

Sumner-Smith G. & Dingwall J.S. (1973) The plating of mandibular fractures in giant dogs. *Vet. Rec.* **92**, 39.

Swaim S.F. (1971) Vertebral body plating for spinal immobilization. *J. Am. Vet. Med. Assoc.* **158**, 1683.

Swaim S.F. (1972) Surgical correction of a spinal fracture in a day. *J. Am. Vet. Med. Assoc.* **160**, 1315.

Swaim S.F. (1975) Evaluation of four techniques of cervical spinal fixation in dogs. *J. Am. Vet. Med. Assoc.* **166**, 1080.

Thomas J.B. & Eger C. (1989) Granulomatous meningoencephalomyelitis in 21 dogs. *J. Small Anim. Pract.* **30**, 287−93.

Umphlet R.C. & Johnson A.L. (1988) Mandibular fractures in the cat, a retrospective study. *Vet. Surg.* **17**, 333−7.

Umphlet R.C. & Johnson A.L. (1990) Mandibular fractures in the dog, a retrospective study of 157 cases. *Vet. Surg.* **19**, 272−5.

Weinmann J.P. & Sicher H. (1955) *Bone and Bones: Fundamentals of Bone Biology*, 2nd edn. Kimpton, London, p. 309.

Wheeler S.J. (1988) Thoracolumbar disc surgery. *In Practice* **November**, 231−40.

Wheeler S.J. & Davies J.V. (1985) Iohexel radiography in the dog and cat, a series of one hundred cases, and a comparison with metrizamide and iopamidol. *J. Small Anim. Pract.* **26**, 247−56.

Whitbread T.J. (1981) Personal communication.

Whitney W.O. & Mehlhaff C.J. (1987) High-rise syndrome in cats. *J. Am. Vet. Med. Assoc.* **191**, 1399−403.

Winstanley E.W. (1976) Fractures of the skull. *Vet. Annual*, **16**, 151. John Wright & Sons, Bristol.

Wolff E.F. (1974) *Vet. Med. SAC* **69**, 859.

Worthman R.P. (1957) Demonstration of specific nerve paralysis in the dog. *J. Am. Vet. Med. Assoc.* **131**, 174.

Chapter 4
The Forelimb

EXAMINATION OF THE DOG WITH FORELEG LAMENESS

The following points should be noted in the history:
1 Breed of dog.
2 Age.
3 Speed of onset of lameness—gradual or sudden. If the onset was sudden, has the animal been involved in an accident, fall or other trauma?
4 Is lameness constant or intermittent? If intermittent, is lameness worse after exercise or rest?
5 Has the dog any other problems?
6 In road traffic accident cases fractures or dislocations may be obvious but it is important not to overlook injuries to the chest or urinary tract.

The history will often give good hints towards diagnosis. The developmental disorders tend to be seen in certain breeds of dog and generally cause a gradual onset of lameness in animals under a year of age. A sudden onset of lameness indicates a traumatic episode; common causes include a sprained joint, foreign body in the foot and bite wounds.

Dogs with fractures or dislocations will usually carry the affected leg. The clinical features of a fracture include:
1 Abnormal mobility of bone where no joint exists.
2 Deformity, i.e. local swelling, angulation and shortening of the limb.
3 Crepitus—a grating noise as the bone ends rub together.
4 Pain.

In a dislocation, unlike a fracture where the limb 'waves in the breeze' from the fracture site, characteristic postures are adopted as a result of joint displacement. Joint mobility is restricted and painful but crepitus is not generally as obvious as in a fracture.

Dislocations and ligamentous ruptures tend to be seen in mature dogs over 1 year of age. The same trauma in immature animals is more likely to cause a fracture or separation of an epiphysis.

The common, or well-recognized causes of foreleg lameness are listed below and should be kept in mind when the clinical examination is carried out.

Developmental disorders causing foreleg lameness

Shoulder	Osteochondritis dissecans	Giant breeds, especially Irish Wolfhounds, Pyrenean Mountain Dogs, Great Danes, but can affect any large dog from Labrador-size upwards
Elbow	Ununited anconeal process Osteochondritis dissecans Ununited coronoid process	German Shepherd, Basset Hound } Labrador, Golden Retriever, Rottweiler
Carpus	Lateral deviation due to growth disturbances of the radius and ulna	Great Dane, Irish Wolfhound
Other cause	Panosteitis	(German Shepherd)

Traumatic conditions of the forelimb

Shoulder	Dislocations	Gross instability — lateral dislocation of humeral head most often
Humeral shaft fractures		Distal third mainly, spiral or oblique, often comminuted
Elbow	Dislocation	Radial head dislocates laterally, forearm swung out laterally, held forward and supinated
	Condylar fractures	Spaniels are particularly prone to this injury. Lateral condyle fractures most

		frequently, also 'Y' and 'T' fractures
	Fracture of the olecranon	
Fractures of shaft of radius and ulna		Generally transverse and involve distal third
Carpus	Fracture of accessory carpal bone	Racing Greyhound
	Hyperextension of carpus due to rupture of plantar ligaments	
Metacarpus		Fractures and crush injuries common
Greyhound toe injuries	Interphalangeal subluxations and dislocations	Left foot most frequently involved
	Fractures — phalanges and sesamoids. 'Knocked up toe'	

Conditions causing a gradual onset of lameness in older dogs
Brachial plexus tumour.
Bicipital tenosynovitis: shoulder.
Osteosarcoma: proximal humerus.
Osteoarthritis: elbow.
Osteosarcoma: distal radius.
Osteoarthritis: carpus.

PHYSICAL EXAMINATION
Look at the dog standing, assess weight bearing and look for evidence of muscle wasting. The spine of the scapula becomes more prominent in chronic foreleg lameness and the greater trochanter of the femur becomes more prominent in chronic hind leg lameness. Note any joint deformity. Observe the animal's gait when walking, trotting and running, both in a straight line and in a circle. Assess the degree of lameness and differentiate lameness from ataxia or paresis.

Most larger dogs feel more secure and behave better if examined on the floor. Small dogs are obviously easier to handle and examine on a table. The owner or assistant should hold the dog's head firmly from the contralateral side to the leg being examined. Run your hands down both front legs, compare the affected leg with the normal one, check for muscle wasting, joint swelling and deformity. Check the nails and pads; in chronic lameness the nails will be long and there will be little wear of the pads compared with the normal foot. Alternatively, the dog with foreleg paresis will often have excessive wear of the nails through dragging the toes or knuckling at the digits. Each joint should be checked systematically. The shoulder is fully extended. The leg should be gripped *above* the elbow with one hand and pulled forward, while the other hand is placed over the anterior aspect of the shoulder and used to push the joint caudally. Remember that extension of the shoulder naturally tends to extend the elbow and it is possible to confuse pain arising from either joint. A sudden onset of shoulder pain is most frequently caused by strain of the shoulder muscles and lameness will resolve provided adequate rest is given. If an immature dog of the larger breeds has pain on extension of the shoulder and the onset of lameness is gradual, then the most likely cause is osteochondritis dissecans. A limited range of shoulder flexion sometimes associated with pain is seen in dogs with bicipital tenosynovitis or contracture of the extensor muscles of the shoulder. A limited range of shoulder movement is also seen in small breeds of dogs with congenital dislocation. The proximal humerus is a common site for osteosarcoma formation and the lesion causes a hard, painful swelling. It is also worth checking the axilla for tumour formation in older animals.

The elbow is checked next. One hand is cupped behind the olecranon and the other is used to grip the forearm and gradually extend the elbow. Pain on extension is a feature of ununited anconeal process, osteochondritis dissecans and ununited coronoid process. If either of the last two conditions are present pain can be increased by supinating the forearm while extending the elbow. Ununited anconeal process causes an increase in synovial fluid production and a fluctuating swelling develops caudal to the humeral condyles. All three conditions if untreated cause osteo-arthritis; the elbow joint becomes thickened with a limited range of flexion, crepitus and there is a varying degree of pain on manipulation.

Condylar fractures of the humerus cause obvious pain and crepitus in the elbow. Fracture of the lateral condyle occurs most frequently. Lateral support for the joint is lost and the distal humerus can be palpated subluxating medially in relation to the radius and ulna. By comparison palpation of the elbow in a dog with an intercondylar fracture ('Y' or 'T' fracture) reveals total disruption in the continuity of the distal humerus. Dislocation of the elbow results in a limited range of painful joint movement and the forearm is held forward abducted and supinated.

The main movements of the carpus are flexion and extension. Hyperextension is seen in German Shepherd puppies occasionally and is associated with laxity of the carpal flexor tendons and ligaments. Traumatic hyperextension is seen in mature dogs with rupture of the plantar ligaments of the carpus. In the racing Greyhound feel the accessory carpal bone; chip fractures are common and give rise to pain on flexion and extension of the joint. Normally there is little medial or lateral movement of the carpus unless there has been damage to the collateral ligaments. Lateral deviation of the carpus and foot (carpal valgus) is seen in immature giant breeds of dog due to growth disturbances of the radius and ulna. Thickening and pain in the carpus is usually due to osteoarthritis. However, the distal radius is a common site for osteosarcoma formation. Feel the metacarpal bones and, in the racing Greyhound, particular care should be taken over the palpation of the toes as injuries are common. Finally, look at the nails for damage and check the pads for cuts, bruising or foreign bodies.

If the physical examination of the lame dog causes obvious pain further manipulation, if necessary, should be done under general anaesthesia. The radiographic examination is undertaken next. The most useful views are:

Shoulder	Lateral radiograph
Elbow	Flexed lateral and craniocaudal radiographs
Carpus	Craniocaudal and lateral radiographs. If joint is unstable the lateral radiograph is taken first with the carpus flexed and secondly with the joint extended.

Other procedures such as (a) the aspiration and examination of synovial fluid, (b) special serological tests for conditions like rheumatoid arthritis, systemic lupus erythematosus or toxoplasmosis, and (c) exploratory arthrotomy may be necessary to determine the cause of lameness.

If the initial findings are negative the dog is rested and treated symptomatically. Radiographic examination is repeated 4−6 weeks later if lameness has not resolved. The repeat radiograph is particularly useful when initial findings were suggestive but not conclusive for osteosarcoma formation.

FORELEG LAMENESS IN CATS

The basic principles of examining the lame cat are the same as the dog. Assessment of the degree of lameness is not so easy and is best observed by allowing the cat to move around the room (keep doors and windows shut to prevent escape). The most common causes of acute lameness in cats are traumatic in origin, i.e. bite wounds from other cats, soft tissue injuries, fractures and dislocations. Cats are relatively free of congenital, developmental and degenerative bone and joint diseases. Lameness caused by nutritional secondary hyperparathyroidism is seen in kittens (p. 29), while in older cats foreleg lameness can be caused by new bone formation particularly around the elbows as a result of hypervitaminosis A (p. 32).

THE SHOULDER JOINT

The shoulder is an enarthrodial joint (Figs 4.1 and 4.2). Although there are weak medial and lateral labio-humeral ligaments present, the joint is mainly supported by the surrounding muscles. Support is provided cranially by the supraspinatus muscle, laterally by the infraspinatus muscle, ventrolaterally by the teres minor muscle and medially by the subscapularis muscle (Fig. 4.3). The tendon of the biceps brachii muscle crosses the anteromedial aspect of the joint and is retained in the bicipital groove of the humerus by the transverse humeral ligament (Fig. 4.2).

The superficial muscles of the shoulder are illustrated in Fig. 4.4.

There are few 'danger points' in the exposure of the shoulder but structures to recognize and avoid include:

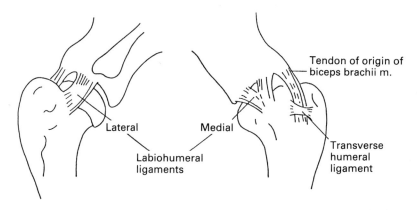

Tendon of origin of biceps brachii m.

Lateral   Medial

Labiohumeral ligaments

Transverse humeral ligament

Fig. 4.1 Shoulder, lateral view.   **Fig. 4.2** Shoulder, medial view.

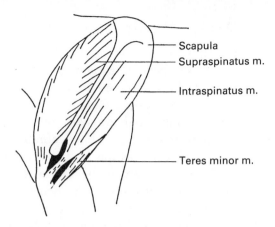

Fig. 4.3 Deep muscles of the lateral shoulder.

Figs 4.1–4.3 Reproduced by permission of Miller M.E. (1952). *A Guide to the Dissection of the Dog*. Edwards Brothers Inc., Michigan.

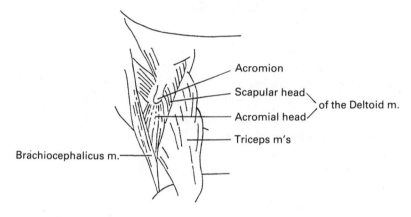

Fig. 4.4

1 A branch of the cephalic vein which runs just cranial to the joint.

2 The circumflex humeral artery and vein and the axillary nerve caudal to the joint.

3 The suprascapular nerve which runs around the neck of the scapula.

Conditions which can affect the canine shoulder joint are summarized in Fig. 4.5.

Traumatic conditions of the shoulder

FRACTURES OF THE SCAPULA (Cheli 1976; Caywood *et al.* 1977; Holt 1978; Piermattei & Greeley 1979)
The scapula with its blade-like structure, lateral supporting muscle mass and proximity to the chest wall is well protected

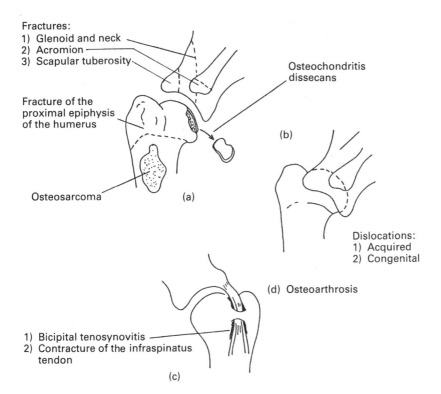

Fractures:
1) Glenoid and neck
2) Acromion
3) Scapular tuberosity

Osteochondritis dissecans

Fracture of the proximal epiphysis of the humerus

(b)

Osteosarcoma   (a)

Dislocations:
1) Acquired
2) Congenital

(d) Osteoarthrosis

1) Bicipital tenosynovitis
2) Contracture of the infraspinatus tendon

(c)

Fig. 4.5 (a) Fractures of the scapula (1,2 and 3); (b) shoulder dysplasia, acquired and congenital dislocation; (c) muscle injuries include bicipital tenosynovitis and contracture of the infraspinatus tendon; (d) osteoarthritis.

against trauma (Fig. 4.6). Consequently, scapular fractures are uncommon. Generally, the fragments are well supported by the adjacent tissues and this, together with the cancellous nature of the bone, ensures that the majority of scapular fractures will heal well with conservative treatment. An Elastoplast support bandage is applied around the shoulder and chest for 4 weeks. The exceptions which should be treated surgically include intra-articular fractures, avulsion fractures and grossly displaced fractures of the blade and neck.

Displaced fractures of the scapular blade and spine
The supraspinatus and infraspinatus muscles are reflected to reveal the fracture site. Wire sutures are a popular method of fixation. However, a plate will provide better stability. If the screws are to achieve maximum purchase in the bone, the plate should be placed in the angle formed between the spine and body (Fig. 4.7). An ASIF semi-tubular plate fits the angle well if it is applied upside down with the convex side of the plate towards the bone.

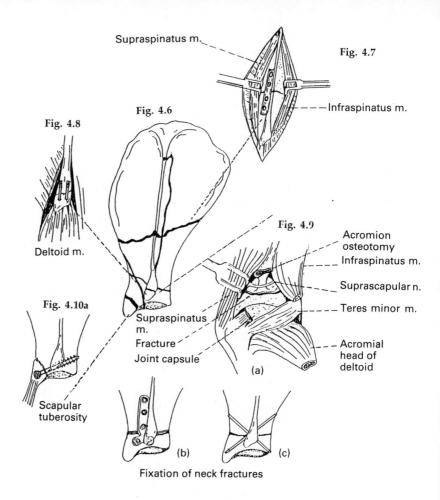

Supraspinatus m.

Fig. 4.7

Infraspinatus m.

Fig. 4.6

Fig. 4.8

Deltoid m.

Fig. 4.9

Acromion
osteotomy

Infraspinatus m.

Suprascapular n.

Teres minor m.

Fig. 4.10a

Supraspinatus
m.

Fracture

Joint capsule

(a)

Acromial
head of
deltoid

Scapular
tuberosity

(b)

(c)

Fixation of neck fractures

Fracture of the acromion
The acromion is distracted by the deltoid muscle following
fracture. Fixation is simply achieved using one of two wire
sutures (Fig. 4.8).

Fractures of the scapular neck and glenoid (Fig. 4.9a, b and c)
Osteotomy of the acromion is carried out to allow ventral
reflection of the acromial head of the deltoid. (The osteotomy
is repaired during wound closure with wire sutures as
shown in Fig. 4.8.) The underlying supraspinatus muscle is
retracted cranially. The tendon of insertion of the infraspinatus muscle is cut and the muscle is reflected caudally
to complete exposure of the scapular neck, suprascapular
nerve and joint capsule. The nerve must be carefully protected during fracture reduction and fixation. Transverse
fractures of the scapular neck are stabilized using a small
ASIF mini 'T' plate (Fig. 4.9b) or two Kirschner wires
(Fig. 4.9c). Lag screw fixation is used for sagittal fractures
of the scapular neck which extend into the glenoid (Fig.

4.10b). The joint capsule should be opened during exposure of the fracture to check that accurate anatomical reduction of the fragments is achieved.

Osteotomy of the greater tuberosity of the humerus for
exposure of scapular fractures
Osteotomy of the lateral tuberosity of the humerus permits an extensive exposure of the scapular tuberosity, neck of the scapula or articular surfaces of the shoulder. The osteotomy is repaired with two lag screws (the screw holes are prepared before osteotomy is undertaken). An osteotome or oscillating saw is used to free the lateral tuberosity which can then be reflected dorsally with the attached supraspinatus and infraspinatus muscles (Fig. 4.10b (i), (ii)).

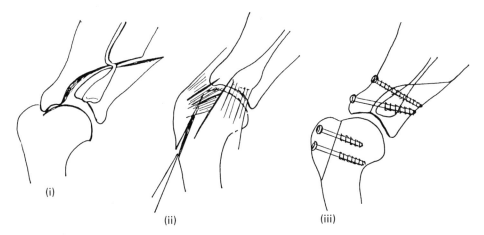

(i)

(ii)

(iii)

Fig. 4.10b (i) Oblique fracture of the scapula with displacement of the articular surfaces; (ii) osteotomy of the lateral tuberosity of the humerus allows the supraspinatus and infraspinatus muscles to be reflected to expose the fracture; (iii) fixation of the fracture and osteotomy with lag screw.

Avulsion of the scapular tuberosity
The scapular tuberosity develops as a separate ossification centre which fuses with the scapula when the dog reaches approximately 5 months of age. Avulsion of the tuberosity occasionally occurs in immature dogs; the fracture extends through the growth plate and the fragment is distracted by the pull of the biceps tendon (Fig. 4.10a). Exposure of the fracture is achieved by retracting the brachiocephalicus muscle cranially to reveal the greater tuberosity of the humerus and the insertion of the supraspinatus muscle. The shoulder is rotated laterally and the scapular tuberosity exposed by blunt dissection medial to the insertion of the supraspinatus muscle. Alternatively use a lateral approach

with osteotomy of the lateral tuberosity of the humerus see above. The fracture is stabilized with a lag screw (preferably cancellous) or a tension band wire (Fig. 4.10a).

In a chronic avulsion fracture, reduction may be impossible due to contracture of the biceps brachii muscle. Under these circumstances, the scapular tuberosity is excised and the biceps tendon sutured to the transverse humeral ligament. Alternatively the origin of the biceps tendon can be anchored in the bicipital groove using a ligament staple (Fig. 4.10b (iv), Veterinary Instrumentation).

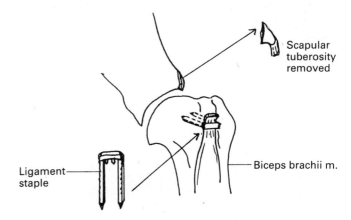

Scapular
tuberosity
removed

Ligament
staple

Biceps brachii m.

Fig. 4.10b(iv) Use of a ligament staple for fixation of the tendon of the Biceps brachii m. following removal of the scapular tuberosity or in the treatment of bicipital tenosynovitis.

Fractures involving the proximal humeral epiphysis and metaphysis

Fractures of the proximal humerus can be divided into intra-articular fractures in which there is involvement of the humeral head and/or tubercles, and extra-articular fractures where fracture occurs either through the proximal growth plate of the humerus with separation of the epiphysis (epiphysiolysis) or through the metaphyseal region.

Intra-articular fractures are rare. They occur in immature animals and the fracture extends through the growth plate. Fixation of the fracture is achieved with two Kirschner wires driven through the lateral aspect of the greater tuberosity and on into the humeral head (Figs 4.11a, b and c). Conversely the wires can be introduced through the articular surface of the humerus but the ends must be countersunk with a nail punch to allow normal shoulder movement.

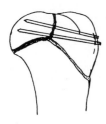

Fig. 4.11a

Fracture-separation of the proximal epiphysis of the humerus

This is a rare injury which occurs in immature animals.

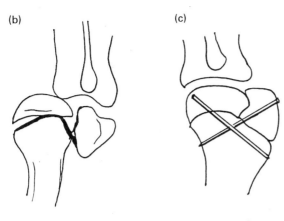

(b) (c)

Fig. 4.11b,c Fracture separation of proximal humeral epiphysis in a cat, fixation with crossed Kirschner wires.

Considerable trauma is needed to separate the epiphysis and there is usually gross anterior displacement of the epiphysis in relation to the metaphysis. Open reduction is necessary in most cases. A longitudinal skin incision is made over the anterolateral aspect of the proximal humerus. The brachiocephalicus muscle is retracted cranially to expose the fracture. The epiphysis is grasped with small AO reduction forceps (Straumann, Great Britain Ltd) and with the aid of a periosteal elevator the epiphysis is levered back into its normal position. Generally, stability is good once reduction is achieved and this can be maintained with a lag screw in dogs approaching maturity (Fig. 4.11d) or an intramedullary pin in puppies (Fig. 4.12). Healing should occur within 4–6 weeks. Premature closure of the growth plate may occur as a result of the initial trauma but this is of doubtful significance unless it happens in a pup under 6 months of age. The lag screw or intramedullary pin is removed as soon as fracture healing is complete.

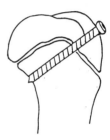

Fig. 4.11d

Dislocation of the shoulder

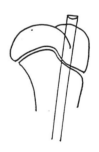

Fig. 4.12

CONGENITAL DISLOCATION
(Vaughan & Clayton-Jones 1969)
The condition is rare and is usually seen in toy breeds of dogs. The humeral head luxates medially in most cases and the glenoid cavity is deformed and convex. Both shoulder joints may be affected. There is no treatment but as these animals are usually small and light they are not greatly incapacitated by the deformity. The shoulder tends to stabilize, and lameness resolves as the dog matures. If lameness persists or develops in later life due to degener-

ative joint disease then arthrodesis of the joint should be recommended (see p. 207).

ACQUIRED DISLOCATION OF THE SHOULDER
(Vaughan 1967; Ball 1968; Campbell 1968; Leighton 1969; De Angelis & Schwartz 1970; Hohn *et al.* 1971)
Acquired dislocation of the shoulder is uncommon. The humeral head may luxate medially or laterally. Lateral dislocation is seen most often. Manipulation of the shoulder reveals gross instability and spontaneous reduction often occurs when the dog is positioned for radiographic examination.

Stabilization of the shoulder to prevent recurrence of the dislocation can be a real problem. In fresh dislocations, closed reduction is readily accomplished; this is followed by application of a body cast (Fig. 4.13) for 3–4 weeks to prevent redislocation. Ideally the body cast is applied with the dog in the natural standing position. The dog is sedated first; pethidine is given to provide analgesia; passive extension of the shoulder will reduce the dislocation in most cases, and then the cast can be applied to maintain reduction. Application of the cast with the dog standing ensures that the cast can be closely applied to the natural contours of the shoulder and chest. A well-fitting body cast is comfortable for the animal to wear and minimizes the risk of redislocation.

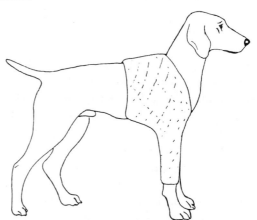

Fig. 4.13

If the shoulder is grossly unstable or should redislocation occur after removal of the body cast then some form of internal fixation will be necessary. Techniques include:
1 Suturing the torn joint capsule and damaged shoulder muscles.

2 Braided nylon, terylene or strip of skin can be threaded through a tunnel in the spine of the scapula and then down through the greater tuberosity on the lateral side of the joint in a figure of eight pattern (Fig. 4.14) to form a prosthetic ligament.

3 The biceps tendon can be transposed medially or laterally (depending on the direction of the dislocation) to serve as a collateral ligament (Fig. 4.15a, b). Osteotomy of the greater tuberosity is necessary to permit lateral transposition of the tendon.

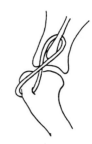

Fig. 4.14

(a)　　　　　(b)

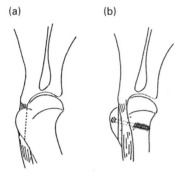

Fig. 4.15

4 A simple and effective method of restabilizing the shoulder following dislocation in any direction is shown in Figs 4.16a–e. Multifilament polyester or carbon fibre is used as a prosthesis to create a medial and lateral collateral ligament for the shoulder (Fig. 4.16b). If neither of these materials is available then a double strand of No. 7 braided nylon can be used. A skin incision is made directly over the joint (Fig. 4.16a). The acromial head of the deltoid is sectioned about 1 cm from its origin and the muscle belly is reflected to reveal the infraspinatus and supraspinatus muscles (Fig. 4.16c). The supraspinatus muscle and the suprascapular nerve are retracted to expose the neck of the scapula. A tunnel is drilled through the scapular neck and a second tunnel is drilled through the proximal humerus. The shoulder is rotated laterally and wire loops are used to thread the prosthesis from lateral to medial through the scapular tunnel and then from medial to lateral through the humeral tunnel. The joint capsule is repaired and then the ends of the prosthesis are tied. A support bandage is applied round the shoulder for 2 weeks following surgery.

Shoulder dysplasia (Evans 1968)
Shoulder dysplasia resulting in excessive joint laxity is

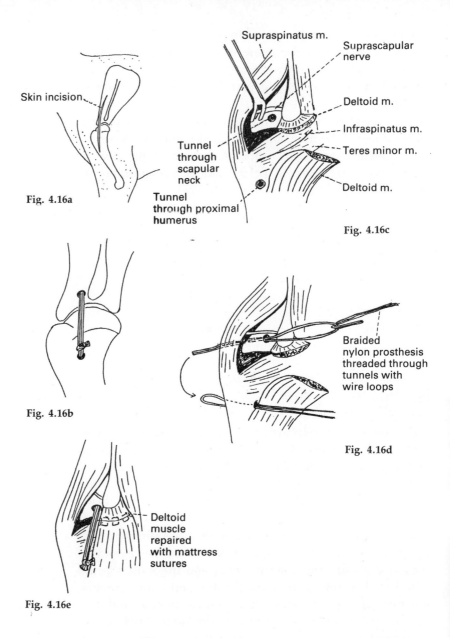

Fig. 4.16a

Skin incision

Supraspinatus m.

Suprascapular nerve

Deltoid m.

Infraspinatus m.

Teres minor m.

Deltoid m.

Tunnel through scapular neck

Tunnel through proximal humerus

Fig. 4.16c

Fig. 4.16b

Braided nylon prosthesis threaded through tunnels with wire loops

Fig. 4.16d

Deltoid muscle repaired with mattress sutures

Fig. 4.16e

occasionally encountered in the dog. The condition has been described in a 3½-year-old Collie (Hanlon 1964) and a 10-month-old Labrador (Evans 1968).

Muscle and tendon injuries

Two specific muscle and tendon injuries of the shoulder are recognized. These are bicipital tenosynovitis and contracture of the infraspinatus muscle or supraspinatus muscle.

Bicipital tenosynovitis is frequently diagnosed as a cause of shoulder lameness, often as a last resort when no other cause of foreleg lameness can be found. Nevertheless bicipital tenosynovitis is a definite condition; it tends to be seen in older dogs of the larger breeds, often working dogs like Labradors. The tendon of origin of the biceps muscle originates on the scapular tuberosity and runs down the craniomedial aspect of the humerus in the bicipital groove. The tendon is retained in the groove by the transverse humeral ligament. The biceps tendon provides cranial support for the shoulder and the muscle flexes the elbow. An extension of the shoulder joint capsule acts as a synovial sheath for the biceps tendon. Trauma to the tendon results in inflammatory changes around the tendon with adhesions to the sheath and later osteophyte formation in the bicipital groove.

Clinically lameness tends to become worse with exercise, there is pain on shoulder flexion and the range of shoulder flexion may be limited. Deep palpation over the bicipital groove causes pain. Radiographs of the shoulder may demonstrate roughening of the groove, osteophyte formation or calcification in the biceps tendon. There may well be concomitant degenerative changes in the shoulder. An arthrogram using positive contrast (Conray 280) may show incomplete filling of the biceps sheath due to the presence of adhesions. Bicipital tenosynovitis causes chronic lameness. Initially there may be a response to rest and analgesics. The next stage in treatment is to inject methylprednisolone (Depo-Medrone, 1–2 ml, Upjohn) into the shoulder or bicipital groove. If there is a good response this tends to confirm the diagnosis. It is preferable to inject Depo-Medrone directly into the bicipital groove; this is done under general anaesthesia under conditions of strict asepsis. The dog is placed on its back. With the shoulder flexed it is easy to palpate the bicipital groove on the craniomedial aspect of the humerus and the injection can be given accurately into the groove. Exercise is restricted for 2 weeks and then gradually increased. If lameness recurs the injection can be repeated two or three times.

If lameness and severe shoulder pain persist then there are several surgical options:

1 Section of the transverse humeral ligament to relieve pressure on the biceps tendon (a possible complication of this procedure is intermittent displacement of the biceps tendon out of the bicipital groove).

2 If it is accepted that pain associated with bicipital teno-synovitis is associated with movement of the biceps tendon, then prevention of tendon movement should alleviate pain. The tendon can be cut close to the scapular tuberosity and a new site of origin provided by fixing the tendon in the bicipital groove using a bone screw and spiked ASIF washer (Brinker *et al.* 1990) or a ligament staple (Fig. 4.10b(iv) (Veterinary Instrumentation).

3 The biceps tendon normally contributes to stability of the shoulder and ideally this function should be preserved. Consequently several dogs with bicipital tenosynovitis have been treated at this clinic simply by fixing the biceps tendon in the bicipital groove using a staple. The staple is inserted while the shoulder is in the flexed position. The initial results have been encouraging.

Technique (Fig. 4.10b(iv)

The dog is placed in dorsal recumbency for surgery with the affected leg pulled caudally. A medial approach is used to expose the bicipital groove. A longitudinal incision is made over the groove and extended through a thin layer of deep pectoral muscle to reveal the biceps tendon. The transverse humeral ligament is incised longitudinally and the biceps tendon displaced medially out of the groove. At this stage any osteophytes are removed from the groove. Next the biceps tendon is returned to its normal position, the shoulder is flexed and a ligament staple is used to anchor the tendon within the bicipital groove. In this way sliding movement of the tendon and hence pain are eliminated but at the same time the tendon remains in its normal anatomical position and continues to maintain shoulder stability.

TRAUMATIC MEDIAL DISPLACEMENT OF
THE BICEPS TENDON

This is a rare injury; it has been recorded in the Border Collie (Bennett & Campbell 1979) and in the racing Greyhound. Clinically there is pain on shoulder manipulation and the biceps tendon can be felt luxating in and out of the bicipital groove. Displacement results from rupture of the transverse humeral ligament. Treatment options include fixing the biceps tendon in the groove with a ligament staple (see bicipital tenosynovitis) or the creation of a new transverse humeral ligament using a wire prosthesis. Eighteen gauge wire is used to act as a prosthetic ligament; the wire is passed through tunnels in the lateral and medial

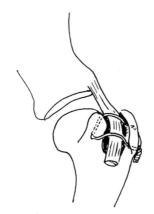

Fig. 4.16f Wire suture placed through lateral and medial tuberosity of the humerus to prevent displacement of the biceps tendon.

tuberosities forming a bridge over the bicipital groove (Fig. 4.16f). Care should be taken to ensure that the wire does not interfere with the gliding motion of the biceps tendon. The most likely complication of this technique is bicipital tenosynovitis.

CONTRACTURE OF THE INFRASPINATUS OR SUPRASPINATUS MUSCLE (Hufford *et al.* 1975; Vaughan 1979)

Contracture of the infraspinatus muscle is an occasional cause of foreleg lameness in the dog. Contracture of the supraspinatus muscle occurs even less frequently and gives similar signs. Working dogs are usually affected and have an acute onset of lameness at exercise. Although use of the affected limb is regained within 2 or 3 weeks, an abnormal action persists characterized by lateral circumduction of the distal limb with a rapid flip-like extension of the paw when the foot is advanced. Range of shoulder flexion is limited and there is atrophy of the supra- and infraspinatus muscles. On full flexion of the leg the forearm swings out laterally from the body instead of moving forward in a straight line. Caudocranial radiographs of the shoulder may show that the gap between the acromion and the greater tuberosity is reduced on the side of contracture (Fig. 4.17b). Normal limb function is rapidly restored by tenotomy of the contracted infraspinatus or supraspinatus tendon of insertion.

Treatment involves tenotomy of the contracted tendon. A lateral approach is made to the lateral tuberosity of the humerus. The cranial edge of the acromial head of the deltoid muscle is retracted caudally (Figs 4.3 and 4.4) to reveal the insertions of the infraspinatus and supraspinatus on the greater tuberosity. The damaged scarred tendon, usually the infraspinatus, is identified and sectioned. The procedure

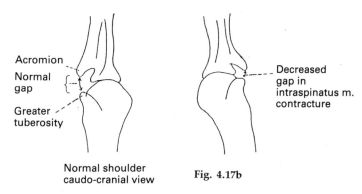

Fig. 4.17a

Fig. 4.17b

should immediately restore a normal range of shoulder movement. As soon as the surgical wound has healed exercise should be encouraged to prevent development of adhesions.

Osteochondritis dissecans (Craig & Riser 1965; Birkeland 1967; Griffiths 1968; Clayton-Jones & Vaughan 1968, 1970; Smith & Stowater 1975; Olsson 1975, 1976)

Osteochondritis dissecans (OCD) is a disease of articular cartilage characterized by focal separation of articular cartilage and subchondral bone. The disease can affect the shoulder, elbow, stifle or hock but it is most frequently diagnosed as a cause of shoulder lameness. The condition is often bilateral but generally only one pair of joints is involved. Olsson (1976) has shown that OCD is due to abnormal enchondral ossification. Typically, the lesion is found in the caudal part of the humeral head (Fig. 4.18a). Here the articular cartilage becomes thicker than normal because enchondral ossification does not keep pace with normal cartilaginous growth. The deeper layers of chondrocytes die and a zone of chondromalacia is formed. Modelling of the joint surface may be delayed giving flattening (Fig. 4.18b) or more typically cleavage occurs through the zone of chondromalacia and the overlying flap of cartilage becomes detached (Fig. 4.18c). The flap eventually comes to lie in the caudal part of the joint below the humeral head. In this position the flap does not interfere with joint function. The flap may survive on synovial fluid, grow and ossify and it is then referred to as a joint mouse (Fig. 4.18c). The erosion in the humeral head heals by fibrocartilage formation.

A number of factors play a part in the development of osteochondritis dissecans lesions. These include genetic

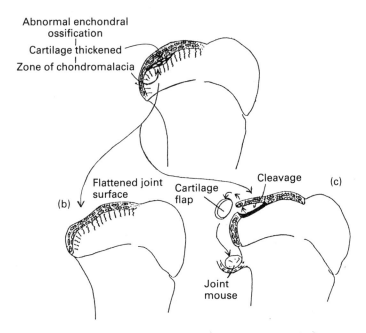

Abnormal enchondral
ossification
Cartilage thickened
Zone of chondromalacia

Flattened joint
surface
(b)

Cartilage
flap

Cleavage
(c)

Joint
mouse

Fig. 4.18

factors, feeding, exercise and trauma. Trauma is thought to
be important in the aetiology of osteochondritis dissecans
because lesions are invariably found in those areas of articular cartilage which are particularly prone to concussion.
It has been shown that the caudal part of the humeral head
where the lesion is found is prone to concussion both
when the shoulder is in the flexed and extended positions.

The large and giant breeds of dog, especially the Pyrenean
Mountain Dog, Irish Wolfhound and Great Dane, are
affected most frequently by osteochondritis dissecans of
the shoulder. Male dogs, presumably because of their greater
weight, are affected more often than females. The condition
is bilateral in just over 50% of cases. OCD is a disease of
the *immature* dog (no matter which joint is involved) and
causes a gradual onset of lameness before the dog reaches
a year of age. The average age at the onset of lameness is 5
months. Lameness tends to be intermittent in nature and
is often worse after exercise or immediately the dog gets
up from rest. The main finding on clinical examination is
pain on extension of the shoulder. Later the shoulder
muscles become wasted and the spine of the scapula becomes more prominent.

A lateral radiograph of the joint will usually confirm the
diagnosis. In doubtful cases two further lateral radiographs
are taken, one with the head of the humerus rotated

medially and the other with the humeral head rotated laterally. Osteochondritis dissecans affects the caudal humeral head and in positive cases flattening or an erosion will be seen in the subchondral bone of this region (Fig. 4.19a). The overlying flap of articular cartilage is radiolucent but with time it becomes calcified and appears as a fine white line over the erosion (Fig. 4.19b). In chronic cases a joint mouse may be seen. There may be irregularity of the humeral head at the site of the original erosion and osteophytes develop especially around the caudal margins of the joint (Fig. 4.20). Although dogs are usually clinically lame on one leg only, the condition affects both shoulders in approximately 50% of cases; consequently both joints are radiographed as a routine.

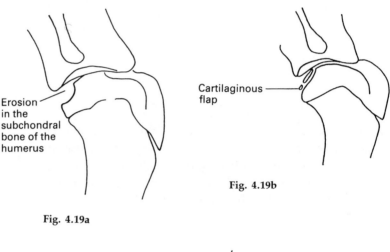

Erosion in the subchondral bone of the humerus

Cartilaginous flap

Fig. 4.19b

Fig. 4.19a

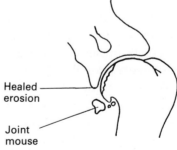

Healed erosion

Joint mouse

Fig. 4.20

TREATMENT

The majority of dogs with OCD of the shoulder would eventually recover with conservative treatment. However, the recovery period is prolonged (several months) and healing may be complicated by osteo-arthrosis in the joint.

Conservative treatment (restricted exercise and analgesics) is used in the early stages of the disease, especially if the lesion is small on radiographic examination. If lameness shows no signs of resolution within 6 weeks and there is definite radiographic evidence of OCD, then surgical treatment should be recommended. An arthrotomy is performed, the cartilaginous flap removed and the erosion in the humeral head curetted. An interesting feature of OCD is that shoulder pain persists until the cartilaginous flap becomes detached. Once this happens, pain rapidly disappears and lameness resolves. Some veterinarians favour an aggressive form of conservative treatment in which the dog is encouraged to exercise, run up and down slopes and the shoulder is forcibly manipulated. The rationale of these manoeuvres is to cause early detachment of the cartilaginous flap.

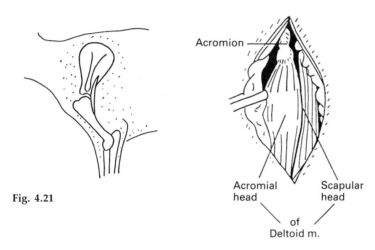

Fig. 4.21

Fig. 4.22

SURGICAL TECHNIQUE

A curved skin incision is made over the shoulder just caudal to the scapular spine (Fig. 4.21). The subcutaneous fat and fascia are retracted to expose the acromion and acromial head and scapular head of the deltoid muscle (Fig. 4.22). The two heads of the deltoid are separated and retracted to expose the infraspinatus and the teres minor muscles (Fig. 4.23).

The infraspinatus and the teres minor muscles are separated and retracted to expose the joint capsule (Figs 4.23 and 4.24). A transverse incision is made in the joint capsule to reveal the articular surface of the humeral head and the osteochondritis dissecans lesion. The flap of cartilage is

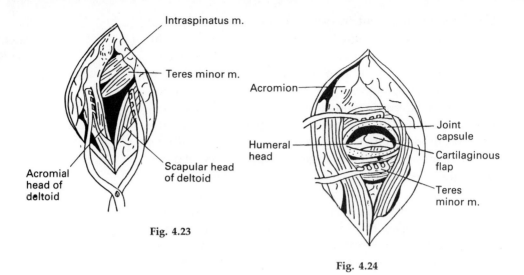

Fig. 4.23

Fig. 4.24

removed and the underlying erosion in the subchondral bone curetted. The joint is flushed out with saline solution to remove any remaining fragments. Closure of the wound is routine.

An alternative approach to the shoulder is illustrated in Figs 4.25–4.27. This approach is more traumatic but provides better exposure and is ideal for the surgeon who only occasionally operates in the shoulder.

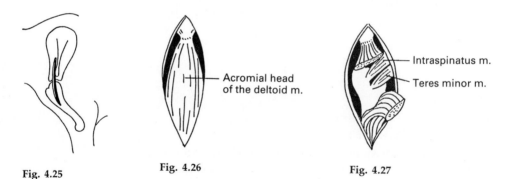

Fig. 4.25

Fig. 4.26

Fig. 4.27

A skin incision is made over the spine of the scapula and extended down over the proximal third of the humerus. The acromial head of the deltoid is exposed and the origin of the muscle is transected approximately 2 cm from the acromion. The muscle is reflected to reveal the infraspinatus and teres minor muscles which are separated to expose the joint capsule. The arthrotomy is then performed as described on p. 203.

After surgery, exercise is restricted to walking on a leash

for 1 month. Most dogs are less lame than before the operation within the month and should be sound within 3 months. In dogs with bilateral lesions a 6-week interval is left between each arthrotomy. The second operation is seldom necessary and is only performed if the dog is lame on the contralateral leg. Lameness often resolves, presumably because the dog takes excessive weight on this leg when the first shoulder is operated on and this results in early detachment of the cartilaginous flap and relief from pain (see p. 203).

COMPLICATIONS
1 Excessive muscle damage during exposure and possibly failure to close the joint capsule may lead to seroma formation within a few days of surgery. The content of the seroma is aspirated with a needle as necessary.
2 Skin overlying the shoulder is very mobile, wound healing may be slower than normal and skin sutures are left *in situ* for at least 10 days to avoid the risk of wound breakdown.

Osteosarcoma
The proximal humerus is a common site for osteosarcoma in older dogs (see p. 34).

BRACHIAL PLEXUS TUMOURS
The clinical features of brachial plexus tumours in dogs have been described by Wheeler *et al.* (1986) with reference to 22 cases. Most of the dogs were medium to large breeds, average age was 7.4 years. Typically cases had a chronic intractable foreleg lameness or paresis which had been present for 6–8 months without a diagnosis having been made. Marked limb muscle atrophy was a feature in 88% of cases and the spinatus muscle group over the scapula were most frequently affected. Pain or hyperaesthesia on palpation of the shoulder and axillary region was another feature (60% of cases). There was a palpable axillary mass in 68% of cases. Axillary masses can be difficult to palpate and this examination is best done under general anaesthesia; palpate both axillae for comparison. Ipsilateral loss of the panniculus reflex and Horner's syndrome may also be present. Plain radiography is usually negative; chest radiographs should always be taken although metastases are rare. Myelography can be useful and may help demonstrate that the nerve root tumour has extended to the neural canal. Surgical exploration of the brachial plexus can be undertaken; a craniomedial approach was described by

Knecht & Greene (1977) and is illustrated in Fig. 4.28a (i–iii). The cranial edge of the superficial pectoral muscle is severed near its insertion on the humerus and then by retraction of the muscle and blunt dissection the brachial plexus is exposed. The tumour mass is identified and then biopsy or excision can be attempted. Even if excision is possible, local recurrence is likely. Amputation with excision by resection of the nerves as far proximal to the mass as possible gives the animal the best chance of survival. Neurofibrosarcomas or neurofibromas are identified in this region most often.

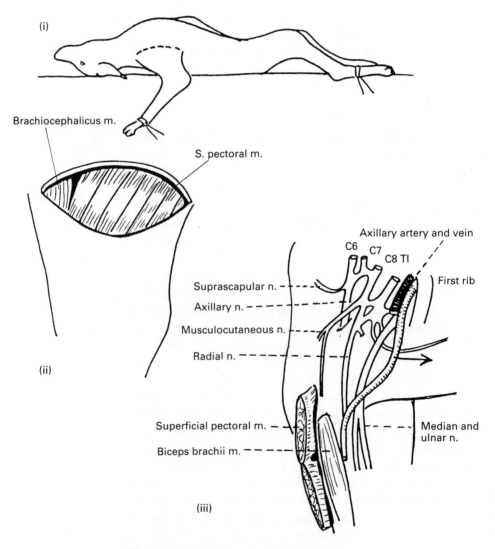

Fig. 4.28a Exposure of the brachial plexus.

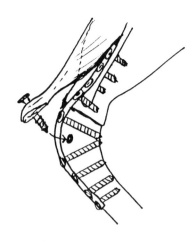

Fig. 4.28b Shoulder arthrodesis in a dog using a plate for fixation on the cranial aspect of the dog. The lateral tuberosity is reattached with a lag screw.

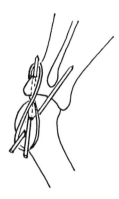

Fig. 4.28c Shoulder arthrodesis in the cat using Kirschner wires and a tension band wire for fixation.

Shoulder arthrodesis

The main indications for shoulder arthrodesis are: chronic dislocations (congenital or acquired), irreparable fractures, and the relief of chronic pain associated with chronic degenerative joint disease. The principles of arthrodesis are described on p. 269.

The shoulder is exposed through a combined cranial and lateral approach (Fig. 4.16a–e). The suprascapular nerve is identified and protected. The joint capsule is opened and the articular surfaces of the joint removed using a high speed burr. Alternatively a saw is used to produce two flat surfaces which can be apposed at an angle of 105–110°. A dynamic compression plate (DCP, Straumann Great Britain Ltd) is used for fixation. The plate is contoured to fit into the angle formed between the cranial junction of the spine and body of the scapula and then brought down over the cranial surface of the proximal humerus (Fig. 4.28b). Ideally the plate should be slid beneath the scapular nerve but most surgeons contour the plate to form a 'small bridge' over the nerve. In small cats and dogs two Kirschner wires and a tension band wire are used for fixation (Herron 1990) (see Fig. 4.28c). Arthrodesis of the shoulder carries a good prognosis. Full limb function should be regained within 3 months and there should be very little change in the animal's gait. The procedure can be done on both shoulders in dogs with bilateral congenital shoulder dislocation (8 weeks between surgeries) and again the functional end results have been excellent (Herron 1990).

FRACTURES OF THE HUMERUS

The majority of fractures of the humerus, with the exception of condylar fractures, are caused in road traffic accidents. As a general rule, humeral fractures are treated by internal fixation because it is difficult to satisfy the main criteria for using external fixation, in particular the immobilization of the joint above and below the fracture. Chest injuries, particularly pneumothorax, are common complications of humeral fractures. Other possibilities include intra-pulmonary haemorrhage, diaphragmatic rupture, rib fractures and occasionally chylothorax. A careful clinical and radiological examination should be done to check for and, if necessary, treat chest injuries before embarking on fracture fixation. Cases with closed pneumothorax or intra-pulmonary haemorrhage are an anaesthetic risk and surgery should be delayed (usually a matter of several days) until resolution occurs. During this period the dog is kept strictly confined in a kennel and the fractured humerus is immobilized with a Thomas extension splint, Velpeau dressing or a body cast. Sometimes early fracture repair must be undertaken in a dog with a pneumothorax, for example, the heavy animal with multiple limb bone fractures. Under these circumstances the pneumothorax can be relieved with a chest drain which is inserted before anaesthesia is induced.

The majority of humeral shaft fractures follow the curvature of the musculospiral groove and are spiral or oblique in nature. The radial nerve lies close to the fracture site and paralysis is a common complication. Fortunately the paralysis is invariably transient and resolves within 2−3 weeks of fracture repair. Nevertheless, the nerve should be inspected during open reduction of shaft fractures and carefully protected during insertion of implants. Fractures of the humerus can be broadly classified (Braden 1975) into three groups:

1 Fractures involving the proximal epiphysis and metaphysis.
2 Fractures of the shaft.
3 Distal humeral fractures (supracondylar, condylar and intercondylar fractures).

The approximate distribution of fractures between these three groups has been quoted as 3%, 40% and 52% (Braden 1975). Methods of repair of humeral fractures have been described (Brinker 1974; Braden 1975).

Fractures of the humeral shaft

The medullary cavity of the humerus is wide proximally and gradually decreases in size towards the supratrochlear foramen. Consequently, although fractures do occur in the proximal shaft the majority involve the distal two-thirds and in particular the distal third. Fractures of the proximal and mid-shaft regions tend to be transverse while the more distal fractures follow the curvature of the musculo-spiral groove and are spiral or oblique in nature. Many are also comminuted.

Methods of fixation

INTRAMEDULLARY PIN

Although an intramedullary pin can be used for fixation of shaft fractures of the humerus, rotational stability is usually poor because of the shape of the medullary cavity which is wide proximally and narrow distally. The method should be reserved for small breeds of dog which have transverse fractures which will impact under weight bearing. Pre-operatively, radiographs are taken of both the fractured humerus and the normal humerus. The normal is used as a guide to select a pin of the correct diameter to fit the medullary cavity as snuggly as possible. If necessary, the length of pin required can be assessed at this stage. The pin is partially transected with a hacksaw; the surgeon is then able to break it off flush with the surface of the greater tuberosity after insertion. The position of the fracture influences the length and diameter of pin required. For fractures involving the proximal or mid-shaft region, the pin is driven down the shaft to a point just proximal to the supratrochlear foramen (Fig. 4.29a). For fractures involving the distal third, a smaller diameter pin is used. The pin should be directed towards the medial side of the shaft so that the tip bypasses the supratrochlear foramen and is embedded in the medial condyle (Fig. 4.29b). A standard

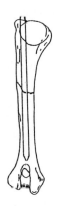
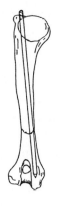
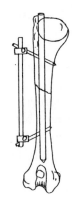

Fig. 4.29a   Fig. 4.29b   Fig. 4.29c

anterolateral approach (p. 211) is used to expose the humeral shaft and fracture site. The method of insertion of the pin is a matter of personal preference, but the author prefers retrograde pinning. The pin is driven up the shaft from the fracture site, keeping the shoulder flexed and the pin directed towards the lateral side of the greater tuberosity. Once the tip of the pin has emerged, it is grasped with the Jacob's chuck and drawn up the shaft sufficiently to permit reduction of the fracture. Reduction of the fracture is maintained with bone-holding forceps while the pin is driven into the distal shaft. When it has been inserted to the correct depth the pin is broken off flush with the bone (or cut with a saw or pin cutters). To minimize the risk of rotation and subsequent non-union, half a Kirschner device can be used to supplement the intramedullary pin (Fig. 4.29c).

PLATE FIXATION

Plate fixation is the preferred method of treatment for fractures of the humeral shaft in dogs. Ideally the plate should be placed on the anterior aspect of the bone; this is the tensile side (see p. 94). However the plate may also be placed on the lateral or medial side of the bone. Choice of site is dependent on the type of fracture and its position. Lag screws are used for the initial fixation of oblique or comminuted fractures and the position of these screws in relation to the plate must be considered in the choice of approach. Figures 4.30–4.45 illustrate some typical fractures of the humeral shaft with surgical approach and mode of fixation.

The prognosis following plate fixation of humeral shaft

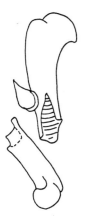

Fig. 4.30

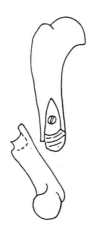

Fig. 4.31

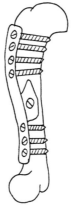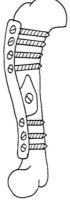

Fig. 4.32

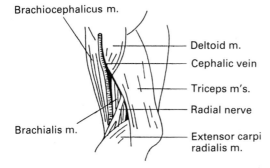

Brachiocephalicus m.

Deltoid m.

Cephalic vein

Triceps m's.

Radial nerve

Extensor carpi
radialis m.

Brachialis m.

Fig. 4.33

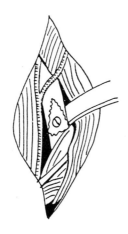

Fig. 4.34

fractures is generally good, but fracture reduction and insertion of the implants, especially in comminuted fractures is not easy. The chances of a successful outcome may be jeopardized through wound infection and osteomyelitis when operating time is prolonged. The likelihood of this complication is minimized by strict asepsis, antibiotic prophylaxis and by keeping surgery time to a minimum. The inexperienced surgeon will be wise to refer comminuted shaft fractures of the humerus to a specialist for treatment.

A COMMINUTED MID-SHIFT FRACTURE OF
THE HUMERUS

A lateral view is shown in Fig. 4.30. Figure 4.31 shows how the butterfly fragment is reduced and fixation achieved with a lag screw; finally (Fig. 4.32) the plate is contoured and applied to the anterior aspect of the humerus.

An anterolateral approach is used to expose this fracture. A skin incision is made from the greater tuberosity to the lateral condyle. The cephalic vein is identified. The brachiocephalicus and brachialis muscles are separated and retracted to expose the shaft of the humerus (Fig. 4.33). The radial nerve is easily identified by separating the brachialis from the lateral head of the triceps. The nerve can then be traced distally as it runs around the brachialis to emerge on its lateral aspect at the level of the extensor carpi radialis muscle (Fig. 4.33).

In exposure of the distal anterior surface of the shaft the brachialis is retracted caudally and used to protect the radial nerve (Fig. 4.34). The proximal surface of the humerus is exposed by subperiosteal elevation between the pectoral and deltoid muscles.

A COMMINUTED FRACTURE INVOLVING THE
DISTAL THIRD OF THE HUMERUS

A lateral view of the fracture appears in Fig. 4.35. In Fig. 4.36 the butterfly fragment has been reduced and fixation achieved with two lag screws. Figures 4.37 and 4.38 show how the plate is contoured and applied to the lateral aspect of the humerus (∗ indicates lag screws).

The anterolateral approach is used to expose the fracture (Figs 4.33 and 4.34). In addition, the brachialis muscle and radial nerve are mobilized so that the plate can be slid beneath them on the lateral aspect of the humerus (Fig. 4.39). The origin of the extensor carpi radialis muscle is freed from the lateral condyle to complete exposure of the distal humerus.

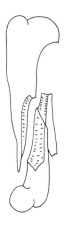

Fig. 4.35

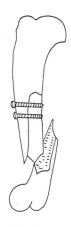

Fig. 4.36

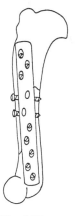

Fig. 4.37

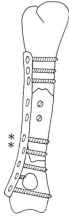

Fig. 4.38

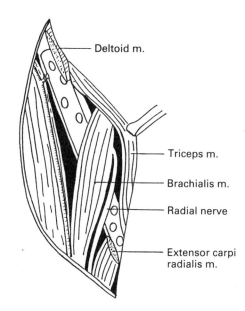

Deltoid m.

Triceps m.

Brachialis m.

Radial nerve

Extensor carpi radialis m.

Fig. 4.39

AN OBLIQUE FRACTURE OF THE DISTAL THIRD OF THE HUMERUS

A lateral view of the fracture is shown in Fig. 4.40. Initial fixation is by interfragmentary compression using two lag screws (Fig. 4.41). Then the plate is contoured and applied to the medial side of the humerus (Figs 4.42 and 4.43).

A skin incision is made over the medial aspect of the humerus. The median nerve and the biceps muscle are retracted cranially and the ulnar nerve and medial head of the triceps caudally to expose the humeral shaft. Branches of the brachial artery and vein run with the nerves and should be protected. The medial side of the humerus is

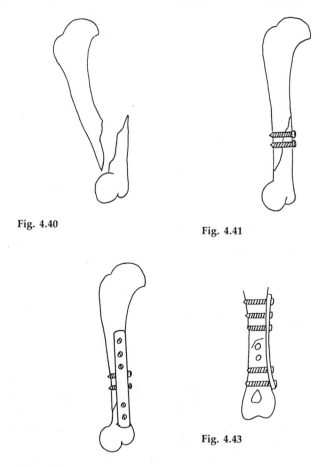

Fig. 4.40

Fig. 4.41

Fig. 4.43

Fig. 4.42

relatively flat and is an ideal surface for the application of a plate. However, exposure of the humerus is limited proximally by the pectoral muscles and the brachial blood vessels.

SUPRACONDYLAR FRACTURES OF THE HUMERUS
In supracondylar fractures, the fracture line passes through the supratrochlear foramen. The fractures tend to be transverse or oblique in nature and some are also comminuted. In immature dogs, the fracture may take the form of a Salter Type II epiphyseal separation.

Supracondylar fractures must be accurately reduced and rigidly stabilized because of their proximity to the elbow joint.

A medial approach is used to expose the fracture (see p. 213). There are several ways of stabilizing the fracture. One of the simplest (Brinker 1974) is to use an intramedullary pin (retrograde introduction, p. 209) which is driven down the shaft into the medial condyle. Rotation is

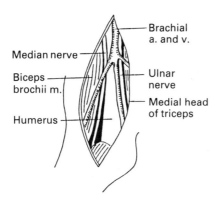

Fig. 4.44

prevented with a Kirschner wire placed obliquely across the fracture site from the lateral condyle (Fig. 4.45).

Rush pins introduced through each of the humeral condyles into the humeral shaft (Fig. 4.46) also provide a satisfactory method of treating supracondylar fractures.

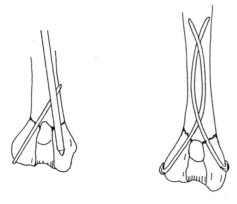

Fig. 4.45

Fig. 4.46

At this clinic three other methods are frequently used. In oblique supracondylar fractures or oblique fractures extending through the distal humeral growth plate, two lag screws are used for fixation (Fig. 4.47). The first screw is placed transversely just proximal to the supratrochlear foramen and the second screw is driven up through the medial condyle. In immature dogs the screws are removed as soon as healing is complete (approximately 4 weeks) to prevent premature closure of the growth plate.

In large dogs, especially those with comminuted supracondylar fractures, a plate is applied to the medial side of the humerus. For adequate stability two screws should be placed in the distal fragment (Fig. 4.48). Braden (1975)

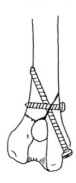

Fig. 4.47

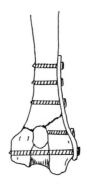

Fig. 4.48

recommends a caudal approach for comminuted supra-condylar fractures in large dogs (see p. 224) with the application of two plates on the posterior aspect of the supratrochlear ridges. This method of fixation is described in more detail under the management of 'T' and 'Y' fractures of the humerus (see p. 224).

Humeral fractures in the cat

The shape of the humerus is similar in the cat and dog, however in the cat the medullary cavity has a more uniform diameter and the diaphysis is straighter. Consequently the majority of shaft fractures in the cat can be treated satisfactorily by the use of an intramedullary pin (Chapter 2). In oblique or comminuted fractures additional fixation can be provided using cerclage wires or by the addition of an external fixator. In the management of distal humeral fractures, it should be remembered that the medial epicondyle in the cat possesses an epicondyloid fossa through which the ulnar nerve passes. The principles of treating fractures in this region are the same as in the dog, although Kirschner wires rather than a plate tend to be used to attach the humeral condyles to the shaft in cats.

Condylar fractures of the humerus

The management of condylar fractures described here is based on a series of 133 cases treated by the author (Denny 1983). There are areas of structural weakness in the distal humerus which predispose to certain types of fracture (Shuttleworth 1938; Walker & Hickman 1958). The humeral trochlea (Fig. 4.49) is separated from the shaft by the supra-trochlear foramen. Main support for the trochlea is provided by the medial epicondyle which is in effect a direct extension of the humeral shaft. Laterally, the trochlea is supported by

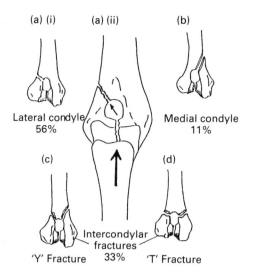

(a) (i)   (a) (ii)   (b)

Lateral condyle   Medial condyle
56%   11%

(c)   (d)

Intercondylar
fractures
'Y' Fracture   33%   'T' Fracture

Fig. 4.49

the lateral epicondyle but this is a far weaker structure than its medial counterpart. Condylar fractures usually result from a violent upward stress transmitted through the head of the radius onto the humeral trochlea, for example, when a dog falls or jumps from a height, taking excessive weight on the leg (Walker & Hickman 1958). It comes as no surprise that the lateral condyle which has the weakest attachments to the humeral shaft fractures most frequently (56% of cases). In the face of even greater stress, the medial condyle is also sheared from its attachments to the main shaft, giving rise to the intercondylar ('Y' or 'T') fracture (Figs 4.49c and d). Intercondylar fractures occurred in 33% of cases; the fracture is referred to as a 'Y' fracture (Fig. 4.49c) if the supracondylar ridges are fractured obliquely, and a 'T' fracture if the ridges are fractured transversely. Solitary fractures of the medial condyle occur in 11% of cases.

Condylar fractures, as with any intra-articular fracture, require accurate anatomical reduction and rigid internal fixation to promote primary bone union if normal joint function is to be restored. Basic methods of fixation were described by Knight (1956, 1959) and Walker & Hickman (1958); a variety of techniques were subsequently proposed (Brinker 1974) and these have been reviewed by Braden (1975) and more recently by Payne-Johnson & Lewis (1981) and Denny (1983).

FRACTURE OF THE LATERAL CONDYLE
The commonest cause of fracture of the lateral condyle is a

fall. The fracture occurs most often in dogs under a year of age (67% of cases) and the peak age incidence is at 4 months. The fracture is stabilized with a single lag screw driven through the lateral condyle into the medial condyle (Figs 4.54b and c). Failure to treat the fracture surgically results in medial luxation of the medial condyle, because lateral support for the joint is lost. Malunion or non-union of the lateral condyle causes permanent joint deformity (Figs 4.50a and b). The range of elbow movement remains limited and varying degrees of lameness persist. The prognosis is obviously better in immature dogs because of their ability to remodel the distal humerus following fracture.

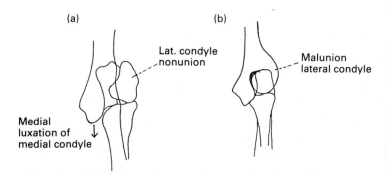

(a)   (b)

Lat. condyle
nonunion

Malunion
lateral condyle

Medial
luxation of
medial condyle

Fig. 4.50

Lag screw fixation (Brinker 1974)

If the fracture of the lateral condyle is less than 12 hours old, there is usually little swelling and the unstable condyle can be easily palpated. Having prepared the leg for surgery the most prominent point of the lateral and medial condyle is grasped between finger and thumb and pressure is exerted while the elbow is extended; initially crepitus may be felt but if reduction is successful the lateral condyle will be felt to slip or click back into its normal position where it is maintained by thumb pressure. The elbow is maintained in the extended position and a condyle clamp (Fig. 4.51) is carefully slid into position. The holes of the clamp fit over the most prominent points of the condyles and the clamp is tightened to maintain reduction. A check X-ray is taken; if reduction is satisfactory the leg is reprepared for surgery and a transcondylar lag screw inserted through a stab incision made over the lateral condyle (details of correct positioning of the screw hole are given below).

If the fracture is more than 24 hours old considerable

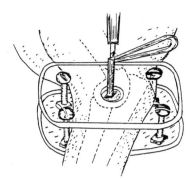

Fig. 4.51 Condyle clamp (constructed from two sheets of perspex plus four bolts), used to maintain reduction of a fractured lateral condyle. This allows a transcondylar lag screw to be inserted through a stab incision.

soft tissue swelling will have occurred and accurate closed reduction may be difficult as a result. Under these circumstances open reduction should be performed. A skin incision is made directly over the lateral condyle (Fig. 4.52a). The lateral head of the triceps muscle is exposed and the deep fascia along its anterior border incised (Fig. 4.52b). The muscle is retracted to expose the condyle (Fig. 4.52c). The radial nerve emerges between the lateral head of the triceps and the brachialis just proximal to the incision, but provided dissection is limited to the soft tissues directly over the

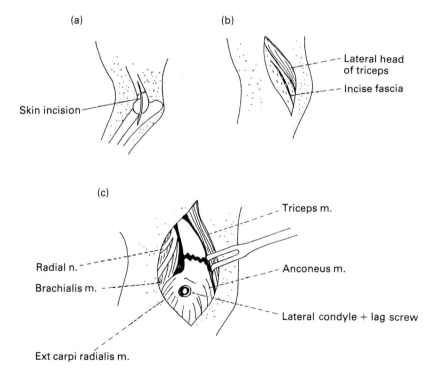

(a)

Skin incision

(b)

Lateral head of triceps

Incise fascia

(c)

Triceps m.

Radial n.

Brachialis m.

Anconeus m.

Lateral condyle + lag screw

Ext carpi radialis m.

Fig. 4.52

lateral condyle and its supracondylar ridge there should be little risk of nerve damage during exposure. Haematoma or granulation tissue is removed from the intercondylar fracture site, the adjacent surfaces of the fractured supracondylar ridge are cleaned of all soft tissue and reduction of the condyle can then be readily achieved by manipulation. If the fracture of the supracondylar ridge is accurately reduced it can be assumed that reduction of the intercondylar fracture site is also adequate. Temporary fixation is achieved with a transcondylar Kirschner wire (Fig. 4.53a). The wire is removed after insertion of the lag screw.

Alternatively, reduction can be maintained in the following ways:

1 By the application of Vulsellum forceps or ASIF reduction forceps to the condyles (Fig. 4.53b).

2 In small dogs the fractured supracondylar ridge can be stabilized with Allis tissue forceps (Fig. 4.53c).

3 In large dogs a Kirschner wire can be placed across the fractured supracondylar ridge.

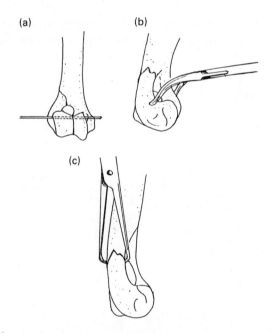

(a) (b)

(c)

Fig. 4.53

The drill hole for the transcondylar lag screw is commenced immediately below and just in front of the most prominent point of the lateral condyle and directed to emerge at the corresponding spot on the medial condyle (Fig. 4.54a). If a cancellous screw is used for fixation, the threaded portion of the screw must grip entirely in the medial condyle (Fig. 4.54b(ii)). If a cortex screw is used then the hole in the lateral condyle must be overdrilled to the same diameter as the screw to ensure that the lag effect is achieved as the screw is tightened giving compression of the fracture site (Fig. 4.54b(i)).

Lateral condylar fractures, provided they are adequately reduced and stabilized, carry a good prognosis and the screw can be left *in situ*. The average recovery period is 4 weeks (range 2–8 weeks). Seventy-seven per cent of dogs regain full limb function and 23% have slight or occasional lameness (Denny 1983).

Management of non-union fractures of the lateral humeral condyle

Non-union fractures of the lateral humeral condyle tend to be seen in mature dogs. The usual causes are:
1 Failure to treat the fracture by internal fixation.
2 Failure to provide adequate internal fixation.
3 Failure to control exercise during fracture healing.
4 Occasionally infection is the cause of non-union.

Lateral condylar fractures should be stabilized with a transcondylar lag screw used in conjunction with a Kirschner to prevent rotation of the fragment. If a lag screw is used alone, the condylar fragment may rotate on the screw and the screw may loosen or fracture before bone union occurs. Dogs treated in this way may have reasonable limb function for several weeks following surgery. Lameness then becomes worse with pain and

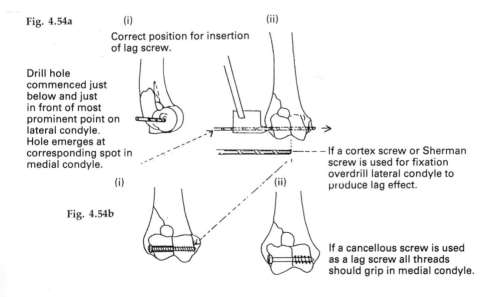

Fig. 4.54a

(i) (ii)

Correct position for insertion of lag screw.

Drill hole commenced just below and just in front of most prominent point on lateral condyle. Hole emerges at corresponding spot in medial condyle.

If a cortex screw or Sherman screw is used for fixation overdrill lateral condyle to produce lag effect.

(i) (ii)

Fig. 4.54b

If a cancellous screw is used as a lag screw all threads should grip in medial condyle.

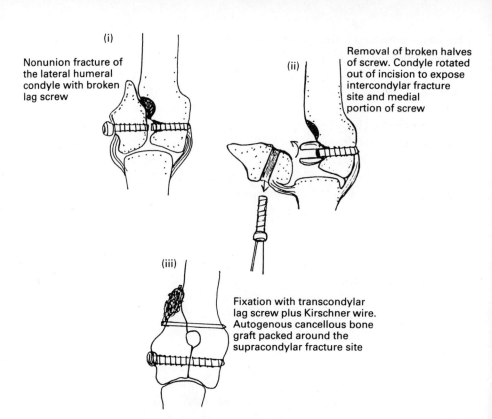

(i) Nonunion fracture of the lateral humeral condyle with broken lag screw

(ii) Removal of broken halves of screw. Condyle rotated out of incision to expose intercondylar fracture site and medial portion of screw

(iii) Fixation with transcondylar lag screw plus Kirschner wire. Autogenous cancellous bone graft packed around the supracondylar fracture site

Fig. 4.54c

crepitus evident on palpation of the elbow. Radiographs (Fig. 4.54c(ii)) show non-union of the condylar fragment and often bone lysis around the screw indicating movement or low-grade infection. In some cases the screw starts to 'back out' of the bone. Fracture of the screw is seen in chronic non-unions (Fig. 4.54c(i)).

Treatment options
1 If the screw is loose it is either replaced by a larger diameter screw or redirected into the medial condyle. A transcondylar Kirschner wire should also be placed to prevent rotation.
2 If the screw has broken then an attempt should be made to remove the broken halves. Removal of the lateral condylar half of the screw should present no problem but retrieval of the tip of the screw from the medial condyle can be awkward. If the tip of the screw is protruding into the soft tissues on the medial side of the medial condyle then a small stab incision is made over it, the tip of the screw is grasped with rongeurs or orthopaedic pliers and the broken end of the screw gradually twisted out of the bone. If this

is not possible because all the screw threads are buried in the medial condyle then a lateral approach is used to remove both halves of the screw. Once the shank of the screw has been removed, the lateral condyle is freed from its dorsal soft tissue attachments and rotated out of the incision to allow inspection of the lateral fracture surface of the medial condyle, from which a few threads of broken screw usually protrude. The broken end of the screw is grasped with rongeurs and removed (Fig. 4.54c(iii)). Once the broken screw has been removed from the lateral condyle, the intercondylar fracture surfaces are 'freshened up' then reduced and fixation achieved with another transcondylar lag screw and Kirschner wire.

In long-standing lateral condylar non-union fractures associated with displacement it is preferable to use the transolecranon approach to the elbow (see 'Y' fractures, p. 224) to permit accurate reduction of the fracture. Often much fibro-cartilaginous callus and perhaps broken implants must be removed before reduction can be achieved. Cancellous bone taken from the proximal humerus and packed around the supracondylar fracture site will speed up fracture healing (Fig. 4.54c(iii)).

FRACTURES OF THE MEDIAL CONDYLE
The commonest cause of fracture of the medial condyle is a fall and there is no specific age incidence for the injury. The same principles of treatment apply as for lateral condylar fractures, however the medial condylar fragment is often large enough to accept two lag screws, one transcondylar and one placed proximal to the supratrochlear foramen (Fig. 4.54d, e). Exposure of the medial condyle is described on p. 215. Medial condylar fractures carry a similar prognosis to fractures of the lateral condyle.

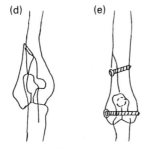

Fig. 4.54d−e Tracing pre- and post-operative radiography of a pointer with a fracture of the medial condyle.

INTERCONDYLAR FRACTURES OF THE HUMERUS

Intercondylar 'Y' or 'T' fractures are caused by falls or road traffic accidents in most cases. There is no specific age incidence. Treatment of these fractures is difficult and can present a real challenge even to the most experienced of orthopaedic surgeons. To permit adequate exposure and accurate anatomical reduction of the fracture a caudal approach to the elbow is recommended (Fig. 4.55a–c). The dog is placed in dorsal recumbency for surgery with the affected leg pulled forward. A skin incision is made over the caudolateral aspect of the elbow, the subcutaneous fat and fascia are incised and undermined to allow reflection of skin from both sides of the elbow. Fascia along the cranial border of the medial head of the triceps is incised and the ulna nerve is identified and retracted (Fig. 4.55b) from the olecranon. The anterior margin of the lateral head of the triceps is also freed from fascial attachments. Transverse osteotomy of the olecranon is performed with an oscillating saw, or hack saw, distal to the tendon of insertion of the triceps on the olecranon and proximal to the anconeal process (Fig. 4.55b). (After repair of the intercondylar frac-

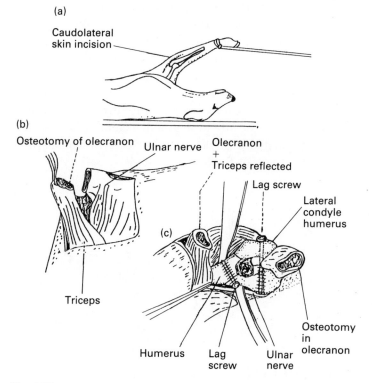

(a)

Caudolateral skin incision

(b)

Osteotomy of olecranon   Ulnar nerve   Olecranon + Triceps reflected

Lag screw

Lateral condyle humerus

(c)

Triceps

Osteotomy in olecranon

Humerus   Lag screw   Ulnar nerve

Fig. 4.55

ture the olecranon is reattached using Kirschner wires or a screw in combination with a wire tension band (see Fig. 4.77). If a screw is used the screw hole should be prepared before the osteotomy of the olecranon is performed.)

The olecranon is reflected with the attached triceps muscle mass and remnants of the anconeus muscle are reflected as necessary to complete exposure (Fig. 4.55c) of the entire caudal surface of the elbow joint. The condyles are reduced first. The easiest way of doing this is to reduce the proximal ends of the condyles and fix them with a Kirschner wire in a 'T' fracture or lag screw in a 'Y' fracture (Fig. 4.56b). Then complete reduction of the articular surface of the condyles and insert a transcondylar lag screw (Fig. 4.56c). Generally the screw is inserted from lateral to medial. The humeral condyles are attached to the shaft of the humerus with a Kirschner wire or lag screw (Fig. 4.56d), then a plate is applied to the posterior aspect of the medial supracondylar ridge (Fig. 4.56e). In large dogs a second smaller plate can be applied to the lateral supracondylar ridge (Braden 1975).

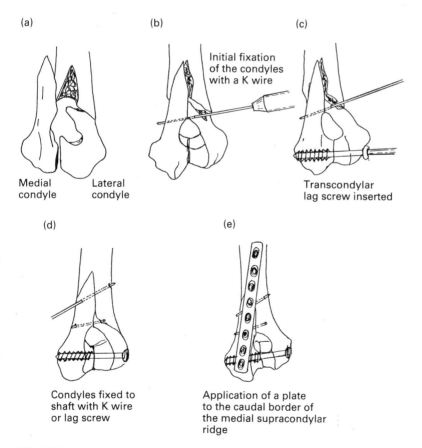

(a)

Medial   Lateral
condyle   condyle

(b)

Initial fixation
of the condyles
with a K wire

(c)

Transcondylar
lag screw inserted

(d)

Condyles fixed to
shaft with K wire
or lag screw

(e)

Application of a plate
to the caudal border of
the medial supracondylar
ridge

Fig. 4.56

The olecranon osteotomy is repaired as described above and subsequent wound closure is routine. A Robert Jones bandage is applied for a week post-operatively to provide support and control post-operative swelling.

Intercondylar fractures carry a moderate prognosis: 46% of dogs regain normal limb function, 36% have slight or occasional lameness and 18% have moderate to severe lameness as a result of deformity and osteoarthritis (Denny 1983). In another series of intercondylar fractures (20 cases) reviewed by Anderson *et al.* (1990), 64% of cases had a satisfactory outcome following internal fixation.

THE ELBOW

Anatomy (Figs 4.57 and 4.58)
The elbow is a composite joint in which the humeral condyles articulate with the head of the radius, the humero-radial joint, and also with the semilunar notch of the ulna, the humero-ulnar joint. The humero-radial joint transmits most of the weight-bearing load on the elbow while the humero-ulnar part maintains joint stability in the sagittal plane. The elbow is a ginglymus joint capable of flexion and extension only. Strong collateral ligaments and the anconeal process which fits deep into the olecranon fossa of the humerus prevent lateral movement of the elbow.

Soft tissue structures of surgical importance are illustrated in Figs 4.58a and b, while the normal radiographic anatomy of the elbow in the immature dog is shown in Fig. 4.59a.

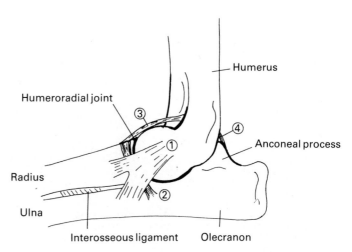

Fig. 4.57a Lateral aspect of the left elbow: (1) lateral collateral ligament; (2) annular ligament; (3) oblique ligament; (4) olecranon ligament.

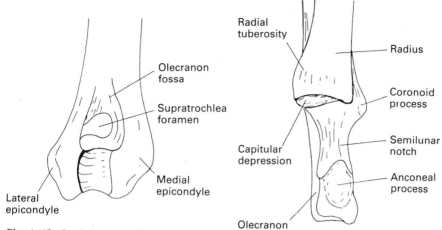

Fig. 4.57b Caudal aspect of left humerus.

Fig. 4.57c Cranial aspect of left radius and ulna.

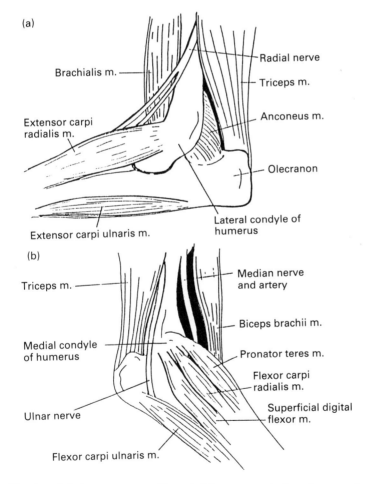

Fig. 4.58 Soft tissue structures of surgical importance, (a) lateral aspect of left elbow; (b) medial aspect of left elbow.

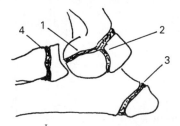

Fig. 4.59a Ten-week-old
Rhodesian Ridgeback puppy.
Lateral radiograph of normal
elbow: (1) growth plate of medial
condyle; (2) growth plate of
medial epicondyle; (3) proximal
ulnar growth plate; (4) proximal
radial growth plate.

The growth plates of the distal humerus, proximal radius
and proximal ulna all close at approximately 7 months
(range 5–8 months) (Sumner-Smith 1966).

Developmental conditions of the elbow (Fig. 4.59b)
include:

1 Osteochondritis dissecans (Olsson 1975; Denny & Gibbs
1980).

2 Ununited medial coronoid process (Olsson 1975; Denny
& Gibbs 1980).

3 Ununited anconeal process (Van Sickle 1966; Grøndalen
& Rørvick 1980).

4 Ununited medial epicondyle (Vaughan 1979; Denny 1983).

5 Congenital dislocation (Campbell 1979).

6 Subluxation secondary to growth disturbances of the
radius and ulna caused by:

(a) Premature closure of the distal ulnar growth plate
(O'Brien *et al.* 1971; Vaughan 1976).

(b) Premature closure of the distal radial growth plate
(Clayton-Jones & Vaughan 1970; Barr & Denny 1985).

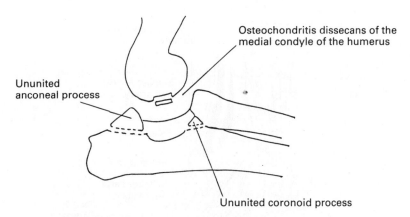

Osteochondritis dissecans of the
medial condyle of the humerus

Ununited
anconeal process

Ununited coronoid process

Fig. 4.59b

Osteochondritis dissecans (OCD), ununited medial coronoid process (UCP) and ununited anconeal process (UAP)

These can all be classed as osteochondritic-type lesions of

the elbow. These conditions result from abnormal endo-chondral ossification of either the articular cartilage in OCD, or of growth plate cartilage in UCP and UAP (Olsson 1975). All three conditions cause chronic lameness in immature dogs; and though the clinical features of each are similar, different breeds are affected by them. Ununited anconeal process is seen most frequently in German Shepherds and in Basset Hounds, while OCD and UCP are seen mainly in Retrievers, Labradors and Rottweilers. In fact both OCD and UCP lesions may be found in the same joint.

All three conditions cause a gradual onset of lameness at 4–5 months of age. Lameness tends to be intermittent in nature and is often most obvious after exercise or when the dog gets up from rest. There is pain on extension of the elbow, and in both OCD and UCP, the degree of pain is increased by supinating the forearm during elbow extension.

The lesions cause osteo-arthrosis; there is increased synovial fluid production which is most obvious in the dog with UAP because a fluctuating swelling develops just caudal to the humeral condyles. The elbow becomes thickened, crepitus may be appreciated and the range of joint flexion decreases as the arthrosis proceeds.

UNUNITED ANCONEAL PROCESS (Van Sickle 1966; Ljunggren *et al.* 1966; Bradney 1967; Corley *et al.* 1968; Hanlon 1969)

Ununited anconeal process is a well-recognized problem in the German Shepherd and the Basset Hound. The condition occasionally occurs in other large breeds. In affected animals the anconeal process develops as a separate ossification centre. The process should unite with the ulna by the time the dog is 5 months old. Non-union results in elbow instability and osteo-arthrosis.

Affected animals present with a gradual onset of lameness at 4 to 5 months of age. There is pain on palpation of the elbow, particularly when it is forcibly extended. There may be obvious crepitus and in long-standing cases, the elbow becomes thickened and the range of joint movement is limited due to osteo-arthrosis. A flexed lateral radiograph of the elbow will confirm the diagnosis (Fig. 4.60). The condition is bilateral in 40% of cases, consequently both elbows should be radiographed.

Treatment is by surgical excision of the anconeal process. A skin incision is made along the posterolateral border of

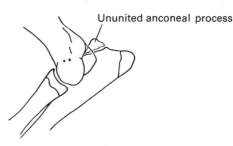

Ununited anconeal process

Fig. 4.60

the humerus (Fig. 4.61). The cranial edge of the lateral head of the triceps is retracted caudally to expose the anconeus muscle. The anconeus muscle together with the joint capsule to which it is closely attached are incised just caudal to the lateral condyle (leaving sufficient muscle on the condylar side to be sutured). Haemorrhage from the muscle may be a problem but this can be controlled by using self-retaining retractors to retract the muscle edges and expose the caudal aspect of the elbow joint. The elbow is flexed to reveal the anconeal process which is prised away from its cartilaginous attachments to the ulna with a periosteal elevator. After removal of the process, the joint is flushed out with normal saline and the anconeus muscle and joint capsule closed together with a continuous vicryl suture. Subsequent wound closure is routine. A support bandage is applied for a week post-operatively and exercise is restricted for 4 weeks. If the lesion is bilateral, a 6-week interval is left between operations.

The anconeal process normally contributes to the stability of the elbow joint. Instability after removal may predispose the dog to intermittent elbow sprains and osteoarthrosis.

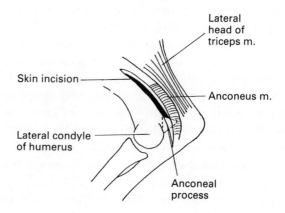

Lateral head of triceps m.

Skin incision

Anconeus m.

Lateral condyle of humerus

Anconeal process

Fig. 4.61

Grøndalen & Rørvick (1980), in a follow up of 37 dogs treated for ununited anconeal process, reported that 39% of the cases were occasionally lame after exercise or were stiff after rest.

It might be expected that the dislocation of the elbow is more likely to occur after removal of the anconeal process. This does not occur, presumably because scar formation after surgery provides sufficient stability.

Dogs with ununited anconeal process may reach maturity without serious lameness problems. They may then present in later life with a sudden onset of lameness. The elbow is painful and radiographs demonstrate advanced osteo-arthrosis and an ununited anconeal process. What should be done in this situation? The osteo-arthrosis has usually been aggravated by an elbow sprain and lameness should resolve with rest and the administration of non-steroidal anti-inflammatory drugs. Surgical removal of the anconeus should only be considered at this late stage if lameness shows no sign of resolving or should the process have become displaced.

OSTEOCHONDRITIS DISSECANS OF THE MEDIAL CONDYLE OF THE HUMERUS (Olsson 1975; Wood *et al.* 1975; McCurnin *et al.* 1976; Leighton 1978; Denny & Gibbs 1980)

Osteochondritis dissecans of the medial condyle of the humerus is a common cause of elbow lameness in the Labrador, Golden Retriever and Rottweiler. There is a gradual onset of lameness at 4–5 months of age. Lameness tends to be intermittent in nature and is often most obvious either when the dog gets up from resting or after exercise. There is pain on forced extension of the elbow and the degree of pain can be increased by supinating the forearm during extension. Elbow thickening may be appreciated, especially in chronic cases, and the range of elbow flexion becomes reduced.

Radiographic diagnosis is not easy in the early stages. A flexed lateral view and a craniocaudal view should be taken of both elbows. Osteochondritis dissecans rapidly causes osteo-arthrosis in the elbow. The first indication of this is osteophyte formation on the caudal aspect of the anconeal process (Fig. 4.62a), giving it a 'fuzzy' appearance. Later similar changes develop on the medial aspect of the elbow (Fig. 4.62b) and on the head of the radius (Fig. 4.62a). The craniocaudal view of the elbow may demonstrate the OCD lesion as a small erosion in the subchondral bone of the

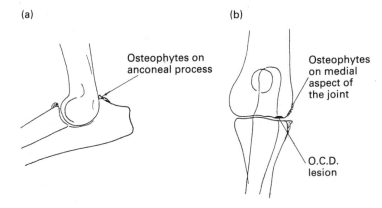

(a)

Osteophytes on
anconeal process

(b)

Osteophytes
on medial
aspect of
the joint

O.C.D.
lesion

Fig. 4.62

medial condyle of the humerus (Fig. 4.62a). However, this feature cannot be demonstrated in every case of osteochondritis dissecans.

Surgical treatment should be undertaken early to prevent the development of osteo-arthrosis. There is little to be gained by surgery once joint changes have become advanced. However if radiographs demonstrate the presence of any loose bodies (joint mice) then surgical removal of these fragments will help reduce the frequency or severity of lameness in chronic OCD cases.

UNUNITED MEDIAL CORONOID PROCESS
(Olsson 1975; McCurnin *et al.* 1976; Denny & Gibbs 1980)
Failure of the coronoid process to unite with the ulna is an osteochondritic-type lesion of the elbow. The condition affects the Labrador, Golden Retriever and Rottweiler and occasionally dogs have both OCD and ununited coronoid process in the same joint. The history and clinical signs associated with ununited coronoid process are identical to osteochondritis dissecans. Ununited coronoid process also causes the rapid development of osteoarthrosis with a similar distribution of osteophytes as described under OCD. A craniocaudal or oblique craniocaudal view of the elbow may demonstrate the ununited coronoid process (Fig. 4.63) but even in positive cases the radiographic findings may not be conclusive. Nevertheless, if a Labrador, Retriever or Rottweiler under a year of age is presented with chronic foreleg lameness, pain can be localized to the elbow and there is radiographic evidence of osteo-arthrosis, then an exploratory medial arthrotomy is justified. The medial approach gives access to both OCD lesions and ununited coronoid process.

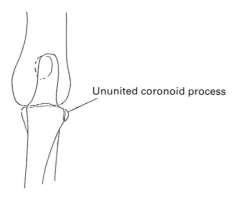

Ununited coronoid process

Fig. 4.63

Elbow—medial arthrotomy technique

After routine surgical preparation, the dog is placed on its side and a bolster is placed beneath the elbow (Fig. 4.64a). A skin incision is made over the medial humeral condyle (Fig. 4.64a). The pronator teres and flexor carpi radialis muscles are separated close to their origin on the medial epicondyle and retracted with a West's retractor (Arnolds Vet. Products Ltd). A vertical incision is made in the joint capsule over the humeral condyle only (Fig. 4.64b). The blades of a pair of straight scissors are then introduced between the articular surfaces of the joint and spread laterally to complete exposure (Fig. 4.64c). The West's retractor is repositioned to include the cut edges of the joint capsule. This method of arthrotomy minimizes the risk of damage to the median nerve and artery which cross the anterior and distal margins of the joint. The articular surfaces are separated with the aid of Hohmann retractors and exposure is improved with the aid of an assistant who exerts pressure on the forearm and 'hinges' the elbow open over the bolster (Fig. 4.64d).

The medial condyle of the humerus (Fig. 4.64d) is inspected for an osteochondritis dissecans lesion. If a cartilaginous flap is present, it is removed and the underlying erosion in the subchondral bone is curetted. In some cases the lesion takes the form of fissures in the cartilage; this area is curetted. If there is no evidence of osteochondritis dissecans the coronoid process is inspected, freed from any remaining cartilaginous or fibrous attachments and removed. The coronoid process will be found either as a discrete triangular fragment of bone and cartilage or it may be in the form of two or three fragments. The coronoid process lies immediately beneath the medial collateral liga-

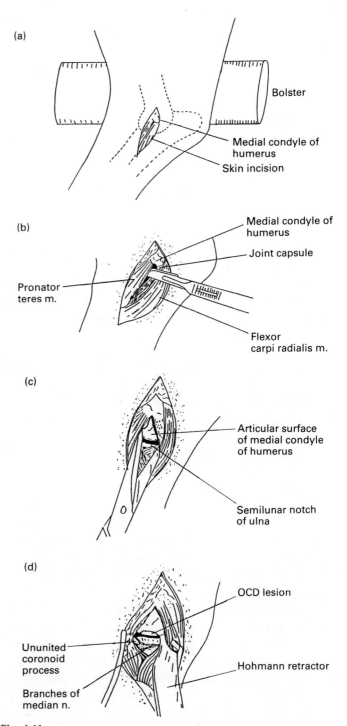

(a)

Bolster

Medial condyle of
humerus

Skin incision

(b)

Medial condyle of
humerus

Joint capsule

Pronator
teres m.

Flexor
carpi radialis m.

(c)

Articular surface
of medial condyle
of humerus

Semilunar notch
of ulna

(d)

OCD lesion

Ununited
coronoid
process

Branches of
median n.

Hohmann retractor

Fig. 4.64

ment and exposure can be improved by cutting the caudal margin of the collateral ligament, however complete section of the ligament should not be necessary.

Osteochondritis dissecans and ununited coronoid process have the same aetiology (Olsson 1975) and consequently it is wise to inspect the coronoid process even when there is an obvious osteochondritis dissecans lesion present as both conditions can co-exist. After the lesion has been dealt with, the joint is flushed out with saline. The muscle bellies are coapted with a continuous suture of vicryl which effectively seals the joint capsule. The rest of the wound closure is carried out in routine fashion.

Complications Osteo-arthrosis present at the time of surgery or secondary to surgical interference may lead to poor exercise tolerance with varying degrees of lameness and a limited range of elbow movement.

Surgical exposure of the osteochondritis dissecans lesion or ununited coronoid process in the elbow can be difficult for the inexperienced surgeon and failure to identify and treat either lesion will result in progressive osteo-arthrosis.

Post-operative care and results The elbow is supported with a bandage for 1 week. Antibiotic cover is given for 5 days and skin sutures are removed at 10 days. Exercise is restricted for 6 weeks and then gradually increased. In dogs with bilateral lesions, a 6-week interval is left between operations. Normal limb function is generally regained within 2 months of surgery and the initial follow-up work (Denny & Gibbs 1980) revealed little increase in the degree of osteo-arthrosis present at the time of surgery and some 70% of surgically treated cases were sound on follow-up. However subsequent follow-up work and radiographic examination of both conservatively and surgically treated cases (Houlton 1984) provides a bleaker outlook for dogs with elbow osteochondrosis caused by OCD, ununited coronoid process or both. Only 68% of dogs were sound at follow up and the results of both conservative and surgical treatment were said to be disappointing in this series. The surgically treated elbows were more likely to have a reduced range of joint movement associated with joint thickening compared with conservatively treated cases. Although surgical treatment of the painful elbow resulted in a considerable improvement in limb function, the degenerative changes were not halted and a significant degree of osteo-arthrosis occurred. Houlton indicated that surgery should be reserved for treatment of the persistently painful elbow and the non-painful joint should be treated conservatively. Read *et al.* (1990) also published the results of treatment in 130 cases of fragmentation of the medial coronoid process. Sixty-eight cases were treated surgically by medial arthrotomy and 62 were treated conservatively (rest and anti-inflammatories). There was no difference between the two groups in the incidence of lameness following treatment. Surgical treatment did not decrease the incidence of post-treatment lameness, but the surgically treated dogs were more active and less severely lame than the conservatively treated group. It was concluded that young dogs with mild lameness due to fragmented coronoid process in the elbow probably do not benefit from surgical treatment but dogs with chronic, moderate to severe lameness have a better prognosis if treated surgically.

Elbow osteochondrosis (ununited coronoid process and osteochondritis dissecans) has been shown to have a high degree of heritability within a population of dogs owned by the Guide Dogs for the Blind Association (Guthrie & Pidduck 1990). They recommended the following guidelines to reduce the incidence of the condition:

1 Never breed from affected individuals.
2 Do not breed again from the sires and dams of affected individuals, that is either by repeating the same mating or putting them to different partners.
3 Do not breed from the siblings of affected individuals.
4 Do not breed from any offspring of affected individuals.

Ununited medial epicondyle (Vaughan 1979; Denny 1983) The distal humerus develops from three centres of ossification: one for the lateral condyle, one for the medial condyle, and one for the medial epicondyle (Fig. 4.59a) (Hare 1961). The medial epicondyle is the point of origin of several carpal and digital flexor muscles; this epiphysis normally fuses with the distal humeral epiphysis and metaphysis by 6 months.

Failure of the medial epicondyle to unite with the humerus is occasionally encountered as a fusion defect in immature Labradors. History and clinical signs are similar to osteochondritis dissecans of the elbow. Radiographic examination shows the ununited epicondyle as a discrete fragment on the medial side of the elbow (Fig. 4.65a). There are numerous muscle attachments to the fragment. If it is large, then it should be reattached to the humerus with a lag screw (Fig. 4.65b). If the fragment is small, lameness

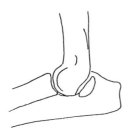

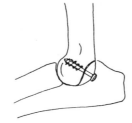

Fig. 4.65a   Fig. 4.65b

will generally resolve by the time the dog reaches 1 year of age provided exercise is restricted.

Congenital dislocation of the elbow (Campbell 1979)
Congenital dislocation of the elbow is uncommon — two types of deformity are recognized:
1 Lateral rotation of the ulna. This condition has been recorded in the Sheltie, Pekingese, Cocker Spaniel, Yorkshire Terrier, Boston Terrier, Miniature Poodle and Miniature Pinscher. Elbow deformity is recognized at or within a few weeks of birth. The olecranon can be palpated lying lateral to the distal humerus and the elbow cannot be fully extended. A lateral radiograph of the elbow will show the radial head in the normal position but the olecranon lying lateral to the humerus (Fig. 4.65c). If the olecranon can be manipulated and rotated back into its normal position, then the joint can be stabilized with a transarticular pin (Fig. 4.65d). The pin is removed after 4 weeks. Campbell (1979) reported good limb function in three out of four dogs treated in this way.
2 Caudolateral luxation of the radial head. Although lateral luxation occurs most frequently in the smaller breeds of dog like the Pekingese, Yorkshire Terrier and Pomeranian,

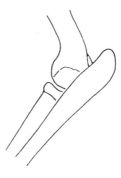

Fig. 4.65c Congenital dislocation of the elbow with lateral rotation of the ulna.

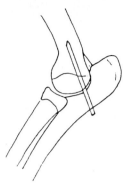

Fig. 4.65d Reduction and fixation with a transarticular pin.

it has also been recorded in larger breeds such as the Staffordshire Bull Terrier, Bulldog, Mastiff and Labrador. Owners of affected animals are often more concerned about elbow deformity than lameness. There is lateral bowing of the elbow and the radial head can be palpated lateral to the joint. The range of elbow movement is limited but there is usually little pain. The characteristic radiographic changes are shown in Fig. 4.65e. Although surgical correction by osteotomy and lag screw fixation of the radius to the ulna can be attempted (Campbell 1979), affected animals manage surprisingly well despite the deformity and require no treatment except restricted exercise until one year of age.

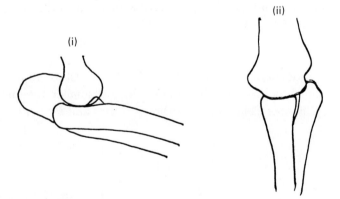

Fig. 4.65e Eight-month-old Labrador with congenital lateral dislocation of the radial head; (i) lateral view, (ii) cranio-caudal view.

Subluxation of the elbow secondary to growth disturbances of the radius and ulna

Premature closure of the distal ulnar growth plate is a common growth disturbance in rapidly growing pups of the larger breeds, especially the Great Dane and the Irish

Wolfhound. Growth of the radius continues at the normal rate, but the direction of growth is impeded by the 'bow string' effect of the ulna; consequently there is first cranial then medial bowing of the radius causing lateral deviation of the foot. Later subluxation of the elbow occurs as the head of the radius pushes the humeral condyles proximally (Fig. 4.65f) (O'Brien *et al.* 1971).

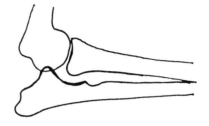

Fig. 4.65f Proximal luxation of the elbow caused by premature closure of the distal ulnar growth plate.

In the growing pup, the bowing of the radius and the carpal valgus deformity are corrected by stapling (Vaughan 1976); however, in the older animal wedge osteotomy is performed. In both procedures, the ulna should be sectioned to relieve its 'bow string' effect. Section of the ulna allows not only growth of the radius to continue unimpeded, but also a gradual reduction of the elbow luxation. In extreme cases (Figs 4.65f, g), the elbow luxation can be corrected by transverse osteotomy of the ulna shaft to allow the olecranon to be moved proximally. Reduction is maintained by fixing the proximal ulnar shaft to the radius with two lag screws (Fig. 4.65g).

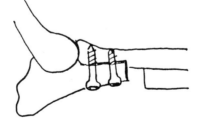

Fig. 4.65g Reduction by osteotomy of the ulna with lag screw fixation.

Subluxation of the elbow in Basset Hounds
Lameness associated with subluxation of the elbow secondary to premature closure of the distal ulnar growth plate is encountered quite often in the Basset Hound. There is usually a gradual onset of unilateral or bilateral

foreleg lameness at 6—8 months of age. There is pain evident on elbow manipulation. Lateral radiographs should be taken of both forearms to confirm the diagnosis (include the elbow and carpus). In positive cases the head of the radius will lie proximal to the distal articular margin of the semi-lunar notch of the ulna (Fig. 4.65h). The proximal luxation of the elbow can be reduced by removing a section of the ulnar shaft (Fig. 4.65i). This will also allow growth of the radius to continue unimpeded. The operation can be done on both forelegs at the same time in dogs with bilateral elbow luxations. Post-operatively exercise is restricted to short walks on a leash only for 6 weeks. Lameness should resolve within this period.

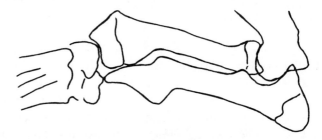

Fig. 4.65h Six-month-old Basset Hound with elbow luxation caused by premature closure of the distal ulnar growth plate.

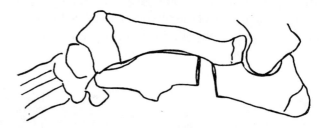

Fig. 4.65i Reduction of elbow luxation by section of the ulnar shaft.

Premature closure of the distal radial growth plate

This is an uncommon growth disturbance (Clayton-Jones & Vaughan 1970; Barr & Denny 1985) and is probably the result of trauma in most cases. The condition causes shortening of the forearm and an increase in the humero-radial joint space (Fig. 4.65j) with elbow instability and pain. The average age at the onset of lameness is 6 months.

Various methods of restabilizing the elbow have been described. Most have concentrated on lengthening the radius in order to achieve stability and maintain limb length. The most promising of these techniques allows a

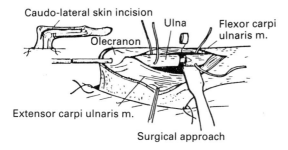

Fig. 4.65j Treatment of elbow instability caused by premature closure of distal radial growth plate: surgical approach.

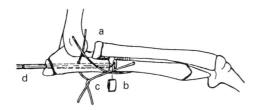

Fig. 4.65k Surgical technique: (a) increased humero-radial joint space; (b) ulnar osteotomy; (c) tension band wire; (d) intramedullary pin.

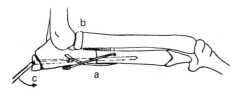

Fig. 4.65l Fixation of ulnar osteotomy using intramedullary pin and wire tension band (a); humero-radial joint space closed (b); intramedullary pin broken off flush with olecranom (c).

gradual reduction of the humero-radial joint space (Mason & Baker 1978; Barr & Denny 1985). Transverse osteotomy of the proximal radial shaft is performed; transfusion pins are placed through the humeral condyles and the head of the radius. Rubber bands are placed externally over the protruding ends of the pins and used to gradually close the humero-radial joint space. The device is removed after approximately 2 weeks.

An alternative method of restabilizing the elbow is to shorten the ulna. Although the technique has the disadvantage of causing further limb shortening, it is quick and easy to carry out, and requires little post-operative care compared with the dynamic reduction technique described above. The caudal aspect of the ulna is exposed. A section of the ulna shaft (equal to the gap between the humeral condyles and the head of the radius) is removed. The interosseous ligament between the proximal radius and ulna is sectioned. The ulna osteotomy site is closed, reducing the humero-radial joint space. The osteotomy is stabilized with an intramedullary pin and tension band wire (Figs 4.65k and 4.65l).

A fairly guarded prognosis should be given, however the degree of lameness is usually much improved following surgery and some cases will become sound provided that the degree of osteo-arthrosis present at the time of surgery is not too severe. The results of various forms of treatment in a series of 17 dogs is shown in Table 4.1 (Barr & Denny 1985).

Table 4.1 Results of treatment

Treatment	Total number of dogs	Sound	Slight intermittent lameness	More severe lameness	No 'follow-up' examination
Conservative	7	2	3	1	1
Radial osteotomy and plate fixation	1		1		
Radial osteotomy with pins and elastic	2	2			
Ulnar osteotomy	7	2	4		1 (Too early to assess)

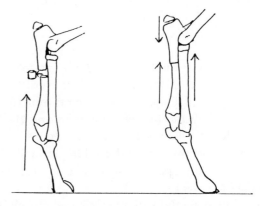

Fig. 4.65m 'Short radius syndrome': section of ulnar shaft removed.

Fig. 4.65n Weight bearing causes closure of the osteotomy and the humero-radial joint space.

The surgical treatment of this condition can be simplified even further: if only a section of the ulnar shaft is removed as in Figs 4.65m and 4.65n and the dog is encouraged to bear weight on the leg by the administration of non-steroidal anti-inflammatory drugs, the ostectomy gap in the ulna will gradually close and heal (Fig. 4.65m) resulting in simultaneous closure of the humero-radial joint space. The results of treatment are the same as the standard ulnar shortening procedure but the recovery period is longer.

Traumatic conditions
Traumatic conditions of the elbow include (Figs 4.66–4.72):
1 Condylar fractures of the humerus (see p. 217).
2 Supracondylar fractures of the humerus (see p. 214).
3 Fractures of the olecranon.
4 Fractures of the radial head.
5 Dislocation of the elbow.
6 Fracture of the ulna with anterior dislocation of the radial head ('Monteggia' lesion).
7 Avulsion or rupture of the triceps tendon of insertion.

Fig. 4.66 Fracture of the lateral or medial condyle.

Fig. 4.67 'Y' fracture.

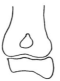

Fig. 4.68 Distal epiphyseal separation.

Fig. 4.69 Supracondylar fracture.

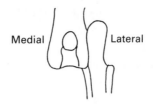

Medial   Lateral

Fig. 4.70 Dislocation of the elbow.

Fig. 4.71 Fracture of the olecranon.

Fig. 4.72 Fracture of the ulna with anterior dislocation of the radial head.

Traumatic dislocation of the elbow joint

Dislocation of the elbow is seen in dogs (and cats) over a year of age. The injury is caused in road traffic accidents or when a dog catches its leg in a fence and is suspended by the limb.

The radial head dislocates laterally and this can only occur if the anconeal process has become disengaged from its fossa between the humeral condyles. Therefore the elbow must be flexed by more than 45° in the accident and twisted for dislocation to occur, and provided this concept is grasped then a rational method of reduction can be employed (see below).

After dislocation of the elbow the affected limb is held forward, abducted and supinated. The elbow joint is painful and flexion and extension are limited.

Reduction is achieved under general anaesthesia by fully flexing the elbow; the radius and ulna are then rotated medially and the elbow joint is slowly extended until the anconeal process is re-engaged in its normal position between the humeral condyles. If the manipulation is successful the radial head and anconeal process 'snap' back into place, a full range of elbow movement is restored and the joint should feel stable. No further treatment should be necessary except to apply a support bandage for a week and restrict exercise for 4 weeks. Occasionally the elbow remains unstable due to stretching or rupture of the collateral ligaments. Stability can be restored by replacing the medial collateral ligament with a wire prosthesis anchored by two screws, one placed in the medial condyle of the humerus and the other in the ulna (Fig. 4.73).

In long-standing neglected dislocations open reduction must be carried out but this can be difficult. The operation is done in two stages. First reduction is achieved through a lateral approach to the elbow. Fibrous adhesions are broken down and the radial head and anconeal process are levered back into their normal position with a periosteal elevator inserted into the joint space. The lateral wound is closed, the dog turned over and the medial aspect of the joint exposed. A wire medial collateral ligament prosthesis is inserted as in Fig. 4.73 to prevent redislocation.

The prosthesis is not removed unless the screws loosen or eventual fracture of the wire leads to soft tissue reaction.

MONTEGGIA FRACTURE DISLOCATION
(Boyd & Boals 1969; Schwarz & Schrader 1984)
Fracture of the ulna with anterior dislocation of the radial head is known as a 'Monteggia fracture'. Anterior dislocation of the radial head occurs when the annular ligament which normally binds the radial head to the proximal ulna ruptures and the ulna fractures just distal to the elbow. The ulna shaft is firmly attached to the radius by the interosseous ligament and consequently moves with the radius in an anterior direction (Figs 4.74 and 4.76). Provided the injury is recent, the dislocation of the radial head can be reduced by manipulation, and, because of the strong interosseous attachments between the radius and ulna, reduction of the dislocation can be maintained by repair of the ulna alone. This is done with an intramedullary pin and tension band wire (Fig. 4.75), or a plate if the fracture is comminuted (Fig. 4.76b).

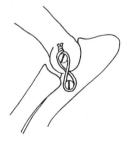

Fig. 4.73

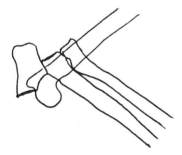

Fig. 4.74 Two-year-old domestic short haired cat with a Monteggia fracture dislocation.

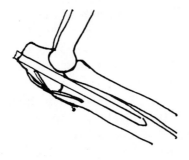

Fig. 4.75 Reduction and fixation with an intramedullary pin and tension wire band.

(a)

(b)

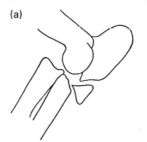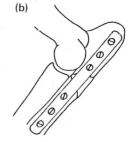

Fig. 4.76 Plate fixation in comminuted Monteggia fracture.

ANTERIOR DISLOCATION OF THE
RADIAL HEAD IN CATS

Anterior dislocation of the radial head associated with rupture of the annular ligament but without fracture of the ulnar shaft is occasionally seen in cats. Open reduction is performed and the radial head fixed to the ulna with a lag screw (Figs 4.77a and b).

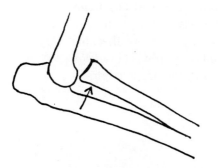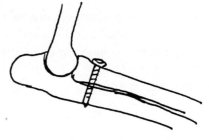

Fig. 4.77b Lag screw fixation.

Fig. 4.77a Cat: anterior dislocation of the radial head.

Fracture of the olecranon

Fracture of the olecranon is illustrated in Fig. 4.77c. The fragment is distracted by the strong pull of the triceps tendon and this can only be overcome by internal fixation.

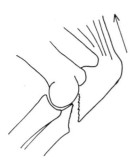

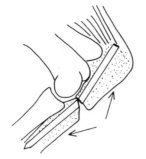

Fig. 4.77c

Fig. 4.77d

Most fractures occur through the semilunar notch. The articular margin of the fracture serves as a fulcrum and if an intramedullary pin or a screw is used for fixation as in Fig. 4.77d it will be subjected to excessive bending forces and will often break before fracture healing is complete unless the elbow is immobilized in a plaster cast. This problem can be overcome and the tensile forces of the triceps used to advantage to compress the fracture by using the wire tension band for fixation (see Figs 4.77h, i, j). Alternatively, a plate can be used for fixation and this method is indicated for comminuted fractures of the olecranon. The plate is applied to the lateral or caudal aspect of the ulna (Fig. 4.77).

Fractures of the proximal olecranon are treated by lag screw fixation or wiring techniques. Exposure of the olecranon is achieved through a curved caudolateral skin incision; the extensor carpi ulnaris muscle and the flexor carpi ulnaris muscle are separated and retracted to reveal the shaft of the ulna (Figs 4.77e, f, g).

Avulsion of the tendon of insertion triceps muscles
This injury is occasionally encountered in the dog. Rupture

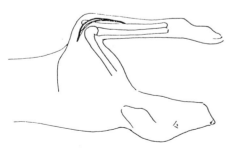

Exposure of the olecranon and ulnar shaft – caudolateral skin incision

Fig. 4.77e

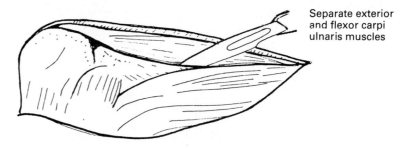

Separate exterior
and flexor carpi
ulnaris muscles

Fig. 4.77f

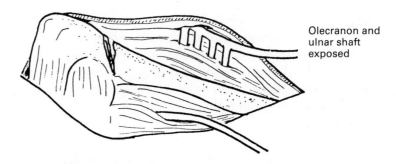

Olecranon and
ulnar shaft
exposed

Fig. 4.77g

(h)

(i)

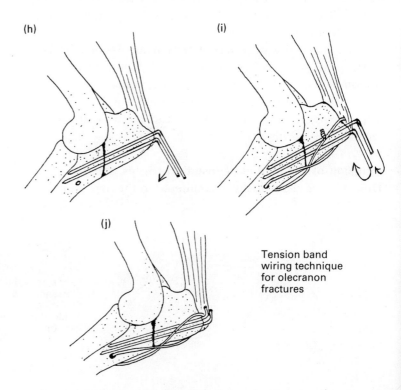

(j)

Tension band
wiring technique
for olecranon
fractures

Fig. 4.77h,i,j Tension band wiring technique for olecranon fractures.

of the triceps tendon can also occur as a complication of local steroid injection (Davies & Clayton-Jones 1982). Following rupture or avulsion the leg is carried semi-flexed, the animal is unable to extend the elbow and there is pain and swelling over the point of the olecranon. The avulsed tendon can be reattached using Kirschner wires and a tension band wire (Fig. 4.77j), while ruptures are repaired with Bunnell or Pennington-type sutures of monofilament nylon (see p. 376). If insufficient tendon remains to suture then a length of filamentous carbon fibre or polyester can be passed through the musculotendinous portion of the triceps. A tunnel is drilled transversely through the proximal olecranon through which the carbon fibre or polyester is passed in a figure of eight pattern and tied. Post-operatively the leg should be kept in extension with a full-length Robert Jones bandage for 4–6 weeks (change bandage at weekly intervals).

Fractures of the radial head
Fractures of the radial head are rare. Management of these fractures has been described by Neal (1975). Open reduction is indicated to restore the integrity of the joint surface and fixation is achieved with a lag screw or Kirschner wire depending on the size of the fragment. If the fracture is comminuted and cannot be stabilized, then excision of the radial head can be performed as a salvage procedure.

Arthrodesis of the elbow
Arthrodesis of the elbow is only occasionally necessary and is used most often for the relief of chronic pain associated with degenerative joint disease. The articular surfaces of the elbow are exposed through a caudal approach with osteotomy of the olecranon. The lateral joint capsule is incised to allow exposure of the humero-radial joint. Articular cartilage is removed from all articular surfaces using a high speed burr or osteotome. Cancellous bone can be collected from the olecranon osteotomy site and packed into the joint. The elbow should be fused at a functional angle of 110° and temporary fixation of the joint at this angle is maintained with a Kirschner wire while a dynamic compression plate is contoured and applied to the caudal surface of the humerus and ulna (Fig. 4.78a and b). The olecranon process is attached to the medial epicondyle of the humerus with a lag screw.

Arthrodesis of the elbow relieves pain but causes a change in gait. Initially the animal may advance the leg by cir-

(a)   (b)

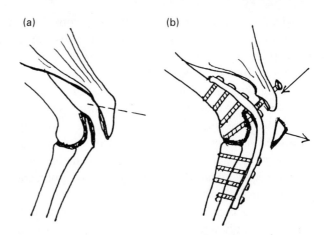

Fig. 4.78 Elbow arthrodesis: (a) osteotomy of olecranon with removal of articular surfaces; (b) application of DCP to caudal aspect of elbow. Reattach olecranon to distal humerus with lag screw.

cumduction and tends to drag the toes. Within 3–6 weeks compensatory movement of the adjacent joints allows a reasonable degree of limb function and a return to 'normal activity'.

A dog which has had an arthrodesis of the elbow is more prone to fracture the radius and ulna than normal because fusion of a major joint produces a much longer lever arm. All the stresses are concentrated at the junction between rigid plate and elastic bone and fracture may occur as a result of trivial trauma. To minimize the risk of this complication, the end screw should penetrate one cortex only and the plate should be removed once bone union is complete.

RADIUS AND ULNA

Growth disturbances of the radius and ulna
(Denny 1976)

Longitudinal growth of the radius and ulna occurs from the proximal and distal growth plates (Fig. 4.79). The distal growth plates contribute approximately 70% of the final length of the radius and 85% of the ulna (Parkes *et al.* 1966). The remaining percentage is derived from the proximal growth plates, however in the ulna this plate contributes more to the length of the olecranon than to the shaft of the bone.

The radius and ulna lie parallel to each other and their rate of growth is closely interrelated. A growth disturbance occurs when there is a discrepancy in the rate of growth

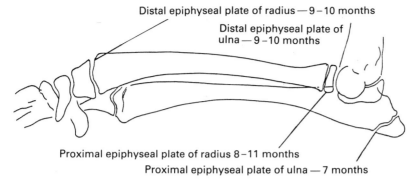

Distal epiphyseal plate of radius — 9–10 months

Distal epiphyseal plate of ulna — 9–10 months

Proximal epiphyseal plate of radius 8–11 months

Proximal epiphyseal plate of ulna — 7 months

Fig. 4.79

between two bones: this is caused by either premature closure or a decrease in the rate of growth at one growth plate while growth at the adjacent plate continues normally.

Growth disturbances of the radius and ulna caused by premature closure of the distal ulnar growth plate are seen most frequently in giant breeds of dog, especially Great Danes and Irish Wolfhounds. It is usually the largest pup in the litter that is affected and predisposing factors are over-feeding and uncontrolled exercise during puppyhood. Growth disturbances can also be precipitated by trauma. A serious potential complication of fracture of the distal third of the radius in puppies is premature closure of the distal ulnar growth plate and if untreated, severe limb deformity will result.

The degree and type of deformity seen depends on the age of the animal at the time of injury and the growth plate involved. The approximate times of closure of the epiphyses of the radius and ulna are given in Fig. 4.79. The radiological features of forelimb growth disturbances have been reviewed and described by O'Brien *et al.* (1971).

PREMATURE CLOSURE OF THE DISTAL
ULNAR GROWTH PLATE

Premature closure of the distal ulnar growth plate causes the following deformities. Growth of the radius continues at the normal rate, but the direction of growth is impeded by the 'bow-string' effect of the ulna; consequently there is firstly anterior and then medial bowing of the radius causing lateral deviation of the foot (carpal valgus deformity). Later, external rotation of the carpus and subluxation of the elbow occurs (Fig. 4.80) as the head of the radius pushes the humeral condyles proximally.

With any growth deformity, radiographs should be taken

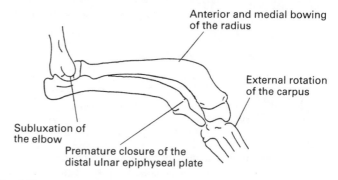

Fig. 4.80

which include the elbow and carpal joints of both limbs for comparison of the growth plates and assessment of the degree of deformity and changes in the joints.

In many Danes and Irish Wolfhounds presented with lateral deviation of the carpus, radiographs show that the ulnar growth plate is still open. The growth plate cartilage is failing to ossify normally and appears as an elongated radiolucent zone. The zone is called a retained cartilaginous core (Fig. 4.81) and it signifies that the ulna growth plate is growing more slowly than its distal radial counterpart.

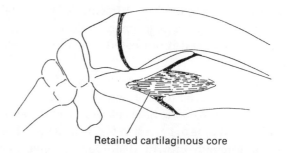

Retained cartilaginous core

Fig. 4.81

The average age of dogs presented with growth disturbances is 5 months and therefore it is necessary to consider what can be done to prevent further deformity during the remaining period of growth. The use of plaster casts or splints to maintain alignment is usually unsuccessful.

If both distal radial and ulnar growth plates are still open lateral deviation of the carpus can be corrected by placing a staple across the medial side of the distal radial growth plate (Fig. 4.83). This temporarily delays growth on the medial side of the leg while continued growth of the ulna and lateral side of the distal radial growth plate straightens the leg. The process usually takes 4–6 weeks.

(Vaughan 1976)

1 The leg is prepared for surgery in routine fashion.

2 A 19 gauge needle is inserted into the medial side of the distal radial growth plate. The needle should slide easily into soft cartilage (Fig. 4.82).

3 Anteroposterior and lateral radiographs are taken to check the position of the needle. The needle is then used as a landmark to decide the correct position for the staple.

4 The dog is taken into the operating theatre, the leg is reprepared and draped. A longitudinal incision is made directly over the growth plate (there is no need to incise the periosteum). The staple is pushed into the bone making sure that the bars of the stable are on either side of the growth plate as judged from the position of the guide needle on the radiographs (Fig. 4.83). The staple is driven into the bone with a hammer. The guide needle is removed and the skin is closed with horizontal mattress sutures. Check X-rays are taken to ensure that the staple is correctly placed and a support bandage is applied for 1 week. The leg generally takes 4–6 weeks to straighten. The staple must then be removed (unless the dog is almost fully grown) otherwise the carpus will tend to deviate medially. Exercise is restricted to short walks while the staple is *in situ*.

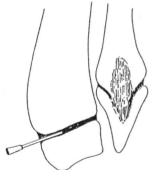

Fig. 4.82

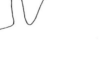

Fig. 4.83

If the distal ulnar growth plate has closed prematurely then in addition to stapling the radius, a 1–2 cm section of the ulnar shaft must be removed to relieve the bow string effect and allow growth of the radius to continue unimpeded (Newton 1974) (Figs 4.84 and 4.85). The gap in the ulnar

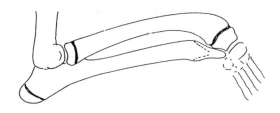

Fig. 4.84

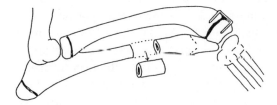

Fig. 4.85

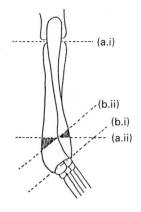

Fig. 4.86

shaft, regardless of size, rapidly fills with callus in 4–6 weeks. Healing of the osteotomy can be delayed by inserting a fat graft in the gap.

Ulnar osteotomy and stapling are designed to prevent further deformity and correct angulation of the radius in the growing dog after premature closure or retarded growth has occurred at the distal ulnar growth plate. Once the distal radial growth plate has closed then the only method of straightening the limb is by wedge osteotomy of the radius and ulna. The method of estimating the position and size of the wedge (Fig. 4.86) is as follows.

A tracing is made of the radiograph of the affected limb. Normally joint surfaces are parallel—draw lines through the elbow (*ai*) and carpus (*bi*), then at the point of greatest deformity of the radius draw line (*aii*) parallel with (*ai*) and (*bii*) parallel with (*bi*). The shaded area indicates the size of the osteotomy.

The ulna must also be sectioned to allow reduction of the radius after removal of the wedge. The radial osteotomy site is stabilized with a plate. The procedure not only straightens the leg but tends to relieve concurrent elbow subluxation (Fig. 4.80).

The wedge (cuneiform) osteotomy will cause a degree of limb shortening; this is not usually of any clinical significance. An alternative method to wedge osteotomy is the oblique osteotomy (Fig. 4.87). This allows correction of angular deformity and any rotational deformity while preserving limb length. An external fixator is used to stabilize the osteotomy (Fig. 4.87).

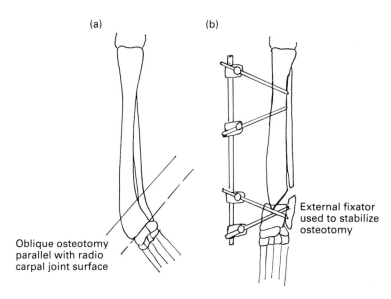

(a) (b)

External fixator
used to stabilize
osteotomy

Oblique osteotomy
parallel with radio
carpal joint surface

Fig. 4.87 Oblique osteotomy.

PREMATURE CLOSURE OF THE DISTAL RADIAL
EPIPHYSEAL PLATE

(Clayton-Jones & Vaughan 1970)

Premature closure of the distal radial epiphyseal plate is fairly uncommon and results in shortening of the radius and forearm with an increase in the humeral–radial joint space, with consequent instability of the joint (Fig. 4.65k). Subluxation of the radiocarpal joint with lateral deviation of the foot may also occur. The aim of surgical treatment is to close the humero-radial joint space and stabilize the elbow; this can be done either by lengthening the radius or by shortening the ulna; the latter is the simpler technique (p. 240).

PREMATURE CLOSURE OF BOTH RADIAL AND
ULNAR DISTAL EPIPHYSEAL PLATES

Premature closure of both the radial and ulnar distal epiphyseal plates results in shortening of the radius and ulna with lateral deviation of both diaphyses. There is a tendency for the carpus to subluxate medially and produce lateral deviation of the foot. The deformity may be corrected by wedge osteotomy of the radius.

Fractures of the radius and ulna

The radius and ulna are long, straight, relatively exposed

bones with little soft tissue cover; consequently, they are more vulnerable to trauma than any other in the forelimb. The majority of fractures, as might be expected, involve the distal radius and ulna and tend to be transverse in nature. However all types of fracture may be encountered and can involve any part of the radius and ulna. It is convenient to classify these fractures into three groups: proximal, shaft, and distal fractures.

PROXIMAL FRACTURES OF THE RADIUS AND ULNA
Possible sites of fracture of the proximal radius and ulna include the olecranon, the head of the radius, and the proximal ulna associated with anterior dislocation of the radial head (Monteggia fracture). These conditions are described on p. 245.

SHAFT FRACTURES OF THE RADIUS AND ULNA
The majority of fractures involve the distal third of the radius and ulna. Shaft fractures can be treated by closed reduction and external fixation using a cast (plaster of Paris is still very popular but lighter stronger materials such as Baycast (Bayer U.K. Ltd) and Vetcast (3M) may be preferred). External fixation is indicated for greenstick fractures, undisplaced fractures and following reduction of displaced transverse fractures provided at least 50% of the fracture surfaces can be brought into contact. The cast should extend from the foot to above the elbow. The pads are left exposed so that they can be checked for warmth and swelling. In young rapidly growing puppies, the cast will need to be changed at 10–14 day intervals while in mature dogs, changes are made every 3–4 weeks once the initial swelling associated with the fracture has subsided.

Although fractures of the distal third of the radius in immature dogs heal rapidly in a cast, a serious potential complication of such fractures is premature closure of the distal ulna growth plate. Owners should be warned of this possibility and it is always worth taking a radiograph at 3 weeks to check the state of the growth plate. If closure occurs, then a section of the ulna must be removed to allow growth of the radius to continue unimpeded, otherwise bowing of the radius and carpal valgus will occur. Although these deformities can be corrected by stapling or corrective osteotomy, they should be prevented from happening.

Poor reduction and/or insufficient immobilization of shaft fractures in casts may lead to malunion, or non-union—

82% of dogs referred to the author's clinic for treatment of non-union fractures had had their fractures plastered initially. It is generally accepted that plate fixation gives consistently good results in the treatment of fractures of the radius and ulna. The method is recommended particularly for mature dogs with overriding transverse fractures, oblique or comminuted fractures. The plate is applied to the anterior surface of the radius (Fig. 4.88). Generally, the distal shaft of the ulna requires no fixation because the radius is the main weight-bearing bone in the forearm and tends to act as a splint for the ulna because of the interosseus attachments between the two bones.

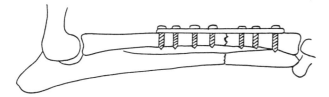

Fig. 4.88

Delayed union and non-union are common complications of fractures of the radius and ulna in Toy Poodles and other miniature breeds of dog. The non-union that develops is characterized by bone lysis and lack of callus and is termed an atrophic type of non-union. Contributory factors are:

1 The small size of these dogs which makes satisfactory immobilization of the fracture difficult, no matter whether external or internal fixation is used.

2 The potential for iatrogenic damage to bone and soft tissues which is much greater in dogs of this size.

Mini-ASIF compression plates used with cortex screws (1.5 mm or 2 mm in diameter) give good results in the treatment of both fresh and non-union fractures in toy and miniature breeds. If non-union is present, fibrous and cartilaginous callus between the fragments is excised, the fracture surfaces are freshened up and a cancellous bone graft is taken from the proximal humerus and packed into the fracture site to stimulate osteogenesis. Fixation is achieved with a mini-plate.

In some miniature dogs the diameter of the radius and ulna is too small to permit the use of a mini-plate and screws and under these circumstances an intramedullary Kirschner wire can be used for the fixation (Fig. 4.89a−c).

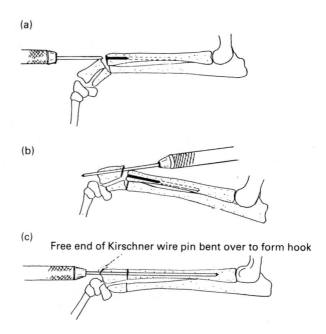

(a)

(b)

(c)

Free end of Kirschner wire pin bent over to form hook

Fig. 4.89

INSERTION OF AN INTRAMEDULLARY
KIRSCHNER WIRE TO STABILIZE A FRACTURE OF
THE RADIUS AND ULNA

This method is illustrated in Fig. 4.89a and b. The fracture
is exposed and the medullary cavity in the proximal fragment is reamed out to a depth of about 1 cm using the tip
of the Kirschner wire (Fig. 4.89a). The wire is then driven
down through the distal fragment, keeping the carpus
flexed so that the wire emerges over the dorsal aspect of
the radial carpal bone (Fig. 4.89b). The chuck is attached to
the protruding end of wire which is withdrawn sufficiently
to allow fracture reduction to be completed. The Kirschner
wire is then directed into the reamed medullary cavity of
the proximal radius (Fig. 4.89c).

The wire is left protruding a little (for easy retrieval after
fracture healing is complete) and it is bent back to form a
hook (Fig. 4.89c) so that the dog's ability to extend the
carpus is not completely inhibited. Excess wire is cut off.
After intermedullary fixation of the fracture, a plaster cast
should be applied for 4 weeks to prevent any rotation at
the fracture site.

It should be stressed that this technique is not an ideal
method of fixation and it should only be used if no better
option is available (e.g. mini-DCP). The Kirschner wire
offers no resistance to rotation at the fracture site and there

is potential for iatrogenic damage to the carpus during insertion and removal of the wire which may lead to degenerative joint disease.

EXTERNAL FIXATOR

The external fixator is a useful way of dealing with radius and ulna fractures, particularly the open, potentially infected fractures. The type 1 configuration is used most often and is applied to the craniomedial surface of the radius with two half pins in the proximal fragment and two in the distal (see section on external fixators, Chapter 2, p. 76).

The common complications of shaft fractures of the radius and ulna have already been mentioned. These are premature closure of the distal ulnar growth plate and delayed union and non-union. The fourth complication is malunion which results from failure to adequately reduce and/or immobilize the fracture during the healing process. Malunion resulting in angular deformity is corrected by wedge osteotomy. The method of estimating the position and size of the wedge is illustrated in Fig. 4.86.

Transverse osteotomy and plate fixation is used for correction of overriding malunions (see Fig. 4.90).

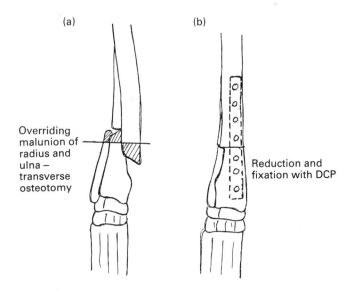

Fig. 4.90 (a) Overriding malunion of radius and ulna-transverse osteotomy; (b) reduction and fixation with DCP.

FRACTURES OF THE RADIUS AND ULNA IN CATS

Radius and ulna fractures in the cat tend to be simple transverse fractures involving the distal third of the shaft. It should be remembered that the cat has a much greater range of supination and pronation of the forearm than the dog and this rotatory movement can lead to non-union if an intramedullary pin placed in the radius is used as the sole method of fixation. Non-union may still occur even if the pin is supplemented by a cast. If intramedullary fixation is chosen then two pins should be used for fixation, one in the radius and the other in the ulna. For best results, a plate (2.7 DCP or mini-veterinary cuttable plate, Straumann Great Britain Ltd) should be used for fixation. The plate is applied to the cranial aspect of the radius.

EXPOSURE OF SHAFT FRACTURES OF THE RADIUS AND ULNA

The dog is positioned in dorsal recumbency with the fractured foreleg pulled caudally by an assistant. In this position it is easy to manipulate the leg during reduction. Both sides of the leg are accessible and it is a comfortable position for the surgeon to work in, particularly if a plate is to be inserted.

If the fracture involves the distal third of the radius, a skin incision is made over the anteromedial aspect of the radius from mid-shaft to carpus. Care is taken to avoid the cephalic vein (Fig. 4.91a–c).

The extensor carpi radialis muscle is retracted laterally to expose the anterior aspect of the radius.

Fractures involving the proximal two-thirds of the radius and ulna are exposed through a skin incision made over the anteromedial aspect of the radius from the elbow to just above the carpus (Fig. 4.92). The deep antebrachial fascia is incised between the extensor carpi radialis muscle and flexor carpi radialis muscle to expose the radial shaft (Fig. 4.92b). Proximally, the bone is covered by the supinator muscle; this is elevated to complete exposure. The radial nerve lies deep to the supinator muscle and must be protected. Distally, the shaft of the radius is covered by the abductor pollicis longus muscle which can be incised to allow application of the plate. The muscle is subsequently repaired with mattress sutures.

DISTAL RADIAL FRACTURES

Fracture separation of the distal radial epiphysis
The injury is seen in immature dogs and the distal radial epiphysis is displaced laterally causing carpal valgus (lateral deviation of the carpus (Fig. 4.93)). Early closed reduction should be carried out and external support provided with

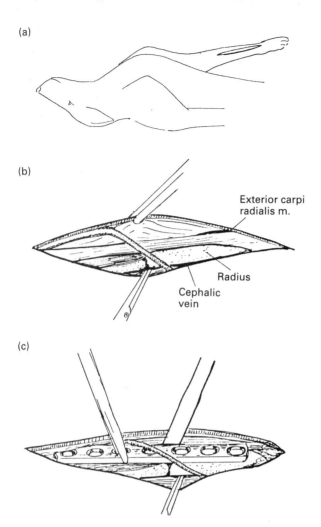

Fig. 4.91 Exposure of fractures involving the distal shaft of the radius and ulna. (a) Cranio-medial approach, skin incision over cranio-medial aspect of the radius; (b) medial surface of radius and the extensor carpi radialis m. exposed; (c) exterior muscles retracted laterally to allow application of plate to the cranial surface of the radius.

a plaster cast for 3 weeks while healing occurs. If treatment is delayed for more than 48 hours then reduction by closed means may prove impossible. Open reduction is carried out using a medial approach and the epiphysis stabilized with two K-wires in dogs under 6 months of age (Fig. 4.94a). The wires are removed after 4 weeks.

The distal radial growth plate normally contributes approximately 70% of the final length of the radius. Premature closure of the distal growth plate may result in serious shortening of the forearm and an increase in the radio-humeral joint space with consequent elbow instability.

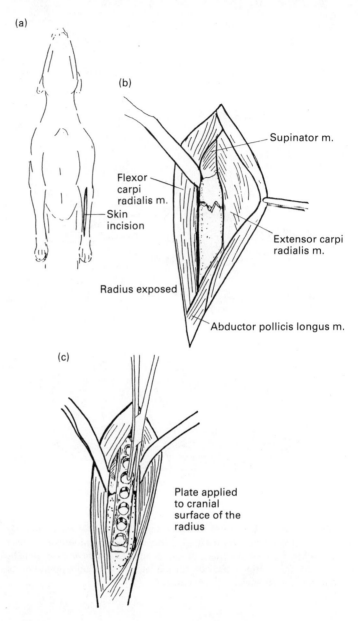

(a)

(b)

Supinator m.

Flexor
carpi
radialis m.

Skin
incision

Radius exposed

Extensor carpi
radialis m.

Abductor pollicis longus m.

(c)

Plate applied
to cranial
surface of the
radius

Fig. 4.92 Cranio-medial approach to the radius and ulna for fractures involving the proximal two thirds of the shaft of the radius.

The management of this complication is described on p. 240. In dogs over 7 months of age with little growth potential left, a wire tension band can stabilize the epiphysis (Fig. 4.94b). External support with a splint or cast is provided for 2–3 weeks following surgery.

Malunion of the distal radial epiphysis is occasionally encountered and this requires wedge osteotomy to correct the resultant carpal valgus deformity. The osteotomy is

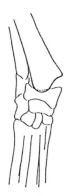

Fig. 4.93

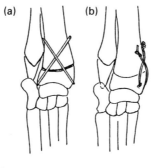

(a) (b)

Fig. 4.94

performed close to the growth plate and, as with more recent separations, a wire tension band and cast are used to stabilize the osteotomy.

FRACTURES INVOLVING THE DISTAL ARTICULAR SURFACE OF THE RADIUS AND ULNA

These are uncommon and are usually seen in dogs that have fallen from a great height. The injury is often bilateral. General principles of dealing with intra-articular fractures apply, open reduction being carried out to allow accurate reduction of the fragments. These are stabilized with lag screws or Kirschner wires and then the area is further supported with a neutralization plate or cast (Figs 4.95 and 4.96).

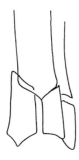

Fig.4.95

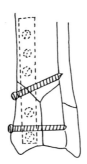

Fig. 4.96

FRACTURE OF THE STYLOID PROCESS OF THE RADIUS

The lateral collateral ligament of the carpus originates from the styloid process and fracture is associated with carpal instability. If the fragment is large enough a lag screw is used for fixation. Smaller fragments are retained in position with a Kirschner wire used in combination with a tension band wire.

FRACTURE OF THE ULNAR STYLOID PROCESS

Fractures of the ulnar styloid process are also associated with carpal instability because the medial collateral ligament of the carpus originates on the process. Intramedullary fixation of the styloid is achieved with a Kirschner wire combined with a tension band wire (Fig. 4.97a and b). Because of the soft tissue injuries and carpal instability associated with styloid process fractures it is important to provide external support with a gutter splint on the caudal aspect of the carpus for 4–6 weeks.

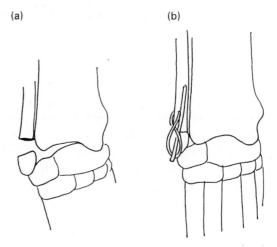

(a)   (b)

Fig. 4.97 (a) Fracture of the ulnar styloid process with subluxation of the radio carpal joint; (b) fixation using a Kirschner wire and a wire tension band.

THE CARPUS

The carpus is a composite joint (Fig. 4.98) supported by multiple intercarpal ligaments.

Fractures of the carpal bones rarely occur with the exception of the accessory carpal bone. A chip fracture of the ventral border of the accessory carpal bone is a common injury in the racing Greyhound which is frequently overlooked (Hickman 1975). The right leg is usually involved and the injury occurs when the dog is rounding a bend and suddenly changes direction (Bateman 1960). The injury may be dismissed initially as a sprain of the carpus and treated conservatively. However, intermittent lameness

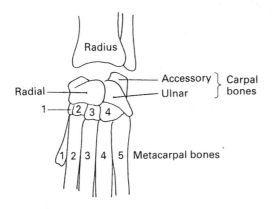

Fig. 4.98

persists especially after severe exercise and there is pain on flexion of the carpus. A lateral radiograph will confirm the diagnosis (Fig. 4.99).

Accessory carpal bone fractures (Fig. 4.100a–e) have been classified into five types (Johnson 1987). Type I fractures from the distal articular surface are the most common and accounted for 68% of cases reported by Johnson *et al.* (1988). The prognosis for a successful return to racing after surgical excision of the fragment is poor, however as a general rule, small fragments are excised while larger frag-

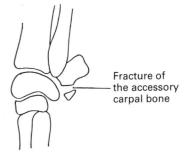

Fig. 4.99

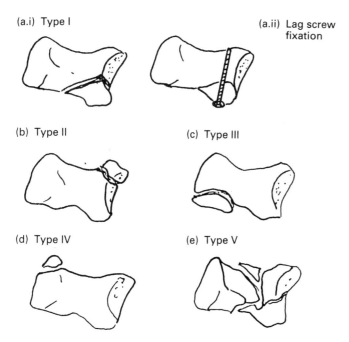

(a.i) Type I

(a.ii) Lag screw fixation

(b) Type II

(c) Type III

(d) Type IV

(e) Type V

Fig. 4.100 Fractures of the accessory carpal bone; classification I–V (Johnson 1987).

ments should be screwed back (Fig. 4.100a(ii)). Brinker *et al.* (1990) recommend lag screw fixation for types I, II and III injuries and claim that 90% of dogs treated in this way return to racing and win races. A carpal flexion cast (see below) should be applied for 6–8 weeks following surgery. Type IV fractures are best treated by surgical excision of fragments with repair of tendinous attachments followed by application of a cast for 6–8 weeks. The cast is applied with the carpus in a moderated degree of palmar flexion which is gradually reduced to a normal position. The same regime of cast application is recommended for dogs with severely comminuted fractures (type V) of the accessory carpal bone (Dee 1991); these carry a guarded prognosis.

Exposure of the accessory carpal bone for screw fixation of type I and type II fractures

The dog is placed in dorsal recumbency with the affected leg pulled forward. A palmar lateral incision is made over the accessory carpal bone. The palmar carpal antebrachial retinaculum is incised lateral to the accessory carpal bone and reflected medially. The abductor digiti quinti muscle is sharply dissected away from the accessory carpal bone and the accessorometacarpal ligaments. The ligaments are retracted to complete exposure of the fracture site.

Fracture of the radial carpal bone

Fractures of the radial carpal bone are rare: small chip fractures are treated by surgical excision of the fragments. Larger fragments are often undisplaced and initial treatment usually consists of immobilization of the carpus in a cast. If delayed union or non-union occur then lag screw fixation of the fracture is undertaken. Screw fixation is used as the primary option if there is displacement of the fragment. Care should be taken to ensure that the screw head does not interfere with carpal movement and if necessary the screw head should be countersunk.

Fracture of the ulnar carpal bone

This fracture is occasionally seen as a complication of lateral dislocation of the radial carpal bone (see Fig. 4.103). Open reduction is performed and the fracture dislocation stabilized with a Kirschner wire or lag screw placed transversely through the radial and ulnar carpal bones.

Chip fractures of individual carpal bones are perhaps seen more frequently and generally the fragments should be removed to prevent carpitis developing.

A prerequisite for accurate surgery of the extremities is a bloodless field and this is best achieved by expressing the blood from the limb with a rubber bandage followed by application of a tourniquet at, or just below, the elbow. A midline skin incision is made over the anterior aspect of the carpus. The deep antebrachial fascia is incised in the midline between the tendons of the extensor carpi radialis and common digital extensor. These tendons are retracted to allow exposure and incision of the joint capsule over the carpal bones. The synovial membrane adheres to the dorsal surfaces of individual carpal bones and must be dissected off the bones as necessary to achieve the required exposure. Following wound closure, a pressure bandage is applied before release of the tourniquet.

Hyperextension of the carpus in puppies

Hyperextension of the carpii is a relatively common problem seen in puppies, often young German Shepherds, and they develop dropping of the carpii which can lead to a plantigrade stance. The condition is due to laxity of the carpal flexor tendons associated with poor muscle tone. The aim of treatment is to improve muscle tone with a regime of short frequent walks (Shires *et al.* 1985). Carpal posture tends to improve by the time the pup reaches maturity. The use of casts or splints should be avoided in these cases as carpal posture becomes worse once the external support is removed.

Dislocation and subluxation of the radiocarpal joint

Dislocations or subluxations of the radiocarpal joint are usually caused by a fall. The radius is displaced cranial to the radial carpal bone and there is often damage to the medial collateral ligament which causes lateral deviation of the foot (Fig. 4.101a).

After closed reduction, joint stability may be restored by immobilizing the carpus in a plaster cast for at least 4 weeks. If instability persists and there is deviation of the foot, then surgical replacement of the medial collateral ligament is carried out using a wire prosthesis (Fig. 4.101b). Occasionally carpal arthrodesis is indicated (see Fig. 4.105) when there has been extensive damage to the collateral ligaments.

Rupture of the plantar ligament of the carpus

Rupture of the plantar ligament of the carpus (Fig. 4.102a)

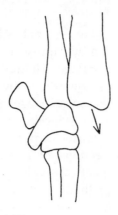

Fig. 4.101a

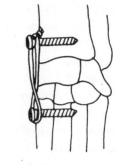

Fig. 4.101b

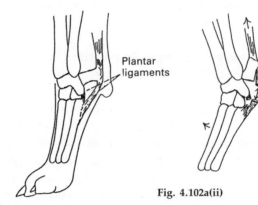

Plantar ligaments

Fig. 4.102a(ii)

Fig. 4.102a(i)

is usually caused by a fall. The carpus 'drops' when the dog takes weight on the affected leg and the joint can be hyperextended on palpation. Carpal posture may improve following external support in a plaster cast but this is usually transient and although techniques for repairing or substituting the plantar ligaments with wire have been described these are not usually successful. Consequently, primary partial, or pancarpal arthrodesis is recommended for treating dogs with hyperextension injuries of the carpus. Partial carpal arthrodesis is used if a stressed lateral radiograph of the carpus reveals hyperextension at the intercarpal or carpo-metacarpal joints. Pancarpal arthrodesis is used if hyperextension occurs at the level of the radiocarpal joint but can be used to treat hyperextension injuries at all levels (see below). The most popular method of partial carpal arthrodesis is that described by Slocum & Devine (1982) using intramedullary pins for fixation (Fig. 4.102b). Alternatively a 'T' plate can be used for fixation (Fig. 4.102c)

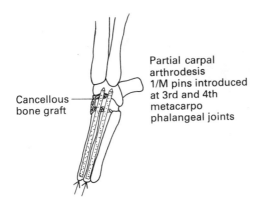

Cancellous bone graft

Partial carpal arthrodesis 1/M pins introduced at 3rd and 4th metacarpo phalangeal joints

Fig. 4.102b

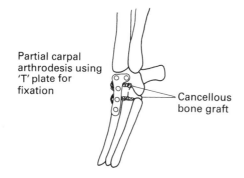

Partial carpal arthrodesis using 'T' plate for fixation

Cancellous bone graft

Fig. 4.102c

(Brinker *et al.* 1983). A gutter splint should be applied to the plantar aspect of the carpus to provide additional support for 6 weeks following surgery. More details of carpal arthrodesis techniques are given below.

Dislocation of the radial carpal bone (Fig. 4.103)

Dislocation of the radial carpal bone is an uncommon injury. Open reduction is usually necessary as the bone tends to rotate on its horizontal axis. Normally a stable reduction is achieved. However, if it is difficult to maintain the bone in position, a small pin can be used for fixation (Fig. 4.104). After reduction the carpus is immobilized in a plaster cast for 4 weeks.

Arthrodesis

The surgical fusion of a joint is called an arthrodesis. Arthrodesis is a salvage procedure and is indicated in the treatment of:

1 Irreparable joint fractures.
2 Chronic joint instability.

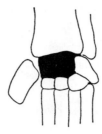 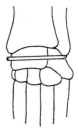

Fig. 4.103   Fig. 4.104

3 The relief of pain associated with chronic degenerative joint disease.
4 Block resection of some bone tumours.

The successful arthrodesis of a joint involves four basic procedures:
1 Removal of all articular cartilage down to bleeding subchondral bone.
2 Where possible flat surfaces should be cut on opposing joint surfaces to ensure optimal contact for bony union. If the contours of the joint are such that this cannot be done then the joint space should be packed with an autogenous cancellous bone graft. Cancellous bone grafts are indicated in most arthrodeses to speed up bony union.
3 The joint should be fused at a normal functional angle.
4 Rigid internal fixation is essential and in the case of the carpus and hock this should be reinforced with an external splint for 6 weeks.

The carpus and intertarsal joint of the hock are arthrodesed most often. Fusion of these joints produces virtually no change in gait. Arthrodesis of the elbow, shoulder or stifle however has a more profound affect on gait. Initially the animal may advance the leg by circumduction and tends to drag the toes. Within 3–6 weeks compensatory movement of the adjacent joints allows a reasonable degree of limb function and a return to 'normal' activity.

Arthrodesis of a major joint creates a much longer lever arm than normal. There is an increased risk of fracture at the junction between plate and bone proximal or distal to the joint as a result of relatively minor trauma. This risk can be minimized by removal of implants as soon as there is radiographic evidence of bony fusion across the joint.

The main indication for carpal arthrodesis is a hyperextension injury which results in chronic instability (Johnson 1980, Parker *et al.* 1981). Pancarpal arthrodesis is the most widely used method of treatment for carpal hyperextension injuries regardless of the joint involved. In a series of 45 cases described by Parker *et al.* (1981), pancarpal arthrodesis was performed using a plate applied to the dorsal aspect of the carpus for fixation. External support was provided for 6–8 weeks following surgery. Seventy-four per cent of the dogs in this series regained normal limb function. External support is essential to protect the plate from excessive bending forces until fusion of the carpus has occurred. Biomechanically it would be preferable to apply the plate to the palmar surface of the carpus where it would be subject to tensile forces only. The palmar approach for pancarpal arthrodesis was described by Chambers & Bjorling (1982).

Hyperextension injuries which involve the intercarpal or carpo-metacarpal joints but not the radiocarpal joint are treated by partial carpal arthrodesis. Techniques for partial carpal arthrodesis include retrograde insertion of intra-medullary pins in the metacarpal and carpal bones (Slocum & Devine 1982, Brinker *et al.* 1983, Willer *et al.* 1990). 'T' plate fixation has also been described (Brinker *et al.* 1983). Willer *et al.* (1990) reviewed a series of 39 dogs with hyper-extension injuries which were treated by partial arthrodesis using intramedullary pins for fixation. Seventy per cent of these cases regained full limb function and 12% had slight lameness after exercise. This result compares favourably with the series treated by pancarpal arthodesis (Parker *et al.* 1981) and allows function of the radiocarpal joint to be preserved.

TECHNIQUE

Pancarpal arthrodesis is performed using a technique similar to that described by Parker *et al.* (1981) but with some differences in positioning and approach. The lower leg is exsanguinated with an Esmarch bandage and a tour-niquet applied at the level of the elbow. The dog is pos-itioned for surgery in dorsal recumbency with the affected leg pulled caudally. A skin incision is made over the medial aspect of the carpus commencing at the distal third of the radius and ending in a mediolateral curve over the distal metacarpus. This skin flap is reflected laterally with the carpal and digital extensor tendons to reveal the dorsal aspect of the carpus. The tendons of insertion of the extensor carpi radialis muscle on the proximal ends of the second and third metacarpal bone are severed and elevated to complete exposure. The joint capsule is removed from the dorsal aspect of the carpus, the joint is flexed and articular cartilage removed at all levels of the carpus using a high speed burr or a small osteotome.

A 3.5 dynamic compression plate (DCP) is generally used for fixation; occasionally a 2.7 or 4.5 DCP is used. Although it has been recommended that the carpus is fused with 10° of extension (Parker *et al.* 1981), in most cases little or no contouring of the plate is necessary to produce this because of the natural angulation of the metacarpus (Fig. 4.105a).

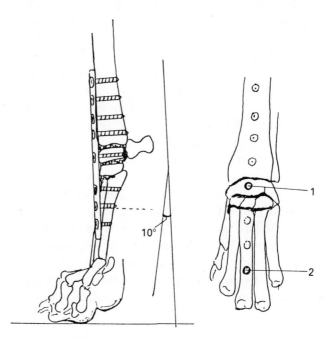

Fig. 4.105a Pancarpal arthrodesis; little or no contouring of the plate is needed to produce 10° of extension because of the natural angulation of the metacarpus.

Fig. 4.105b Pancarpal arthrodesis; position of the first two screws.

The plate is applied to the dorsal aspect of the carpus with a minimum of seven screws; one in the radial carpal bone, three in the third metacarpal bone and at least three in the distal radius. The screw hole in the radial carpal bone is prepared first, followed by the distal screw hole in the third metacarpus. A cancellous bone graft is collected from the proximal humerus and packed into the carpal joint spaces. The graft is held in place by the plate using two screws at the prepared sites, and a third screw in the distal radius. The remainder of the screws are placed in routine fashion. The carpus is supported with a gutter splint for 6 weeks following surgery.

Plate fixation for partial carpal arthrodesis

The use of a 'T' plate for partial carpal arthrodesis was described by Earley (1981) and Brinker *et al.* (1983). Alternatively a five or six hole 2.7 or 3.5 DCP can be used for fixation. The surgical approach is as described for pancarpal arthrodesis. Articular cartilage is removed from the intercarpal and carpometacarpal joints. Autogenous cancellous bone is packed into the joint spaces. The plate is applied to the dorsal aspect of the radial carpal bone and third metacarpal bone taking care that the proximal end of the plate does not interfere with movement of the radiocarpal joint. The proximal two screws are directed into the radial carpal bone and the distal three or four screws are placed in the third metacarpal bone. The carpus is supported with a gutter splint for 6 weeks following surgery.

In dogs which require bilateral carpal arthrodesis the minimum interval between each operation is 5 weeks. The untreated carpus is splinted during this period.

Follow-up radiographs are routinely taken 3 months after surgery to assess carpal fusion. Plates are generally left *in situ* and are only removed if lameness or soft tissue reaction is caused by implant loosening or low grade infection.

Results of treatment

The results of treatment by carpal arthrodesis in a series of 50 dogs were published by Denny & Barr (1991). Fifty-six carpal arthrodesis were carried out in the dogs. Six of these had bilateral arthrodeses. A DCP (Straumann Great Britain Ltd), placed on the dorsal aspect of the carpus, was used for fixation in all cases. The main indication for pancarpal arthrodesis was a hyperextension injury of the radiocarpal joint. Forty-three pancarpal arthrodeses were performed in 40 dogs (a bilateral procedure was performed in three). Hyperextension injuries of the intercarpal and carpometacarpal joints were treated by partial carpal arthrodesis in 10 dogs; three of these had bilateral procedures. Seventy-four per cent of dogs treated by pancarpal arthrodesis regained full limb function. Only 50% of cases treated by partial carpal arthrodesis had a similar result.

The most common complication of pancarpal arthrodesis was loosening of one or more of the distal screws. This was invariably associated with lameness which rapidly resolved once the loose implant had been removed. In three cases the distal screw was removed at 4 months and in another the distal two screws were removed at 1 year.

Plate removal was necessary in eight cases. This was carried out 4–6 months post-operatively in five cases and in the other three at 10 months, 1 year and 4 years. Soft tissue reaction over the plate and persistent lameness caused by implant loosening or low grade infection was the main indication for plate removal. Carpal instability after plate removal occurred in two dogs; one of these fractured its plate 1 year after surgery. Both animals were subsequently treated by external coaptation.

A gutter splint should be used to support the carpus for 6 weeks after removal of the plate to minimize the risk of fracture at one of the levels of carpal arthrodesis. If there is any doubt about the completeness of carpal fusion at the time of plate removal then pack an autogenous cancellous bone graft over the cranial aspect of the carpus after removal of the plate.

In conclusion, pancarpal arthrodesis has proved a useful salvage procedure for the management of carpal disorders particularly carpal hyperextension injuries. Based on these results the management of hyperextension injuries by partial carpal arthrodesis using a plate for fixation is questionable. Hyperextension injuries of the intercarpal or carpometacarpal joints should be managed by pancarpal arthrodesis or by partial arthrodesis using pins for fixation.

CARPAL ARTHRODESIS IN THE CAT
The indications for carpal arthrodesis in the cat are the same as the dog. Crossed Kirschner wires (Fig. 4.105c) can be used for fixation in most cases, but additional external support should be provided with a gutter splint on the

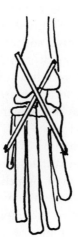

Fig. 4.105c Carpal arthrodesis in the cat using crossed Kirschner wires for fixation.

caudal aspect of the carpus for 6 weeks. The carpus is fixed with about 10° of extension except in cases of radial nerve paresis. Carpal arthrodesis is said to be useful in cats with low radial nerve paresis (Herron 1990, personal communication). Here the carpus should be fixed in a hyperextended position to minimize trauma to the toes. If the carpus is hyperextended then the crossed Kirschner wire technique is no longer possible and under these circumstances an AO veterinary cuttable plate (VCP, Straumann Great Britain Ltd) is used with 1.5 mm or 2 mm diameter cortical screws. External support should be provided for 6 weeks following surgery.

Fractures of the metacarpal bones
Fractures of the metacarpal bones are common in dogs and are usually caused when the foot is crushed by a car wheel. Consequently the fractures may be multiple, comminuted or compound. However, the prognosis is invariably good and the fractures heal well following closed reduction and immobilization in a plaster cast. In grossly displaced fractures of the metacarpal (or metatarsal) bones intramedullary fixation using pins or Kirschner wires (see Fig. 4.102b) is used (Whittick 1974). In the racing Greyhound, plate fixation is recommended and the AO VCP has proved very suitable (Dee 1991).

Fractures of the phalanges
Fractures of the phalanges occur in the racing Greyhound due to a rapid or incoordinate turn placing torsional stress on the phalanx but in other breeds the fracture is more commonly caused by a crush injury. Closed reduction and external support in a plaster cast is a satisfactory form of treatment for all dogs except the racing Greyhound. If the Greyhound is to regain its form best results are obtained by treating the fracture by open reduction and fixation with a lag screw or wire sutures. If lameness persists after the fracture has healed performance may improve after amputation of the distal phalanx to relieve pressure on the fracture site.

Dislocation of the interphalangeal joints — 'knocked-up toe' (Davies 1958; Bateman 1960; Hickman 1975)
Dislocation of the interphalangeal joints is an injury which is frequently encountered in the racing Greyhound. The digits of the left forefoot, particularly the fifth, are usually affected.

Dislocation and subluxations of the interphalangeal joints seldom remain stable following reduction in the Greyhound. Although attention has been directed to affecting stabilization by internal fixation the results are disappointing and consequently the trend is to relieve pressure on the joint.

Treatment of a dislocation or subluxation of the distal interphalangeal joint comprises reduction followed by removal of the nail. The dog is given 4 weeks' rest before training is resumed. If lameness persists then amputation is performed through the distal end of the second phalanx and the third phalanx is removed. Care is taken to conserve the pad.

Dislocations and subluxation of the proximal interphalangeal joint are best treated by arthrodesis of the joint in the normal standing position. Arthrodesis is achieved by removal of the articular surfaces followed by fixation with a Kirschner wire and tension band wire (Dee *et al.* 1990) (Fig. 4.105d and e) or by the application of a plate. The nail is also removed to relieve stress on the joint. If lameness persists complete amputation of the third phalanx is carried out.

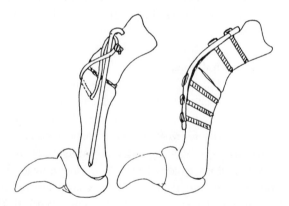

Fig. 4.105d P1, P2 arthrodesis using a Kirschner wire and tension band wire.

Fig. 4.105e P1, P2 arthrodesis using a plate for fixation.

Fractures of the proximal volar sesamoid
(Davies *et al.* 1969)
These fractures are seen mainly in the racing Greyhound and the second and seventh sesamoid on the right fore are most frequently fractured. The fracture tends to be transverse but can be comminuted. It may heal if the foot is immobilized in a cast with the digits in flexion but fibrous

non-unions often persist and Bateman (1959) recommends surgical excision of the fractured sesamoid to prevent lameness.

Abnormalities of the volar sesamoids bones in Rottweilers
In a survey of 50 unselected Rottweilers examined by Vaughan & France (1986), 44% had lesions, deformity, calcification or fragmentation of the sesamoids, particularly the second and seventh in the foreleg. These lesions are often asymptomatic but if the lesion is thought to be significant, this can be tested by infiltration of local anaesthetic around the sesamoid in question. If the sesamoid is the cause of lameness then the local nerve block should abolish lameness. Bennett & Kelly (1985) also described the condition as a degenerative disease of the volar sesamoids characterized by degenerative changes in the articular cartilage of the sesamoid bones and by calcification within ligamentous attachments. They also pointed out that the lesion can be asymptomatic but if associated with pain and lameness surgical excision of the affected sesamoid should provide relief.

Section of the digital flexor tendons
The injury is most frequently caused by the dog stepping on broken glass. The wound occurs between the digital pads on the caudal aspect of the metacarpus or metatarsus. There is profuse haemorrhage and the natural tendency is to control this with sutures and bandage and the important tendon injury is missed. Section of the superficial digital flexor tendon is of little significance but if the deep digital flexor is cut, then flattening of one or more digits occurs. The severed tendon should be repaired (see p. 376) and post-operatively a cast is applied for 3–4 weeks to maintain the foot in a semi-flexed position to ease tension on the sutures.

APPLICATION OF FLEXION BANDAGE
(Fig. 4.105f and g)
A soft conforming bandage, e.g. Soffband is applied first. Next a layer of Elastoplast is applied leaving the central toes exposed. Take a strip of Elastoplast in which two holes have been cut; these will form an anchor point around the nails of digits 3 and 4. This Elastoplast strip is used to bend the foot into the flexed position so that tension is eased on the tendon repair. A final layer of Elastoplast is applied completing the bandage.

(f)

(g)

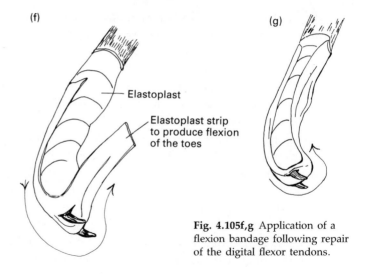

Elastoplast

Elastoplast strip
to produce flexion
of the toes

Fig. 4.105f,g Application of a
flexion bandage following repair
of the digital flexor tendons.

AMPUTATION OF THE FORELIMB

The indications for amputation of the forelimb include:
1 Gross trauma.
2 Gangrene.
3 Paralysis.
4 Osteomyelitis.
5 Neoplasia.

Although complete amputation of the forelimb including
the scapula can be performed (Harvey 1974) it is simpler
to amputate the limb through the proximal third of the
humerus (Hickman 1964).

A semicircular skin incision is made on the lateral aspect
of the limb (Fig. 4.106). The limb is then lifted by an
assistant and a similar incision is made on the medial side
of the limb. The skin flap is reflected and the brachial
artery and vein identified between the triceps and the
biceps muscle (Fig. 4.107). Both vessels are ligated and

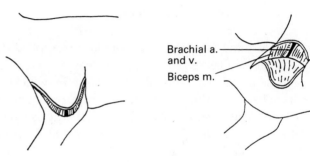

Brachial a.
and v.

Biceps m.

Fig. 4.106   Fig. 4.107

severed. (Early ligation of these vessels reduces the amount of haemorrhage during the operation.)

The limb is lowered, the lateral skin flap is elevated and the cephalic vein ligated (Fig. 4.108). The common tendon of insertion of the triceps is severed and the muscle mass reflected proximally to expose the brachialis and radial nerve (Fig. 4.108). The nerve and brachialis muscle are severed to complete exposure of the distal humerus (Fig. 4.109).

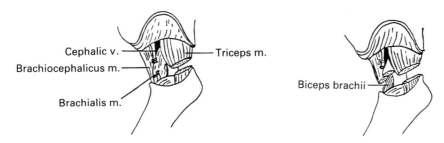

Fig. 4.108   Fig. 4.109

The muscles are then bluntly pushed back from the shaft with a swab until the proximal third is exposed. Amputation is completed by sawing through the humerus at this level (Fig. 4.110a).

Dead space between the muscle bellies is closed with a series of purse string sutures started close to the cut end of the bone and working towards the severed ends of the muscles (Fig. 4.110b). Finally the ends of the muscles are sutured together with horizontal mattress sutures and the skin flaps closed in the same manner.

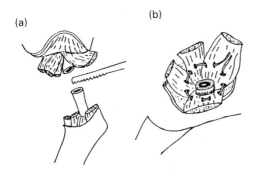

Fig. 4.110

Anderson T.J., Carmichael S. & Miller A. (1990) Intercondylar humeral fracture in the dog: a review of 20 cases. *J. Small Anim. Pract.* **31**, 437–42.

Ball D.C. (1968) A case of medial luxation of the canine shoulder joint and its surgical correction. *Vet. Rec.* **83**, 195.

Barr A.R.S. & Denny H.R. (1985) The management of elbow instability caused by premature closure of the distal radial growth plate in dogs. *J. Small Anim. Pract.* **26**, 427.

Bateman J.K. (1959) Fracture of the sesamoid bones in the dog. *Vet. Rec.* **71**, 101.

Bateman J.K. (1960) The racing Greyhound. *Vet. Rec.* **72**, 895.

Bennett D. & Campbell J.R. (1979) Unusual soft tissue orthopaedic problems in the dog. *J. Small Anim. Pract.* **20**, 27–39.

Bennett D. & Kelly D.F. (1985) Sesamoid disease as a cause of lameness in young dogs. *J. Small Anim. Pract.* **26**, 567–79.

Birkeland R. (1967) Osteochondritis dissecans in the humeral head of the dog. *Nord. Vet. Med.* **19**, 294.

Boyd H.B. & Boals J.C. (1969) The Monteggia lesion. *Clin. Orthop. Relat. Res.* **66**, 94.

Braden T.D. (1975) Surgical correction of humeral fractures. In: Bojrab M.J. (ed.) *Current Techniques in Small Animal Surgery*. Lea & Febiger, Philadelphia.

Bradney J.W. (1967) Non-union of the anconeal process in the dog. *Aust. Vet. J.* **43**, 215.

Brinker W.O. (1974) Fractures of the humerus. In: *Canine Surgery*, 2nd Archibald ed. American Vet Publications Inc. Drawer KK, Santa Barbara, California, p. 1019.

Brinker W.O., Piermattei P.L. & Flo G.L. (1983) *Handbook of Small Animal Orthopaedics and Fracture Treatment*. W.B. Saunders Company, Philadelphia.

Brinker W.A., Piermattei D.L. & Flo G.L. (1990) Fractures of the carpus, metacarpus and phalanges. In: *Handbook of Small Animal Orthopaedics and Fracture Treatment*, 2nd edn. W.B. Saunders, Philadelphia, pp. 216–17, 530–6.

Campbell J.R. (1968) Shoulder lameness in the dog. *J. Small Anim. Pract.* **9**, 189.

Campbell J.R. (1979) Congenital luxation of the elbow of the dog. *Veterinary Annual*, 19th edn. Scientechnica, Bristol.

Caywood D., Wallace L.J. & Johnston G.R. (1977) The use of a Plastic Plate for repair of a comminuted scapular body fracture in a dog. *J. Am. Anim. Hosp. Assoc.* **13**, 176.

Chambers J.N. & Bjorling D.E. (1982) Palmar surface plating for arthrodesis of the canine carpus. *J. Am. Anim. Hosp. Assoc.* **18**, 875–82.

Cheli R. (1976) Surgical treatment of fractures of the scapula in the dog and cat. *Folia Vet. Lat.* **6**, 189.

Clayton-Jones & Vaughan L.C. (1968) Osteochondritis disease in the dog. *J. Small Anim. Pract.* **9**, 283.

Clayton-Jones D.G. & Vaughan L.C. (1970) Disturbances of the growth of the radius in dogs. *J. Small Anim. Pract.* **11**, 453.

Cockett P.A. & Clayton-Jones D.G. (1982) Triceps tendon rupture in the dog following corticosteroid injection. *J. Small Anim. Pract.* **23**, 779.

Corley E.A., Sutherland T.M. & Carlson W.D. (1968) Genetic aspects of canine elbow dysplasia. *J. Am. Vet. Med. Assoc.* **153**, 543.

Craig P.H. & Riser W.H. (1965) Osteochondritis dissecans in the proximal humerus of the dog. *J. Am. Vet. Rad. Soc.* **6**, 40.

Davies J.J. (1958) Greyhound injuries. *Vet. Rec.* **70**, 660.

Davies J.V. & Clayton-Jones D.G. (1982) Triceps rupture in the dog following corticosteroid injection. *J. Small Anim. Pract.* **23**, 779–87.

Davis P.E., Bellenger C.R. & Turner D.M. (1969) Fractures of the sesamoid bones in the Greyhound. *Aust. Vet. J.* **45**, 15.

De Angelis M. & Schwartz A. (1970) Surgical correction of cranial dislocation of the scapulohumeral joint in a dog. *J. Am. Vet. Med. Assoc.* **156**, 435.

Dee J.F., Dee L.G. & Eaton-Wells R.D. (1990) Injuries in high performance dogs. In: Whittick W.G. (ed.) *Canine Orthopaedics*, 2nd edn. Lea & Febiger, Philadelphia, pp. 519–70.

Dee J. (1991) Peak performance patients, current surgical therapy. *Waltham Int. Focus* **1**(2), 2–10.

Denny H.R. (1976) The treatment of growth disturbances of the canine radius and ulna. *The Veterinary Annual* 16th edn. Wright Scientechnica, Bristol, p. 170.

Denny H.R. (1983) Condylar-fractures of the humerus in the dog: a review of 133 cases. *J. Small Anim. Pract.* **24**, 185.

Denny H.R. & Barr A.R.S. (1991) Partial and pancarpal arthrodesis in the dog: a review of 50 cases. *J. Small Anim. Pract.* **32**, 329–34.

Denny H.R. & Gibbs C. (1980) The surgical treatment of osteochondritis dissecans and ununited coronoid process in the canine elbow. *J. Small Anim. Pract.* **21**, 323.

Earley T.D. (1981) Partial arthrodesis of the carpus. Presented at Canine Carpus and Tarsus Shortcourse, University of Tennessee, Knoxville, Tennessee. Reference cited by Brinker, W.O., Piermattei, D.L. & Flo, G.L. (1983) In: *Handbook of Small Animal Orthopaedics and Fracture Treatment*, 1st edn. W.B. Saunders, Philadelphia, p. 404.

Evans P.J. (1968) Shoulder dysplasia in a labrador. *J. Small Anim. Pract.* **9**, 189.

Griffiths R.C. (1968) Osteochondritis dissecans of the canine shoulder. *J. Am. Vet. Med. Assoc.* **153**, 1733.

Grøndalen J. & Rørvick A.M. (1980) Arthrosis in the elbow joint of young rapidly growing dogs IV. Ununited anconeal process. A follow up investigation of operated dogs. *Nord. Vet. Med.* **32**, 212.

Guthrie S. & Pidduck H.G. (1990) Hereditability of elbow osteochondrosis within a closed population of dogs. *J. Small Anim. Pract.* **31**, 93–6.

Hanlon G.F. (1969) Additional radiographic observations on elbow dysplasia in the dog. *J. Am. Vet. Med. Assoc.* **155**, 2045.

Hare W.C.D. (1961) The ages at which the centres of ossification appear roentgenographically in the limb bones of the dog. *Am. J. Vet. Res.* **22**, 825.

Harvey C.E. (1974) Complete forequarter amputation in the dog and cat. *J. Am. Anim. Hosp. Assoc.* **10**, 125.

Herron M.R. (1970) Ununited anconeal process. A new approach to surgical repair. *Mod. Vet. Pract.* **51**, 30.

Herron M. (1990) Shoulder arthrodesis in dogs and cats. Personal communication.

Hickman J. (1964) *Veterinary Orthopaedics*. Oliver & Boyd, Edinburgh and London.

Hickman J. (1975) Greyhound injuries. *J. Small Anim. Pract.* **16**, 455.

Hohn R.B. *et al.* (1971) Surgical stabilization of recurrent luxations. *Vet. Clin. N. Am.* **1**(3), 537.

Holt P.E. (1978) Longitudinal fracture of the scapula in a dog. *Vet. Rec.* **102**, 311.

Houlton J.E.F. (1984) Osteochondrosis of the shoulder and elbow joints in dogs. *J. Small Anim. Pract.* **25**, 399–413.

Hufford T.J., Olmstead M.L. & Butler H.C. (1975) Contracture of the infraspinatus muscle and surgical correction in 2 dogs. *J. Am. Anim. Hosp. Assoc.* **11**, 613.

Johnson K.A. (1980) Carpal arthrodesis in dogs. *Aust. Vet. J.* **56**, 565–73.

Johnson K.A. (1987) Accessory carpal bone fractures in the racing Greyhound. *Vet. Surg.* **16**, 60.

Johnson K.A., Piermattei D.L., Davis P.E. & Bellenger C.R. (1988) Characteristics of accessory carpal bone fractures in 50 racing Greyhounds. *Vet. Comp. Orthop. Traumatol.* **2**, 51/104–54/107.

Knecht C.D. & Greene J.A. (1977) Surgical approach to the brachial plexus in small animals. *J. Am. Anim. Hosp. Assoc.* **13**, 592–4.

Knight G.S. (1956) The use of transfixion screws for internal fixation of fractures in small animals. *Vet. Rec.* **68**, 415.

Knight G.S. (1959) Internal fixation of the fractured lateral humeral condyle. *Vet. Rec.* **71**, 667.

Leighton R.L. (1969) Open reduction of the canine shoulder joint. *J. Am. Vet. Med. Assoc.* **155**, 1987.

Leighton R.L. (1978) Osteochondritis dissecans of the elbow in a dog. *Vet. Med. Small Anim. Clin.* **73**, 311.

Ljunggren G., Cawley A.J. & Archibald J. (1966) The elbow dysplasias in the dog. *J. Am. Vet. Med. Assoc.* **148**, 887.

Mason T.A. & Baker M.J. (1978) The surgical management of elbow joint deformity associated with premature growth plate closure in dogs. *J. Small Anim. Pract.* **19**, 639.

McCurnin D.M., Slusher R. & Grier R.L. (1976) A medical approach to the canine elbow joint. *J. Am. Anim. Hosp. Assoc.* **12**, 475.

Neal T.M. (1975) Fractures of the radius and ulna. In Bojrab M.J. (ed.) *Current Techniques in Small Animal Surgery.* Lea & Febiger, Philadelphia.

Newton C.D. (1974) Surgical management of distal ulnar physeal growth disturbances in dogs. *J. Am. Vet. Med. Assoc.* **164**, 479.

O'Brien T.R., Morgan J.P. & Suter P.F. (1971) Epiphyseal plate injury in the dog: a radiographic study of growth disturbance in the forelimb. *J. Small Anim. Pract.* **12**, 19.

Olsson S.E. (1975) Lameness in the dog. *Proc. Am. Anim. Hosp. Assoc.* **42**, 363.

Olsson S.E. (1976) *Gaines Progress Symposium 1976.* Gaines Dog Research Centre, White Plains NY.

Parker R.B., Brown S.G. & Wind A.P. (1981) Pancarpal arthrodesis in the dog. A review of 45 cases. *Vet. Surg.* **10**, 35–43.

Parkes L.J., Riser W.H. & Martin C.L. (1966) Clinicopathologic conference. *J. Anim. Vet. Assoc.* **149**, 1086.

Payne-Johnson M. & Lewis D.G. (1981) A technique for fixation of intercondylar humeral fractures in immature small dogs. *J. Small Anim. Pract.* **22**, 293.

Piermattei D.C. & Greeley R.G. (1979) *An Atlas of Surgical Approaches to the Bones of the Dog and Cat*, 2nd edn. W.B. Saunders Company, Philadelphia.

Read R.A., Armstrong S.J., O'Keefe J.D. & Eger C.E. (1990) Fragmentation of the medial coronoid process of the ulna in dogs: A study of 109 cases. *J. Small Anim. Pract.* **31**, 330–4.

Schwarz, P.D. & Schrader S.C. (1984) Ulnar fracture and dislocation of the proximal radial epiphysis (Monteggia lesion) in the dog and cat: A review of 28 cases. *J. Am. Vet. Assoc.* **185**, 190.

Shires P.K., Hulse D.A. & Kearney M.K. (1985) Carpal hyperextension in two-month-old pups. *J. Am. Vet. Med. Assoc.* **186**, 49–52.

Shuttleworth A.C. (1938) Condylar fractures of the humerus in the dog. *Vet. J.* **94**, 275.

Slocum B. & Devine T. (1982) Practical carpal fusion in the dog. *J. Am. Vet. Med. Assoc.* **180**, 1204–8.

Smith C.W. & Stowater J.L. (1975) Osteochondritis dissecans of the canine shoulder joint. A review of 35 cases. *J. Am. Anim. Hosp. Assoc.* **11**, 658.

Sumner-Smith G. (1966) Observations on epiphyseal fusion in the canine appendicular skeleton. *J. Small Anim. Pract.* **7**, 303.

Van Sickle D.C. (1966) The relationship of ossification to canine elbow dysplasia. *J. Am. Anim. Hosp. Assoc.* **2**, 24.

Vaughan L.C. (1967) Dislocation of the shoulder joint in the dog and cat. *J. Small Anim. Pract.* **8**, 45.

Vaughan L.C. (1976) Growth plate defects in dogs. *Vet. Rec.* **98**, 185.

Vaughan L.C. (1979) Muscle and tendon injuries in dogs. *J. Small Anim. Pract.* **20**, 711−36.

Vaughan L.C. & Clayton-Jones D.G. (1968) Osteochondritis dissecans of the head of the humerus in dogs. *J. Small Anim. Pract.* **9**, 283.

Vaughan L.C. & Clayton-Jones D.G. (1969) Congenital dislocation of the shoulder joint in the dog. *J. Small Anim. Pract.* **10**, 1.

Vaughan L.C. & France C. (1986) Abnormalities of the volar and plantar sesamoids bones in Rottweilers. *J. Small Anim. Pract.* **27**, 551−8.

Walker R.G. & Hickman J. (1958) Injuries of the elbow in the dog. *Vet. Rec.* **70**, 1191.

Wheeler S.J., Clayton-Jones D.G. & Wright J.A. (1986) The diagnosis of brachial plexus disorders in dogs: a review of 22 cases. *J Small Anim. Pract.* **27**, 147−57.

Whittick W.G. (1974) *Canine Orthopaedics*. Lea & Febiger, Philadelphia.

Willer R.L., Johnson K.A., Turner T.M. & Piermattei D.L. (1990) Partial carpal arthrodesis for third degree carpal sprains: A review of 45 carpi. *Vet. Surg.* **19**, 334−40.

Wood A.K.W., Bath M.C. & Mason T.A. (1975) Osteochondritis dissecans of the distal humerus in a dog. *Vet. Rec.* **91**, 489.

Chapter 5
The Hindlimb

EXAMINATION OF THE DOG WITH HINDLEG LAMENESS

A protocol for examination of the lame dog has already been given at the beginning of Chapter 4. Common or well-recognized causes of hindleg lameness are listed below. These should be kept in mind when the examination is carried out.

Traumatic conditions of the hindleg

PELVIS
Fracture.

HIP
Acetabular fractures.
Fractures of the femoral head or neck ± trochanteric fractures.
Hip dislocation.

FEMUR
Fractures of the proximal femur (see above).
Fractures of the shaft.
Supracondylar and condylar fractures.

STIFLE
Rupture of:
1 Anterior cruciate ligament ± damage to medial meniscus.
2 Collateral ligament.
3 Straight patellar ligament.
Traumatic dislocations of the patella.
Traumatic dislocations of the stifle.
Avulsion of the tendon of origin of the long digital extensor muscle.
Fractures of the distal femur (see above).
Fractures of the patella.
Fractures of the proximal tibia
   avulsion of the tibial crest
   separation of the proximal epiphysis of the tibia.

Fractures of the proximal tibia (see above)
Fractures of the shaft.
Distal tibial fractures
  malleolar fractures
  separation of distal epiphysis.

HOCK

Malleolar fracture.
Rupture of collateral ligaments.

Severe abrasion injury.

} Dislocation of the
  tibiotarsal joint.

Fractures of the os calcis.
Injuries of the Achilles tendon.
Intertarsal subluxation (rupture of plantar ligaments —
  Shelties, Collies).
Fracture of the central tarsal bone.
Fractures of the metatarsus and digits.

Developmental disorders causing hindleg lameness

HIP

Hip dysplasia	Most large breeds, German Shepherds, Labradors, Golden Retrievers especially
Legge Perthes disease	Terriers

STIFLE

Congenital medial luxation of the patella	Small breeds, Cavalier King Charles Spaniels currently seen most frequently.
Osteochondritis dissecans	Wolfhounds, Labradors, Golden Retrievers, German Shepherds Greyhounds
Genu valgum	Giant breeds

HOCK

Osteochondritis dissecans	Labradors, Golden Retrievers, Rottweilers, Wolfhounds

Gradual onset of hindleg lameness in older dogs

1 Lumbosacral lesions — 'cauda equina syndrome'.
2 Osteoarthritis of hip.
3 Osteosarcoma distal femur.

4 Osteo-arthritis of stifle.

5 Bilateral anterior cruciate ligament rupture in overweight dogs.

6 Osteosarcoma proximal tibia.

Physical examination for hindleg lameness

TRAUMATIC CONDITIONS OF THE HIP

The owner or an assistant should steady the dog's head while examination of the hindquarters is being carried out. The stages in the examination given here relate to specific injuries or conditions and obviously do not have to be carried to these lengths in every case, however, each joint should be palpated systematically and both legs carefully compared. Do not omit the rest of the examination when the diagnosis appears obvious. For example, a young Labrador may have hip dysplasia but it is quite possible for that animal to have osteochondritis dissecans in its hock joints as well.

The palpable areas of the pelvis and hip are illustrated in Fig. 5.1a. The external landmarks include the iliac crests, the greater trochanter and the tuber ischii. On rectal examination, the ischium, medial acetabulum and pelvis can be palpated. When traumatic injuries of the pelvis and hip are suspected, i.e. pelvic fractures, dislocation of the hip, fractures of the femoral head and neck, then feel the external palpable landmarks of the pelvis. Compare their relationship with the greater trochanters (Fig. 5.1a) and check for differences between each side of the pelvis. Rectal examination can also be useful to confirm pelvic fractures. These fractures are occasionally complicated by bladder rupture or injury to the urinary tract. If there is any doubt about the integrity of the bladder or urethra then cystography and/or

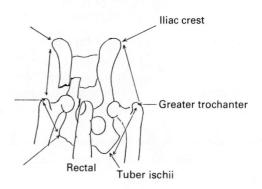

Fig. **5.1a**

urethrography should be undertaken as necessary.

Compare the length of both hindlegs by gripping them just proximal to the stifles, then extend them. Most hip dislocations result in craniodorsal displacement of the femoral head in relation to the acetabulum so the affected leg will be shorter.

Remember that the dog with a fracture of the femoral neck will also have apparent shortening of the affected leg but there is more pain and crepitus evident on manipulation than in a dislocation.

DEVELOPMENTAL DISORDERS OF THE HIP

The clinical signs associated with hip dysplasia include poor muscling of the hindquarters with laxity, pain and crepitus on manipulation of the hips. There are specific tests for hip laxity. Make the dog walk while your hands are held firmly over each greater trochanter. If the hips are very loose, crepitus will be felt as the femoral head slips in and out of the acetabulum. Lie the dog on its side, grip the uppermost leg proximal to the stifle with one hand and try to raise the femoral head out of the acetabulum while keeping the leg parallel to the ground. At the same time place the other hand firmly over the greater trochanter and try and bounce the femoral head in and out of the acetabulum. A definite 'clunking' sound will be appreciated if the hip is loose.

Try and elicit the Ortolani sign. This can be done with the dog standing or lying on its side. Grip the stifle, adduct the leg and then push the femur towards the hip joint. If there is laxity of the joint the femoral head will ride up on the dorsal rim of the acetabulum and then click back into its normal position as pressure on the lower leg is released.

Dogs with hip dysplasia often have taut pectineus muscles. Lie the dog on its back and abduct both hindlegs. It should be possible to bring the stifles almost in contact with the ground. Check the pectineus muscle during the procedure (it is the most prominent muscle over the medial side of the hip) — does it become excessively taut or painful? Although many older German Shepherd dogs presented with hindleg weakness will have radiographic evidence of hip dysplasia, their clinical signs are not usually due to this but are caused by a spinal disorder, chronic degenerative radiculomyelopathy (see p. 127).

Chronic hip pain particularly on abduction of the joint in Terrier breeds under a year of age is generally due to Legge Perthes disease.

THE FEMUR

Femoral shaft fractures should be obvious on clinical examination. Supracondylar fractures of the femur are not always unstable and are sometimes missed on a cursory examination. If there is swelling and pain following trauma, take a radiograph and this should confirm the fracture if present.

The gradual development of a painful swelling involving the distal femur or proximal tibia in larger breeds is most likely to be caused by an osteosarcoma.

THE STIFLE

The palpable areas of the stifle are the distal femur, proximal tibia, tibial crest, patella and straight patellar ligament. Compare both stifles for differences in size. In chronic anterior cruciate ligament injuries the medial side of the stifle over the proximal tibia becomes thickened. Crepitus on manipulation of the stifle is usually due to osteo-arthritis. Distinct 'clicking' noises coming from the stifle are heard in dogs with anterior cruciate ligament rupture when the femoral condyles slip in and out of their normal position on the menisci. Check the stability of the stifle joint; the commonest cause of lameness is rupture of the anterior cruciate ligament and this diagnosis is confirmed by demonstration of the anterior draw movement (Fig. 5.1b).

The collateral ligaments of the stifle can also be damaged and give instability. If, for example, the medial collateral ligament is ruptured it is possible to displace the tibia laterally on the femur. The stifle joint can also be hinged open on the medial side (Fig. 5.1c).

The position of the patella should be checked. Upward displacement or laxity of the straight patellar ligament is associated with injuries to the ligament or fractures of the patella.

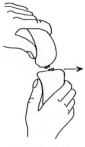

Anterior draw
movement

Fig. 5.1b

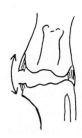

Rupture of
medial collateral
ligament

Fig. 5.1c

The most common developmental disorder of the stifle is congenital medial luxation of the patella. Dogs with intermittent patella luxation walk normally until the patella luxates; the leg may then be carried in a semi-flexed position for a few paces. The dog stretches the leg and is generally able to reduce the luxation itself and consequently resumes a normal action. Permanent medial luxation gives a crouching hindleg action with lateral bowing of the stifle. Check if the patella is riding in the trochlea; can it be displaced medially. The best position to attempt displacement is with the stifle extended or slightly flexed. Compare the position of the tibial crests.

Dogs with permanent medial luxation of the patella will generally have a tibial crest which is rotated 15–90° medial to the long axis of the stifle.

THE HOCK

Most areas of the hock can be palpated. Check the range of hock flexion; it should be possible to touch the anterior aspect of the tibia with the tips of the toes when the joint is fully flexed. A straight hock with a limited range of flexion is a feature of osteochondritis dissecans. If the hock is 'dropped' giving a plantigrade stance, check the Achilles tendon for rupture or avulsion from the os calcis. Also check the os calcis for fracture.

Dropping of the hock with caudal bowing of the intertarsal region is seen in overweight Shelties and Collies when rupture of the plantar ligaments causes an intertarsal subluxation.

Fractures of the central tarsal bone are seen in the racing Greyhound and cause marked swelling and pain. If the clinical and radiological examination fails to reveal a cause of hind leg lameness, it is always worth checking the lumbosacral junction. Palpate this area and extend the junction by extending the hindlegs (does this cause pain?). Take a lateral radiograph of the lumbosacral junction to check for the lesions of the cauda equina which can cause a hindleg lameness (see p. 171).

ORTHOPAEDIC CAUSES OF EXERCISE INTOLERANCE AND COLLAPSE

The conditions which cause exercise intolerance and collapse all impede the function of two or more limbs. Most of the conditions are described in more detail in other sections of the book. They are listed here as a guide to diagnosis.

1 One of the earliest is the *Swimmer syndrome* in puppies.

2 *Spinal conditions*:

(a) Congenital defects, e.g. hemivertebrae — screw tail breeds, Bulldogs, etc. Hindleg ataxia + collapse at 3–4 months.

(b) Cervical spondylopathy (wobbler syndrome) — Great Danes (4 months onwards), Dobermans (1–12 years).

(c) Spinal haemorrhage.

(d) Infarction due to fibrocartilaginous emboli.

(e) Spinal trauma.

(f) Atlanto-axial subluxation — Yorkshire Terriers, Pomeranians under 1 year.

(g) Discs — Dachshunds especially.

(h) Cauda equina lesions — older dogs, larger breeds.

(i) Chronic degenerative radiculomyelopathy — CDRM (older German Shepherds especially).

Peripheral neuropathies

Giant-axonal neuropathy — young German Shepherds.

Distal denervating disease — young dogs, larger breeds.

Progressive axonopathy — Boxers.

3 *Nutritional bone diseases*. Juvenile osteoporosis (nutritional secondary hyperparathyroidism) — pups 3–4 months of age, pain, lameness, reluctance to move.

Skeletal scurvy (hypertrophic osteodystrophy)

Large and giant breeds, 4–6 months.

Metaphyses of long bones enlarged and painful. Intermittent pyrexia.

4 *Developmental disorders*:

(a) Hip dysplasia.

(b) Legge Perthes disease.

(c) Patella luxation.

(d) Osteochondritis dissecans.

5 *Degenerative joint disease*:

(a) Secondary to developmental joint disorders.

(b) Secondary to joint injury, e.g. bilateral anterior cruciate ligament rupture.

(c) Polyarthritis, e.g. rheumatoid.

6 *Bilateral fractures*, e.g. avulsion of tibial crests. *Bilateral ligamentous injury*, e.g. avulsion of straight patellar ligament. Avulsion of gastrocnemeus tendons. Rupture of plantar ligaments of hocks.

7 *Myopathies*.

The cat is an ideal orthopaedic patient having a remarkable ability to survive and recover fully after the most appalling accidents. Healing of bone and soft tissues in this species is invariably good and because the cat is light and agile, it accommodates to some joint injuries which might seriously incapacitate a heavier animal. Examination of the lame cat has already been mentioned under foreleg lameness.

Developmental causes of hindleg lameness in the cat include hip dysplasia and congenital medial luxation of the patella. Acquired causes of lameness include the various traumatic lesions listed in the dog (p. 284). In addition, bite wounds from other cats are common and iliac thrombosis (p. 130) is a specific cause of hindleg dysfunction in this species.

PELVIC FRACTURES

The majority of pelvic fractures in the dog will heal satisfactorily with conservative treatment (Grondalen 1969). However, in some cases malalignment and/or instability of the fragments may result in a prolonged recovery period, narrowing of the pelvic canal or limited hip movement.

In recent years there has been growing interest in the open reduction and internal fixation of pelvic fractures (Leighton 1968; Robins *et al.* 1973; Morris 1970; Kirkbride & Carter 1970; Wheaton *et al.* 1973; Whittick 1974; Brown & Biggart 1975; Brinker 1975; Pond 1975; Hauptman *et al.* 1976).

The open reduction of pelvic fractures is not without hazard and it has been said 'that no other type of fracture lends itself to iatrogenic trauma with so little to show for surgical interference as does the fractured pelvis' (Whittick 1974).

In 1978 the author reviewed a series of pelvic fracture cases. The purpose of the review was to classify pelvic fractures, compare the results of conservative and surgical treatment and establish criteria for adopting either method of treatment.

One hundred and twenty-three dogs had pelvic fracture and the cause of the injury was a road traffic accident in all cases. The majority of dogs were under 3 years of age. Trauma is haphazard in its effects and extent and this is reflected in the great variety in the position and number of pelvic fracture sites recorded. There was a total of 66 combinations of fracture site and no fixed pattern of fracture could be predicted.

The most common complications associated with fracture of the pelvis were: dislocation of the hip in 11% of cases, fracture of the femur in 8% and sciatic nerve paralysis in 2%. Only one dog had a ruptured bladder, while two had rupture of the urethra.

The results of treatment of pelvic fractures were assessed with reference to 40 cases which were managed conservatively and 28 surgically. The follow-up period ranged from 1 to 5 years. Of the dogs treated conservatively, 75% made complete recoveries while the other 25% were either occasionally lame or a slight limp persisted. A slightly higher percentage (78%) of dogs managed surgically made complete recoveries. The recovery period was considerably reduced in most cases. The other 22% were either occasionally lame or had a slight limp, while one dog was severely lame with a permanent sciatic nerve paralysis.

It is difficult to make accurate comparisons between the results of treatment for specific fracture sites because of the number of variable factors, particularly with regard to site and combination of other pelvic fractures. The results of conservative and surgical treatment for sacro-iliac separation or fracture were virtually identical. All the animals except one in the conservative group which had a slight limp made full recoveries in an average time of 6 weeks. Intense pain associated with the injury was rapidly alleviated by surgery.

The duration of lameness after the accident in dogs with fractures of the ilium was reduced by surgical treatment to an average of 3 weeks as compared to 8 weeks for conservative treatment. All the surgical cases made complete recoveries as did the dogs in the conservative group, except for two animals which remained slightly lame.

The recovery period for undisplaced fractures of the acetabulum was slightly reduced by surgical treatment to an average of 6 weeks as opposed to 7 weeks for conservative management. Of cases treated surgically 70% made complete recoveries compared with 55% treated conservatively.

Some dogs with multiple pelvic fractures, particularly those with marked displacement of the iliac or acetabular fragments, had prolonged recovery periods of 6–9 months when managed conservatively; this period was greatly reduced by surgical treatment to an average of 6 weeks.

In conclusion, the majority of dogs with pelvic fractures will recover with conservative treatment. However, the recovery period can be reduced by surgical treatment especially in dogs with multiple bilateral fractures, dogs with fractures of the ilium associated with fracture of the ipsilateral pubis and ischium, and in dogs with displaced fractures of the acetabulum.

Conservative treatment of pelvic fractures

Owners are instructed to rest the dog for a period of 1 month. If it is unable to take weight on the hindlimbs a foam rubber mattress should be provided for the animal to lie on. Massage and regular turning should be encouraged to prevent the development of decubitus ulcers. Owners are also advised to observe that the dog continues to urinate and defaecate and what measures to take to assist it to do so.

The surgical treatment of pelvic fractures

The weight-bearing areas of the pelvis are the sacro-iliac joints, the ilium and the acetabulum. These are the areas that may require internal fixation. The pubis and ischium are non-weight-bearing areas in which fractures do not require fixation as a general rule. Simultaneous reduction of pubic and ischial fractures tends to occur once fractures of weight-bearing areas of the pelvis are reduced and fixed.

The criteria for surgical treatment are pelvic fractures characterized by one or more of the following:

1 Fracture of the acetabulum with displacement of the articular surfaces.
2 Fracture of the ipsilateral ilium, ischium and pubis with resultant instability of the hip joint.
3 Marked displacement of fragments into the pelvic canal.
4 Multiple bilateral fractures of weight-bearing areas of the pelvis.
5 Multiple fractures of the pelvis and hindlimbs.

The open reduction and internal fixation of pelvic fractures is difficult. Reduction should be undertaken as soon as the animal is considered to be in a fit state for surgery. If surgery is delayed for more than a week, reduction of the fragments may prove impossible due to muscle contraction.

SACRO-ILIAC SEPARATION OR FRACTURE

A sacro-iliac separation or fracture (Fig. 5.2) may be stabilized after open or closed reduction by the use of an intramedullary pin driven transversely through the wing of the ilium into the contralateral ilium (Fig. 5.4). The pin is

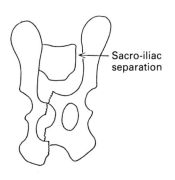

Sacro-iliac separation

Fig. 5.2

passed over the dorsal surface of the sacrum (Leighton 1968; Whittick 1974). Lag screws (Fig. 5.3) can also be used for fixation of the sacro-iliac junction and provide optimal stability (Brinker 1975; Pond 1975; Hauptman *et al.* 1976).

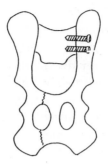 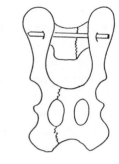

Fig. 5.3   Fig. 5.4

The surgical approach to the sacro-iliac joint and wing of the ilium has been described by Piermattei & Greeley (1966). A skin incision is made directly over the crest of the ilium (Fig. 5.5). The cutaneous trunci muscle and gluteal fascia are incised to reveal the middle gluteal muscle and iliac crest. The wing of the ilium is exposed by elevating the origin of the middle gluteal muscle (Fig. 5.6). The muscles which cover the sacro-iliac joint and insert on the medial surface of the crest and wing of the ilium (iliocostalis and longissimus groups) are usually severely damaged and little elevation is required to expose the joint.

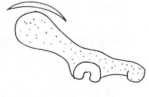

Fig. 5.5

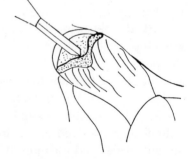

Fig. 5.6

The sacro-iliac joint is reduced and maintained in position with reduction forceps gripping the lateral surface of the ilium and medial dorsal aspect of the wing of the sacrum; alternatively a small Kirschner pin is temporarily driven through the wing of the ilium into the sacrum. The wing of the ilium is then lagged to the sacrum with one or, preferably, two screws. Careful reference is made to the ventrodorsal radiograph of the pelvis to ensure that the screws chosen are of the correct length and do not penetrate the neural canal.

Lag screws are preferred for simple sacro-iliac separation, but when the separation is associated with a sagittal fracture of the sacrum (Fig. 5.4), the fracture is stabilized by trans-fixing the wings of the ilium with a pin because there is usually insufficient bone left on the medial aspect of the sacral fracture to permit the use of a screw without penetration of the neural canal.

FRACTURES OF THE ILIUM

A variety of methods of internal fixation have been used for the treatment of fractures of the ilium (Brinker 1965; Leighton 1968; Brown & Biggart 1975; Robins et al. 1973; Whittick 1974; Brinker 1975).

Fractures of the wing of the ilium are exposed through a lateral skin incision (Fig. 5.7). The middle gluteal muscle is then split in the direction of its fibres to reveal the fracture (Fig. 5.8). Although two pins can be used to stabilize the fracture (Brinker 1975) (Fig. 5.9), a plate is the preferred method of fixation (Fig. 5.10).

Fractures of the shaft of the ilium may be stabilized with a plate (Robins et al. 1973; Brown & Biggart 1975) or alternatively lag screws or Kirschner pins and a wire suture may be used for the fixation of oblique fractures (Brinker 1975).

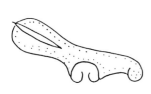

Fig. 5.7

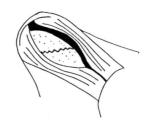

Fig. 5.8

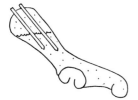

Fig. 5.9

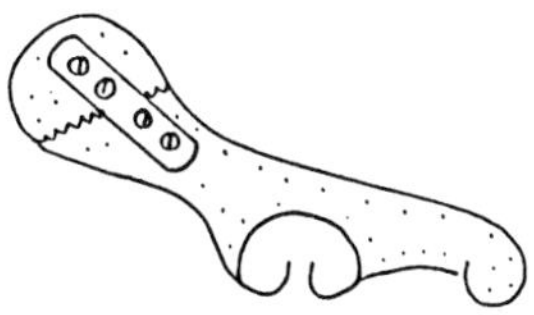

Fig. 5.10

Exposure of the shaft of the ilium is illustrated in Figs 5.11–5.14. A lateral approach with dorsal reflection of the gluteal muscles is used to expose the ilium (Brinker 1975) (Figs 5.11–5.14). A skin incision is made from the iliac crest and extended caudally over the greater trochanter (Fig. 5.12). The incision is continued through the subcutaneous fat and gluteal fascia to expose the aponeurosis between the middle gluteal muscle and the tensor fascia lata (Fig. 5.13). The two muscles are separated and the lateral surface of the body and wing of the ilium exposed by dorsal reflection of the middle and deep gluteal muscles (Fig. 5.14). The application of bone-holding forceps should be done with care to avoid crushing the sciatic nerve which runs close to the medial aspect of the ilium.

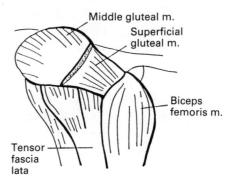

Fig. 5.11

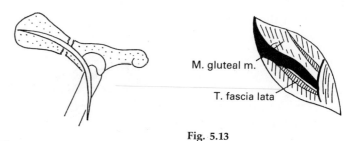

Fig. 5.12

Fig. 5.13

If a plate is used for fixation, it should be carefully contoured to the shape of the ilium, using the radiograph of the contralateral, intact ilium, as a guide (Fig. 5.15). This is important because fracture of the ilium is frequently associated with fracture of the ipsilateral pubis and ischium. However, as the iliac fracture is reduced and its normal contour maintained with the plate, simultaneous reduction of the other fractures usually occurs (Fig. 5.16).

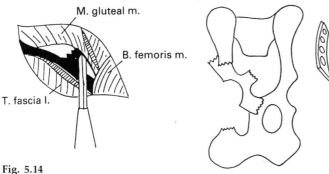

M. gluteal m.

B. femoris m.

T. fascia l.

Fig. 5.14

Fig. 5.15

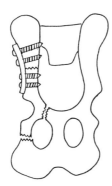

Fig. 5.16

FRACTURES OF THE ACETABULUM
(Wheaton *et al.* 1973; Brinker 1975)

Fractures of the acetabulum must be accurately reduced and primary bone union strived for if normal joint function is to be restored. Undisplaced fractures of the acetabulum are generally treated conservatively, exercise being severely restricted for 6 weeks. Fractures of the caudal acetabulum even if associated with some displacement can also be treated conservatively with a satisfactory outcome. However the cranial acetabulum is the main weight-bearing area of the hip and fractures in this area, particularly if displaced, and especially those in which the femoral head is impacted through the fracture site, should be treated surgically. Special AO/ASIF plates are available for the management of acetabular fractures. These include the acetabular plate designed to curve around the acetabular rim and the reconstruction plate which can be contoured in any direction and cut if necessary. The latter is particularly useful for comminuted or multiple pelvic fractures (Fig. 2.60a p. 101).

A dorsal approach to the hip is used to expose the fracture (Piermattei & Greeley 1966). A skin incision is made directly over the hip (Fig. 5.17). The tensor fascia lata is separated from the biceps femoris to expose the greater trochanter and the gluteal muscles (Figs 5.18 and 5.19). A transverse osteotomy of the trochanter is carried out using a saw or osteotome. (N.B. If a lag screw is to be used to reattach the trochanter, the screw hole should be drilled before the osteotomy is performed.) The trochanter is reflected dorsally to expose the joint capsule and dorsal rim of the acetabulum (Fig. 5.20). An alternative to osteotomy is transection of the tendons of insertion of the gluteal muscles but this is a more traumatic procedure and closure is time consuming. The joint capsule is opened to reveal the femoral head and to allow inspection of the articular surface of the acetabulum. When the fracture involves the caudal part of the joint, it is necessary to expose the body of the ischium; this is achieved after reflection of the gluteal and retraction of the biceps femoris muscles, by severing the insertion of the internal obturator and gemellus muscles close to the trochanteric fossa. These muscles are reflected and used to protect the sciatic nerve to complete the exposure (Fig. 5.20). After the acetabular fracture has been stabilized the trochanter is reattached to the femur using either a lag screw, wire tension band or two wire sutures.

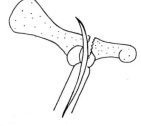

Fig. 5.17

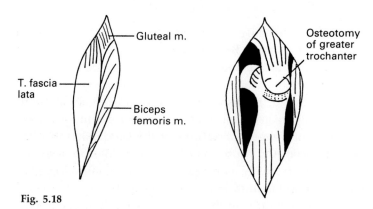

T. fascia lata

Gluteal m.

Biceps femoris m.

Osteotomy of greater trochanter

Fig. 5.18

Fig. 5.19

Oblique fractures of the cranial acetabulum can be stabilized with lag screws (Fig. 5.21). Transverse fractures of the acetabulum can be stabilized in a number of ways, the application of a plate to the dorsal rim of the acetabulum being the preferred method (Fig. 5.22). Alternatively fixation can be achieved by inserting two screws in the dorsal rim, one on either side of the fracture. A wire figure of eight tension band is then placed around the screw heads to

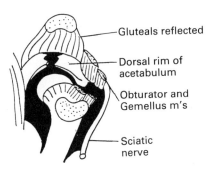

Gluteals reflected

Dorsal rim of acetabulum

Obturator and Gemellus m's

Sciatic nerve

Fig. 5.20

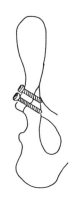

Fig. 5.21

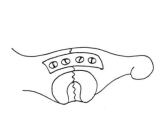

Fig. 5.22

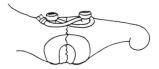

Fig. 5.23

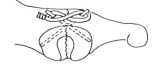

Fig. 5.24

compress the site (Fig. 5.23). Pins can be used instead of screws (Fig. 5.24).

MULTIPLE PELVIC FRACTURES AND MULTIPLE PELVIC FRACTURES COMPLICATED BY HINDLIMB BONE FRACTURES

Dogs having multiple pelvic fractures with or without hindlimb bone fractures are not always good surgical risks in view of the haemorrhage and extensive soft tissue trauma incurred in the accident. However, surgery is undertaken as soon as the animal has recovered from the initial shock and having treated any concomitant injuries to the chest, urinary tract or other soft tissues. The surgical procedures for dogs with multiple fractures are elected to allow pain-free movement while subjecting the animal to a minimum of surgical trauma. Both sides of the pelvis may be repaired in one operation if the animal is considered fit enough. Alternatively repair may be carried out in two operations. The management of a typical case is illustrated in Figs 5.25–5.27.

Pelvic fractures in cats

In practice the majority of pelvic fractures encountered in cats tend to be managed conservatively, the cat being given cage rest for 4–6 weeks. The functional end results tend to be good, however a late complication is chronic

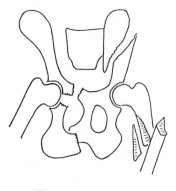

Fig. 5.25 Trace made from the pre-operative radiograph of the pelvis of a three-year-old Labrador with fractures of the left wing of ilium, left femur, right pubis, ischium, acetabulum and a separation of the right sacro-iliac joint.

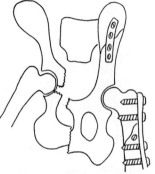

Fig. 5.26 In the first operation the fractures of the left femur and wing of ilium were reduced and plated.

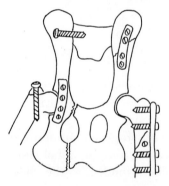

Fig. 5.27 The second operation was performed five days later when the fracture of the right acetabulum was stabilized with a plate and the right sacro-iliac joint with a lag screw.

constipation associated with stenosis of the pelvic canal. This seems to be a far more common problem in cats than dogs. Surgical treatment of pelvic fractures can be undertaken using the same indications and techniques as described in the dog. Recovery periods are greatly reduced by internal fixation of pelvic fractures and reduction of the fragments minimizes pelvic canal stenosis.

Stenosis of the pelvic canal
Malunion of pelvic fractures can result in stenosis of the pelvic canal and cause chronic constipation. This complication is seen most often in cats. The stenosis can be

relieved by splitting the pelvic symphysis and spreading the symphysis open with an allograft (Brinker *et al*. 1983) or a steel insert (Ward 1967; Leighton 1969). An alternative technique, used in cats, is resection of the ventral pelvis. The pubis and ventral ischium are resected with rongeurs (Fig. 5.28a) and the ventral musculature closed in the midline. A ventral midline approach is used to expose the pelvic symphysis. During resection of the ventral ischium care should be taken to protect the obturator nerves which runs through the obturator foramina. Resection of the ventral pelvis (Fig. 5.28b) is a simple technique and has given good results with permanent relief from constipation in a series of six cats treated by the author. The operation does not cause pelvic instability provided the sacro-iliac joints are stable and the other pelvic fractures have healed. Some hindleg weakness may be noticed for a few days following surgery.

(a)   (b)

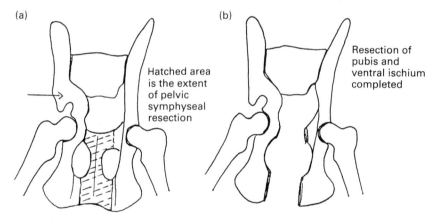

Hatched area is the extent of pelvic symphyseal resection

Resection of pubis and ventral ischium completed

Fig. 5.28 Cat with malunion fracture of ilium causing stenosis of pelvic canal.

SURGERY OF THE HIP

The hip joint is an enarthrosis and the main movements in the dog are flexion and extension. The anatomy of the joint is illustrated in Figs 5.29–5.32. In the skeletally immature dog the main blood supply to the femoral head is derived from the epiphyseal vessels associated with the joint capsule while a small amount is derived from vessels running through the round ligament. In the mature dog the femoral head receives an additional blood supply through the metaphyseal vessels but this source becomes available only after fusion of the epiphyseal plate at 8–11 months. The

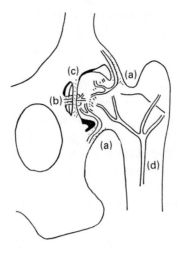

Fig. 5.29 Ventral view of left hip showing: (a) the joint capsule and the epiphyseal blood vessels; (b) the round ligament; (c) the trans-acetabular ligament; (d) the metaphyseal blood vessels.

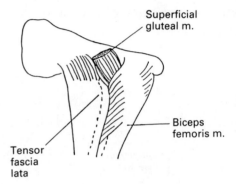

Fig. 5.30 Superficial lateral muscles of the left hip.

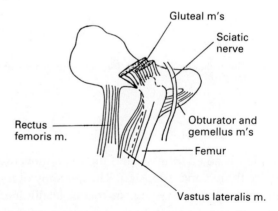

Fig. 5.31 Deep lateral muscles of the left hip.

soft tissue structures which are of surgical importance are shown in Figs 5.30–5.32. Conditions affecting the hip which are amenable to surgical treatment include hip dysplasia, Legge Perthes disease, recurrent or long-standing dislocations of the hip, fractures of the femoral head and fracture of the acetabulum.

Surgical approaches to the hip
There are four basic approaches to the hip: cranial, dorsal, caudal and medial. The dorsal approach (Figs 5.17–5.20) is perhaps the simplest and most versatile. The cranial approach is described on p. 317, Fig. 5.33e(i–iii) and the caudal approach on p. 323, Fig. 5.34.

HIP DYSPLASIA

Hip dysplasia (abnormal development of the hip) is common in most large breeds of dogs, the exception being the Greyhound. Hip dysplasia is a multifactorial disease in which genes, exercise, feeding and other factors play a part (Henricson *et al.* 1972).

Dogs are presented for treatment either during the acute growth stage between 4 and 8 months of age, or later in life when secondary osteo-arthritic changes have occurred in the hip. History includes pain on rising, poor exercise tolerance and a 'rolling' gait. On clinical examination the hindquarters are often poorly muscled. Pain, crepitus and excessive laxity may be evident on manipulation of the hips.

Ventrodorsal pelvic radiographs are taken under general anaesthesia with the dog on its back, its hindlegs fully extended and the stifles inwardly rotated. The radiographic changes in hip dysplasia have been described by Lawson (1976) and Riser (1973). Primary changes seen in the young dog are:

1 Flattening of the femoral head.
2 Lateral displacement of the femoral head with respect to the acetabulum.
3 Luxation or subluxation of the femoral head is seen in severe cases.

These primary changes are followed by degenerative joint disease in older dogs and the associated radiographic changes include:

1 Subchondral erosion of the acetabular margin with osteophyte formation.
2 Flattening of the femoral head due to subchondral eburnation.
3 New bone formation along the articular margin of the femoral head and around the attachments of the joint capsule on the femoral head and trochanteric fossa.

Hip dysplasia causes joint pain and lameness in young dogs. It may also cause osteo-arthrosis and result in continued problems in the mature animal. It is well known that a spontaneous improvement in limb function often occurs as the dysplastic dog reaches maturity and only some 30% of these cases will require treatment in later life. Pain and lameness associated with hip dysplasia are usually most obvious during the last few months of growth. A conservative approach is used initially in most cases. Management is aimed at encouraging the hips to stabilize by limiting exercise to short walks preferably on a leash until the dog is 14 months of age. The animal's weight should be carefully controlled and only non-steroidal analgesics used to control hip pain. The long-term results of conservative management of hip dysplasia in a series of 68 dogs were described by Barr *et al*. in 1987. The average follow-up period was 4.5 years and 76% of the dogs had an acceptable outcome and were able to take normal exercise, average 3 miles per day, without lameness, despite radiological evidence of moderate to severe osteo-arthrosis. The follow-up radiographic examination in these cases showed that the degree of hip subluxation did not become worse as the dogs matured, in fact it was reduced in 42% of cases, i.e. the hips 'tighten up' as the dog matures. The degree of peri-articular new bone increased in all cases but there was no change after 2 years of age. There was no statistical association between the degree of peri-articular new bone formation and clinical outcome which supports the long-standing view that there is no strict correlation between the severity of clinical signs and the radiographic changes associated with hip dysplasia. Some dogs with severe radiographic changes show no evidence of lameness while others with quite minor radiographic changes may have quite marked episodes of lameness.

If the dog does not appear to be responding to this regime of conservative treatment then there are several surgical options:

1 Pectineus myectomy.
2 Triple pelvic osteotomy.
3 Femoral or intertrochanteric osteotomy.
4 Total hip replacement.
5 Excision arthroplasty.

Pectineus myectomy
Considerable attention has been focused on the part played by the pectineus muscle in the aetiology of hip dysplasia.

Bardens & Hardwick (1968) observed that in dogs with hip dysplasia hindleg abduction was limited and the pectineus muscle in such dogs became more prominent and taut as the hip was abducted. Abduction could be increased when the pectineus muscle or its tendon were sectioned. The theory arose that a tight pectineus muscle causes excessive adduction and subluxation of the femoral head. Bardens & Hardwick (1968) claimed that hip dysplasia could be prevented in puppies if the pectineus muscle was sectioned before they reached 4 weeks of age. This point has been disputed by other workers. However, there have been several reports on the effectiveness of pectineus myectomy or tenotomy in the relief of pain associated with hip dysplasia and this leads to improved locomotion (Wallace 1971; Bowen *et al.* 1972; Lust *et al.* 1972; Henry 1973; Vaughan *et al.* 1975). Why should this procedure relieve pain? Perhaps the pain is due to spasm of the hip muscles and this is relieved when the pectineus muscle is cut, or there is a sudden change in the mechanical forces acting on the upper end of the femur and this stimulates the potential of the deep chondrocytes for proliferation and repair (Nissen 1971). Nevertheless, although pectineus myectomy relieves pain the osseous changes associated with hip dysplasia continue unaltered.

TECHNIQUE FOR PECTINEUS MYECTOMY
With the dog in dorsal recumbency and the hindlegs fully abducted, the pectineus muscle can be palpated as a prominent, taut band lying directly over the medial aspect of the hip. A skin incision is made over the line of the muscle and the subcutaneous fat is retracted to complete exposure. The muscle is bluntly dissected from the surrounding tissues taking care to avoid the femoral vessels on the cranial aspect, and a neurovascular bundle which crosses the pectineus near its myotendinous junction (Fig. 5.32). The distal end of the muscle is clamped with artery forceps just proximal to the neurovascular bundle. Using diathermy or scissors the muscle is transected close to its origin, and then just proximal to the artery forceps (which prevent retraction following the initial transection). After removal of the muscle belly, care is taken to ensure that all haemorrhage is controlled; minor ooze may be arrested by packing the wound with a swab while the operation is being performed on the other hip. The subcutaneous fat and fascia is co-apted with a continuous catgut suture and the skin with nylon. Post-operative management consists of con-

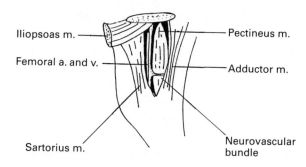

Fig. 5.32 Muscles of the right hip, medial aspect.

trolled exercise which, in the case of puppies, should be continued until they are mature. Complications include persistent haematoma formation and recurrence of symptoms due to scar tissue joining the ends of the muscle after inadequate resection.

SECTION AND REFLECTION OF THE PECTINEUS MUSCLE (Herron 1990)

A simpler quicker alternative to pectineus myectomy is to mobilize the muscle as described above and then section the pectineus through its origin as close to the pubis as possible. The muscle belly is then reflected and pushed as far down the leg as possible to prevent it joining up again. Routine wound closure is carried out.

Pectineus myectomy should be avoided in the pup with marked subluxation of the hips (grade IV hip dysplasia). These pups may have a weak hindleg action but hip pain is not usually a problem. If pectineus myectomy or section is done on one of these cases the hip tends to become increasingly unstable and complete dislocation may occur. It is perhaps safer to use the procedure to relieve pain in cases with mild to moderate degrees of dysplasia (grade II or III), where the degree of subluxation is not so severe. In older dogs with advanced osteo-arthrosis pectineus myectomy is useful to relieve pain but it may be 2−3 months before an improvement in the dog's action is seen, unlike young dogs where an improvement may occur within days.

There is some variation in the results of treatment. Wallace (1971) records a 94% success rate, an improvement being obtained within 24−72 hours of surgery. Vaughan *et al.* (1975) followed up 100 cases; 80% improved but only 35% had a high standard of recovery, while 20% did not improve or became worse.

Pelvic and femoral osteotomies

Pelvic and femoral osteotomies (Brinker 1971; Henry & Wadsworth 1975) have been used in dogs between 4 and 8 months of age to improve stability of the hip. The procedures result in the femoral head being seated more deeply in the acetabulum.

Although the procedures were described in the early 1970s, it is only in recent years that any large series have been undertaken.

FEMORAL OR INTERTROCHANTERIC VARUS OSTEOTOMY

The femoral osteotomy known as intertrochanteric osteotomy (Prieur 1987) is technically the easiest to perform. Ideally it is used in dogs with hip dysplasia between 9 and 15 months of age. The normal angle of the femoral neck in relation to the femoral shaft is $146 \pm 5°$. If the angle is above this, as in hip dysplasia, the dog is said to have coxa valga. This abnormal angulation contributes to further subluxation and instability of the hip. In the intertrochanteric osteotomy a wedge of the proximal femur is removed (Fig. 5.33a) giving the femoral neck an inclination of approximately 135° (i.e. coxa vara) so that the femoral head tilts further into the acetabulum. The procedure is of benefit not only in young dysplastic dogs but also in older animals with degenerative joint disease because the loading of the damaged articular cartilage is more evenly distributed allowing repair to occur. A special hook plate has been developed (Prieur 1987) (Straumann, Great Britain Ltd) for fixation of the osteotomy (Fig. 5.33b(i)). The osteotomy heals rapidly and the opposite hip can be operated on 6–8 weeks later if necessary.

An alternative to the hook plate is to use a narrow 7 or 8 hole 3.5 dynamic compression plate. The plate is contoured

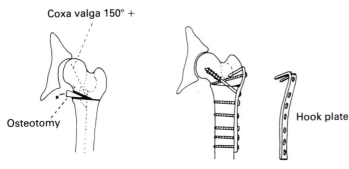

Coxa valga 150° +

Osteotomy

Hook plate

Fig. 5.33a   Fig. 5.33b(i)

right around the greater trochanter to allow three screws to be placed proximal to the osteotomy and four or five distally (Fig. 5.33b(ii, iii)). Temporary fixation of the femoral osteotomy is achieved with a Kirschner wire while the plate is contored and applied to the femur.

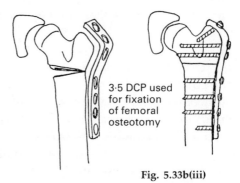

3·5 DCP used
for fixation
of femoral
osteotomy

Fig. 5.33b(iii)

Fig. 5.33b(ii)

TRIPLE PELVIC OSTEOTOMY

The main indication for triple pelvic osteotomy is the management of dogs between 5 and 9 months of age which have moderate to severe grades of hip dysplasia (grades III and IV) in which the acetabulum is shallow but the conformation of the femoral head and the femoral neck angle are normal. If these dogs are becoming increasingly lame and are not responding to conservative treatment then the pelvic osteotomy is used to improve the conformation and stability of the hip.

Pelvic osteotomy is a procedure used to improve stability of the hip in the immature dog with hip dysplasia (Hohn & Janes 1969; Brinker 1971; Schrader 1981; Hohn 1982). Osteotomy of the pelvis permits lateral rotation of the acetabulum to cover the femoral head more effectively and increase contact between the articular surfaces of the hip. Surgery should be done on dogs between 5 and 9 months of age, while they still have potential to remodel the hip once 'normal' contact has been restored (Hohn 1982). Excellent results have been reported using the technique for dogs with mild to moderate degrees of hip dysplasia. In a series of 33 cases described by Hohn & Janes (1969), 91% were reported to have regained normal limb function after surgery. However, it is difficult to assess the functional results of any form of surgical treatment for hip dysplasia in the immature dog because there is no strict correlation between the radiographic changes and the clinical signs.

In most cases managed conservately the hips tend to stabilize by 12–14 months of age, gait improves and only some 30% of dogs with hip dysplasia will require treatment after 2 years of age.

Pelvic osteotomy is a major surgical procedure. Although the operation has been recommended for use in dogs with only mild (grade I) or moderate (grade II) dysplasia with no secondary changes (Brinker *et al.* 1983), Slocum (1984) described good results in 22 cases with grade III and 29 cases with grade IV (severe) dysplasia.

The three stages in triple pelvic osteotomy are:
1 Osteotomy of the pubic ramus (1 cm section removed).
2 Osteotomy of the ischium (wire placed for stabilization).
3 Osteotomy of the ilium with application of a plate to produce lateral rotation of the acetabulum. The wire suture in the ischium is tightened.

Pubic osteotomy
The dog is placed in lateral recumbency with the affected hip uppermost. The leg is raised by an assistant to allow the surgeon to make a standard approach to the pectineus muscle and pubic area of the pelvis (Fig. 5.33c(i)). The pectineus muscle is severed close to its origin on the iliopectineal eminence and is reflected distally. The adductor muscle and a large branch of the deep femoral vein are retracted away from the pubic ramus and exposure is maintained with a Hohmann retractor placed on either side of the ramus. A section of the ramus (about 1 cm) is removed with an oscillating saw or bone rongeurs. Care should be taken to protect the obturator nerve with a retractor while the ostectomy is performed. The surgical wound is closed, the leg is lowered and an approach is made to the caudal ischium.

Ischial osteotomy
A skin incision is made directly over the tuber ischium and extended to the obturator foramen by subperiosteal elevation of the muscle attachments to the dorsal and ventral aspects of the table of the ischium (Fig. 5.33c(ii)). An embryotomy wire is passed through the obturator foramen (Fig. 5.33c(ii)) with the aid of a curved pair of artery forceps. The ischium is sectioned with the wire. A hole is drilled on either side of the ischial osteotomy and a length of 18 or 20 gauge wire passed through these. The wire is not tightened at this stage. The wound is covered with a moist swab and next an approach is made to the ilium.

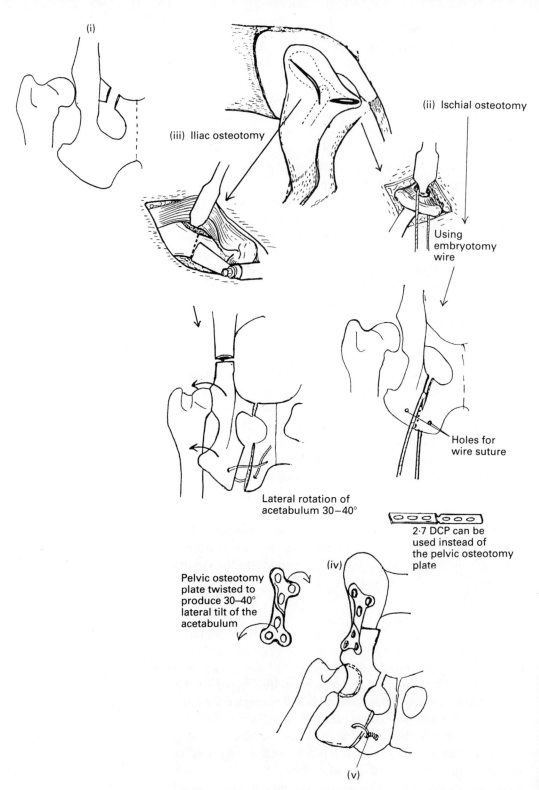

(i)

(iii) Iliac osteotomy

(ii) Ischial osteotomy

Using embryotomy wire

Holes for wire suture

Lateral rotation of acetabulum 30–40°

2·7 DCP can be used instead of the pelvic osteotomy plate

Pelvic osteotomy plate twisted to produce 30–40° lateral tilt of the acetabulum

(iv)

(v)

Fig. 5.33c Stages in triple pelvic osteotomy: (i) pubic osteotomy; (ii) ischial osteotomy; (iii) iliac osteotomy; (iv) acetabulum tilted laterally, plate fixation of ilium; (v) wire suture in ischium tightened.

Iliac osteotomy

A curved skin incision is then made over the ilium and proximal femur (Fig. 5.33c(iii)). The tensor fascia lata is reflected ventrally and the ventral edge of the middle gluteal muscle identified. The middle and deep gluteal muscles are retracted dorsally with the aid of a periosteal elevator and Hohmann retractors to expose the iliac shaft (Fig. 5.33c(iii)). An oscillating saw is used to make a transverse osteotomy incision through the iliac shaft (Fig. 5.33c(iii)).

The tip of a Hohmann retractor is placed on the medial side of the ilium to protect the sciatic nerve while the saw is being used. A pelvic osteotomy plate (Fig. 5.33c(iv)) (Veterinary Instrumentation) is twisted to give about 30−40° of lateral tilt of the acetabulum when attached to the ilium. Alternatively a notched 2.7 DCP (Straumann, Great Britain Ltd) is twisted in the same way (Fig. 5.33c(iv)). The plate is attached to the caudal ilium first and then by screwing the other end of the plate to the cranial ilium the contour of the plate should cause lateral rotation of the acetabulum (Fig. 5.33c(iv)). It is important to try to place at least one of the cranial screws into the body of the sacrum for optimal stability. The gluteal muscles are repositioned and routine wound closure carried out.

The ischial osteotomy site is uncovered again and the wire suture tightened to stabilize the ischial osteotomy (Fig. 5.33c(v)). After closure of this wound a light pressure bandage is placed over the operation sites. Most dogs are weight bearing within a few days with a rapid improvement in limb function over the next 6 weeks. If necessary pelvic osteotomy can be performed bilaterally with a 6−8 week interval between operations. In a series of 26 cases with grade III and IV dysplasia treated by pelvic osteotomy at this clinic, there were good results in all but two dogs.

Total hip replacement (THR)

Total hip replacement is the ultimate treatment for the mature dog with hip pain and osteo-arthosis. The basic criteria for using this procedure are:

1 The dog should be mature, over 14 months of age. However hip replacements have been successfully undertaken in dogs as young as 11 months.

2 The dog should be large, 30 kg plus. The dog should otherwise be fit and well and not have other orthopaedic problems.

3 Ideally one hip should be worse than the other. The dog must have hip pain and be in constant need of medication.

4 The procedure should not be done on dysplastic dogs that are asymptomatic.

Olmstead *et al.* (1981) described the technique for total hip replacement which was used in a series of 132 cases. The procedure gave satisfactory results in 92.5% of cases. The main indication is the treatment of hip dysplasia and the procedure can be done bilaterally. The total hip prosthesis consists of a plastic acetabular cup and a stainless steel femoral component (Richards Canine Total Hip Prosthesis, Richards Manufacturing Inc., Memphis, Tennessee, and imported by Alfred Cox Ltd). The two components are retained in position using polymethyl-methacrylate bone cement. The total hip prosthesis is expensive. The operation must be done under conditions of strict asepsis which cannot be achieved in most practice situations. Special instrumentation and a high degree of technical skill are necessary for correct insertion of the prosthesis. Dislocation of the prosthetic hip can occur at any stage during the first 3 weeks following surgery and exercise must be carefully restricted during this period to prevent this complication arising. Once the joint capsule has healed the hip will remain stable. The more accurate the insertion of the prosthesis, the less the chances of dislocation occurring. Loosening of the acetabular cup may occur as a late complication but it is usually possible to revise this situation and re-cement the cup (loosening is invariably due to technical faults during insertion). Loosening of the femoral component is not a common problem in dogs and when it occurs it is most likely to be associated with infection. This is the most serious potential complication of THR and removal of the prostheses will be necessary. A failed total hip replacement can always be converted back to an excision arthroplasty by removal of the implants.

PEROT HIP PROSTHESIS
At this clinic the Perot hip prosthesis (Veterinary Instrumentation) is routinely used. The Perot prosthesis has a self-retentive acetabular cup so that the risk of dislocation is minimized. The femoral prosthesis is available in three sizes, small, medium and large, and can have either a long or short femoral neck. The two larger femoral prostheses can be used with the same acetabular cups as the femoral head diameter is the same in each. The cups come in two sizes, medium (24 mm diameter) and large (28 mm diameter). The medium size femoral prosthesis is

the most useful and can be used with either the medium or large acetabular cup. A rapid setting bone cement is used (CMW type 2, CMW Laboratories, Dentsply).

A course of antibiotics (Ceporex, Glaxo) is commenced 2 days before the dog is admitted for surgery and is continued for 5 days post-operatively. Total hip replacement must be carried out under conditions of strict asepsis.

Perot recommends the dorsal approach to the hip with osteotomy of the greater trochanter for insertion of his prosthesis. The osteotomy is repaired with a lag screw and the screw hole is prepared before the osteotomy of the trochanter. This approach gives excellent exposure and makes the subsequent reaming and cementing procedures much easier; certainly this approach is ideal for the surgeon carrying out his or her THR for the first time. However in many dogs, especially the large German Shepherds, adequate exposure can also be achieved using the cranial approach with ventral reflection of the origin of the vastus lateralis (Fig. 5.33e). Large bone-holding forceps are used to grip the proximal femur so that it can be rotated or elevated readily during surgery. The joint capsule is incised transversely, the round ligament is cut (if not already ruptured), the femoral head is then rotated out of the acetabulum and all soft tissue reflected from the cranial aspect of the femoral neck. The femoral prosthesis is lined up against the proximal femur and the angle of section of the femoral neck planned. An oscillating saw is used to section the femoral neck and the femoral head is removed. A rasp is used to ream out the proximal femur until the stem of the prosthesis can be slid easily into the medullary cavity and the collar of the prosthesis rests against the remnant of the femoral neck (Fig. 5.33d). The medullary cavity is flushed out with ice cold saline and packed with a ribbon bandage. The femur is retracted caudally and two pairs of self-retaining retractors placed at right angles to each other are used to give a wide exposure of the acetabulum. An acetabular burr is used to ream away all the articular cartilage down to bleeding subchondral bone. A 4.5 mm drill bit is then used to prepare four or five holes in the wall of the acetabulum. These are essential to key in the bone cement; one hole is drilled in the caudal acetabulum extending into the shaft of the ischium, one is drilled cranially extending into the shaft of the ilium and the other two or three holes are spaced out in the more central regions of the acetabulum (Fig. 5.33d). These holes should not penetrate the medial cortex of the acetabulum. The

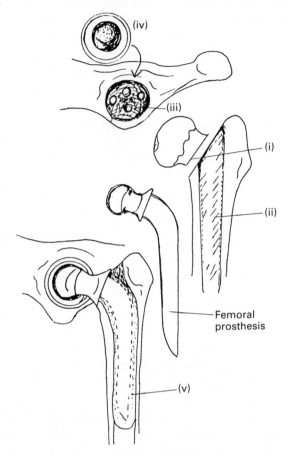

Fig. 5.33d Stages in total hip replacement using Perot prosthesis:
(i) excision of femoral head; (ii) femoral shaft reamed out to take stem of
the femoral prosthesis; (iii) acetabulum reamed out to take cup. Holes
drilled to key in bone cement; (iv) acetabular cup cemented into
acetabulum; (v) femoral prosthesis cemented into femoral shaft and the
femoral head inserted into the self retentive acetabular cup.

acetabulum is flushed out with ice cold saline and pressure
applied with a swab until all bleeding has ceased. The
appropriate sized acetabular cup is selected and a trial
insertion carried out. The cup should be seated in the
normal longitudinal axis of the acetabulum with about 10°
of lateral tilt of the dorsal edge of the cup. Having checked
that the cup can be easily inserted and the correct position
assessed, the cup is removed and the bone cement mixed
according to the manufacture's instructions. Having ensured
that the acetabulum is dry, it is filled with a soft bolus of
bone cement. The acetabular cup is slowly pushed into the
cement and orientated with an acetabular pusher. Excess
cement is removed; do not be in a great hurry to push the

cup immediately into its correct position otherwise all the bone cement will be squeezed out — do the procedure slowly and then press hard on the pusher just as the cement begins to harden.

Once the cement has set hard, the final position and stability of the acetabular cup is checked and any loose tags of bone cement removed. The next stage is the choice of femoral prosthesis — should it have a long or short neck? In most cases the long-necked prosthesis is most suitable. The proximal femur is elevated and rotated to allow easy access to the reamed medullary cavity, the ribbon bandage is removed, and a trial insertion of the femoral prosthesis is made. The prosthesis is usually set in the femur with its head and neck in the neutral position. The prosthesis is removed and a second pack of bone cement mixed. If CMW 2 is used this is allowed to assume a malleable consistency. A slim sausage of cement is made and this is introduced into the medullary cavity. It is pushed down into the cavity as quickly as possible with a small rod (there is only 3 or 4 minutes before the cement goes hard so speed is essential). The femoral prosthesis is then pushed into the proximal femur and seated in the neutral position. Extruded cement is packed into any defect around the collar of the prosthesis and any excess is removed. (An alternative is to use low viscosity cement CMW 1 which is introduced into the femur with a syringe.) Once the cement is hard the femoral head is pushed into the acetabular cup; the cup is self-retentive so a satisfying 'clunk' is usually heard as the head snaps into the cup. The range of hip movement is checked and routine wound closure is carried out. If the dorsal approach has been used, the trochanter is reattached with a cancellous screw. A screw alone may bend or break before healing of the osteotomy is complete. This complication can be prevented by supplementing the screw with a tension band wire.

Post-operatively an oblique lateral check radiograph of the pelvis is taken. This is safer than a conventional ventro-dorsal view which can result in dislocation of the prosthesis if the anaesthetized animal is not positioned with extreme care at this stage. The hip is bandaged with a large bolster made of plastic 'bubble' paper and cotton wool which is strapped to the inner side of the thigh. This bolster minimizes the range of hip movement but allows the animal to use the operated leg. Most dogs are weight bearing on the affected leg the day after surgery with good function within 3 or 4 days. The bolster is worn for 2 weeks and exercise is restricted to short walks only for 6 weeks. After this period extended and flexed ventrodorsal radiographs are taken of the hips and provided everything looks satisfactory a gradual increase in exercise is allowed with a return to normal exercise within 6 weeks.

Results with Perot prosthesis

Eighty-five per cent of dogs treated by the author have had a successful outcome and been able to take normal exercise again. The longest follow-up period is 4 years.

COMPLICATIONS OF TOTAL HIP REPLACEMENT

Limb function following total hip replacement is usually excellent but if the dog suddenly stops using the leg it generally means that a serious complication has arisen. The main complications of THR are listed below:

1 Dislocation of the prosthesis tends to happen within the first 6 weeks and is usually due to incorrect angle of placement of the acetabular cup. Closed reduction is easily achieved in most cases by caudoventral traction on the leg. A bolster is reapplied for 2 weeks after reduction and exercise is restricted for a further 6 weeks. If further dislocation occurs then the options are either a hip revision with a change in position of the cup or removal of the entire prosthesis with conversion to excision arthroplasty.

2 Loosening of the acetabular cup. This is the commonest complication encountered and is usually seen within 4 months of surgery. Loosening at this stage is probably the result of technical faults in insertion of the cup, i.e. not seated deep enough in the acetabulum, wrong angle, too little cement. It is possible to revise this situation and have a satisfactory end result. Exposure is not quite so easy because the femoral prosthesis tends to get in the way. A dorsal approach is used to expose the loose cup. It is removed together with existing cement. The acetabulum is reamed again. Further drill holes are made in the acetabular wall and the new cup cemented *in situ*. Post-operative care is as for a routine THR.

3 If a THR becomes infected the animal gradually stops using the leg and radiographs show areas of osteolysis at the bone—cement interface. Prolonged antibiotic therapy may improve the situation but eventually removal of the prosthesis is unavoidable as loosening occurs.

4 Fatigue fracture of the proximal stem of the femoral prosthesis has been encountered in two cases at 8 months and 1 year respectively. Removal of the proximal end of

the prosthesis and the acetabular cup was done to salvage
the situation.

Excision arthroplasty

Excision arthroplasty is a salvage procedure and may be
used for the treatment of hip dysplasia when conservative
methods and/or pectineus myectomy have failed to control
the pain. The operation is also indicated in the treatment
of Legge Perthes disease and for certain fractures of the
femoral head and acetabulum. Duff & Campbell (1977)
reviewed the literature on excision arthroplasty and
described the long-term results of the operation. Removal
of the femoral head and neck is followed by the development
of a pseudo-arthrosis. There is some shortening of the leg,
and the range of movement, primarily in extension and
abduction, is limited. The gluteal muscles are essential for
the support of the joint after excision and ideally an
approach (cranial or medial) should be used which avoids
damage to these structures. The cranial approach is shown
in Figs 5.17–5.19 and Fig. 5.33e(i–iii).

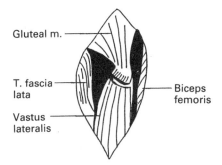

Gluteal m.

T. fascia lata

Biceps femoris

Vastus lateralis

Fig. 5.33e(i)

Fig. 5.33e(ii)

Fig. 5.33e(iii)

CRANIAL APPROACH TO THE HIP

The cranial approach to the hip is as in Figs 5.17–5.19. The
joint is then exposed by blunt dissection within the triangle
bounded by the rectus femoris cranially, the gluteals dorsally
and the vastus lateralis caudally (Fig. 5.33e(i)). Such an
exposure is limited but can be greatly improved by severing
the origin of the vastus lateralis on the femoral neck and
reflecting it ventrally (Fig. 5.33e(i–iii)). The joint capsule
is incised, the round ligament cut and the femoral head
dislocated and rotated laterally. The femoral neck is cut
flush with the shaft using an osteotome or bone cutters
and the head is removed (Fig. 5.33e(iii)). The vastus lateralis

is reattached to the gluteals with horizontal mattress sutures of fine catgut.

After removal of the skin sutures, exercise is encouraged. Most dogs regain 'full use' of the leg within 3 months. The most common cause of failure is inadequate resection of the femoral neck. If bilateral excision is performed a 6–8 week interval should be left between operations.

It has been indicated that the results of excision arthroplasty are not so satisfactory in large dogs. Bone to bone contact and osteophyte formation have been blamed for this. Consequently techniques were developed for interposing muscle between the bone surfaces after excision of the femoral head. In 1987 two papers were published on the results of excision arthroplasty techniques. Mann *et al.* compared standard excision with excision plus interposition of a biceps muscle sling. Montgomery *et al.* also compared these two techniques together with a third method, wedge resection of the femoral head and neck. It was concluded from this work that:

1 There were no significant differences in the recovery periods or end results in the three groups.
2 There was no increase in the post-operative problems associated with increased body weight, however results were poorer in hunting dogs.
3 Consequently the standard excision arthroplasty technique described below is recommended. It is simpler and less time consuming than the others.

Hip dysplasia in cats
The radiological features of feline hip dysplasia resemble those found in the dog. The condition is said to be most common in the Siamese cat and is sporadically encountered in other breeds. Literature on feline hip dysplasia was reviewed by Holt in 1978 and he described the successful treatment of the condition in a Persian cat. The animal was initially treated by bilateral pectineus myectomy. This produced only a temporary improvement in function and bilateral excision arthroplasty was subsequently performed. This resulted in complete remission of lameness.

LEGGE PERTHES DISEASE (AVASCULAR NECROSIS OF THE FEMORAL HEAD) (Spreull 1961; Riser 1963; Ljunggren 1966, 1967; Paatsama *et al.* 1967, 1969; Lee & Fry 1969; Lee 1970; Smith 1971)

Legge Perthes disease is a disease of young dogs between 3 and 9 months of age. The small breeds, in particular the

Terriers, are usually affected. There is interference with the blood supply to the femoral head which results in avascular necrosis. The factors which interfere with the blood supply are not completely understood but several reasons have been postulated and are listed below:

1 Trauma to the epiphyseal blood vessels (Fig. 5.29) resulting in thrombosis.

2 Imbalance of sex hormones. Legge Perthes disease has been reproduced experimentally by the administration of high levels of oestrogen or androgen. The result is premature closure of the proximal epiphyseal plate of the femur and a disturbance in the circulation (Ljunggren 1967).

3 Genetic factors. There is evidence for a genetic predisposition as a high incidence of the disease follows certain breed lines. Pidduck & Webbon (1978), in an analysis of the pedigrees of Toy Poodles affected with Legge Perthes disease from one kennel obtained results consistent with the hypothesis that Perthes' disease is caused by homozygosity for an autosomal recessive gene.

The histological and radiographic changes associated with Legge Perthes disease have been described (Lee 1970). The initial change is ischaemic necrosis of the femoral head. There may be little clinical evidence of lameness or radiological abnormality at this stage. Continued weight bearing causes trabecular fragmentation, deformity and cavitation and a radiograph reveals uneven femoral head density with deformity.

Next, highly vascular granulation tissue penetrates the growth plate and results in revascularization and replacement of the dead tissues by a process of 'creeping substitution'. The removal of bone and deposition of foci of closely trabeculated bone and areas of fibrous tissue gives the femoral head an uneven density on radiographic examination.

Although the femoral head is revascularized and remodelled, deformity inevitably persists and this is associated with osteophytic proliferation around the femoral neck and acetabular rim.

The clinical signs are a gradual onset of unilateral or bilateral hindleg lameness over a period of 3–4 months. The degree of lameness becomes gradually worse until the dog only uses the leg intermittently or carries it. There is obvious muscle wasting and pain on manipulation of the hip, particularly when it is abducted. This degree of lameness remains static for a further 1 or 2 months and then there is gradual improvement.

Excision arthroplasty is considered to be the best method

of treating most cases of Legge Perthes disease (Ljunggren 1966). In a group of 36 cases treated in this way, 30 regained good use of the affected leg. By comparison, of 62 cases treated by conservative methods, only 15 regained use of the leg and a longer period of convalescence was required. Conservative treatment involves complete rest during the first 3 months after the onset of lameness, followed by the encouragement of exercise and passive manipulation of the hip to prevent muscle atrophy and help mould the head of the femur to the shape of the acetabulum and limit the degree of deformity.

VON WILLEBRAND HETEROTOPIC OSTEOCHONDROFIBROSIS OF DOBERMANNS
(Leighton & Ferguson 1987; Dueland *et al.* 1989)

Von Willebrand's disease is the commonest inherited bleeding disorder of man and the dog (Littlewood *et al.* 1987). The condition has been reported in many breeds of dog but in the Dobermann it has also been associated with hindleg lameness. Typically the dogs present with a moderate to severe progressive hindleg lameness, there is muscle atrophy, marked limitation in the range of hip movement, particularly extension, and often pain evident on hip extension. Radiographs initially may show very little except for some subluxation of the affected hip. Later periosteal bony reactions develop on the ischium and/or proximal femur and a mass containing calcified tissue develops close to the hip. The mass usually involves the caudal hip muscles, gemelli, internal/external obturator, quadratus femoris, and can also affect the pectineus and iliopsoas muscles. The condition probably results from trauma with haemorrhage and an initial fibrous reaction with progression to a chondro-osseous response. The lesion may be misdiagnosed as neoplasia. Affected dogs test positive for Von Willebrand's factor.

Some cases respond reasonably well to treatment with prednisolone but in others it may prove necessary to remove the mass of osteochondrofibrotic tissue and section the affected muscles to restore a more normal range of hip movement. The response to surgery has been good and Dueland *et al.* (1989) report complete recoveries in four cases.

TRAUMATIC CONDITIONS OF THE HIP

Dislocation of the hip

Dislocation of the hip is a common injury in the dog. Affected animals are usually over 1 year of age. The femoral head is dislocated in a craniodorsal direction in 85–90% of cases, cranioventral in 2–3% of cases, while caudoventral and caudodorsal dislocations are rare.

In craniodorsal dislocations the dog carries the leg semi-flexed and adducted under the body. If both hindlegs are extended and their length compared, then the affected leg will appear shorter and the distance between the greater trochanter and tuber ischii will be greater than on the normal side. Radiographs should be taken of the hips to confirm the diagnosis and eliminate the presence of fractures.

Closed reduction should be attempted within 48 hours. The dog is anaesthetized and placed on its side with the dislocated hip uppermost. A towel is placed under the leg and used to anchor it to the edge of the table or alternatively, it is held by an assistant. Traction is exerted on the limb in a caudal direction and at the same time it is slightly abducted so that the femoral head is lifted over the rim of the acetabulum. At the same time thumb pressure is applied to the greater trochanter to stop the femoral head slipping ventrally around the rim of the acetabulum. If reduction is successful the femoral head should be forced down into the acetabulum to express any blood clot and the joint flexed and extended several times to check the stability of the reduction. If the joint tends to redislocate when the leg is extended the limb is strapped with the stifle and hock in flexion for 3–5 days (see Fig. 2.1f).

If the hip redislocates or is grossly unstable then there are several surgical options:

1 The De Vita pin is illustrated in Fig. 5.33f. This method can be used to stabilize the hip following either closed or open reduction. A Steinmann pin is introduced beneath the tuber ischiium and driven forward over the neck of the femur and on into the wing of the ilium. The pin is left *in situ* for 3 weeks. Some cases have been reported of iatrogenic damage to the sciatic nerve during insertion of the pin.

2 The acetabulum is exposed (cranial approach), cleared of organized haematoma, the hip is reduced and the joint capsule sutured. The leg is strapped in flexion for 5 days following surgery.

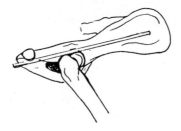

Fig. 5.33f De Vita pin.

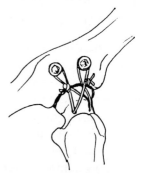

Fig. 5.33g Reinforcement of the joint capsule to prevent dislocation.

3 If the joint capsule is too damaged for a simple suture repair then there are techniques for reinforcing the joint capsule (Fig. 5.33g) (Allen & Chambers 1986). Two screws are placed in the dorsal rim of the acetabulum, a hole is drilled through the dorsal aspect of the femoral neck, heavy non-absorbable suture material (7 m braided polyester, Ethibond, Ethicon) is placed through this hole and around the screws and used to reinforce the joint capsule.

4 A dorsal approach can be used to reduce the hip. Then the greater trochanter is relocated 2–3 cm distal to its original position using Kirschner wires and a tension band wire. This procedure places the gluteal muscles under increased tension forcing the femoral head into the acetabulum (De Angelis & Prata 1973).

5 Pre-articular stabilization using mattress sutures (Mehl 1988). The technique prevents dislocation by limiting the range of rotatory movement of the femoral head. Double mattress sutures of heavy non-absorbable material (Ethibond) are placed between the tendons of insertion of the iliopsoas and the middle gluteal muscle. The sutures lie on the craniolateral side of the hip and are tied while the femoral head is rotated into the acetabulum.

6 Transarticular pinning (Bennett & Duff 1980). Placement of a Steinmann pin across the articular surfaces of the hip can be done as a closed or open procedure. The latter allows more accurate placement of the pin. The pin is removed after 3–4 weeks by which time it is hoped that the joint capsule will have healed sufficiently to maintain stability (Bennett & Duff 1980).

7 Hip toggle procedure. This is the technique favoured at this clinic and is described in detail below. Knowles *et al.* (1953) were the first to describe a satisfactory method of

fixation by replacing the ligamentum teres with a strip of
fascia which was anchored in the acetabular fossa by a
toggle pin. Similar techniques have been described by
Lawson (1965) and Denny & Minter (1973a) using braided
nylon as a substitute for the ligament, by Leonard (1971)
employing stainless steel wire or a heavy plastic suture,
and by Zakiewicz (1967) using skin.

STABILIZATION OF THE HIP USING A TOGGLE PIN
AND A BRAIDED NYLON ROUND LIGAMENT
PROSTHESIS

The majority of hip dislocations occur in a craniodorsal
direction and consequently the gemellus and obturator
muscles which insert on the caudal aspect of the proximal
femur are often torn or stretched over the acetabulum thus
providing a ready-made approach (Fig. 5.34).

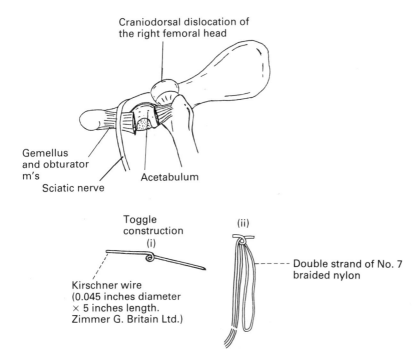

Craniodorsal dislocation of
the right femoral head

Gemellus
and obturator
m's

Sciatic nerve

Acetabulum

Toggle
construction
(i)

(ii)

Kirschner wire
(0.045 inches diameter
× 5 inches length.
Zimmer G. Britain Ltd.)

Double strand of No. 7
braided nylon

Fig. 5.34

Technique
A skin incision is made directly over the greater trochanter
and continued distally over the femur to the midshaft
region (Fig. 5.35). The fascia lata is separated from the
biceps femoris muscle using scissors (Fig. 5.35). The biceps
femoris is retracted to reveal the greater trochanter. The

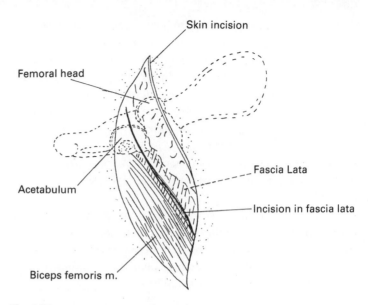

Fig. 5.35

sciatic nerve is identified caudal to the femoral shaft in the loose fascia between the biceps femoris and the semi-membranosus muscle. The path of the nerve is traced proximally around the hip (Fig. 5.36). The nerve is carefully protected while exposure of the acetabulum is completed from the caudal aspect. The insertion of the superficial gluteal muscle is transected and the caudal muscles of the hip (obturator and gemelli), if not already ruptured, are transected close to their insertion on the proximal femur

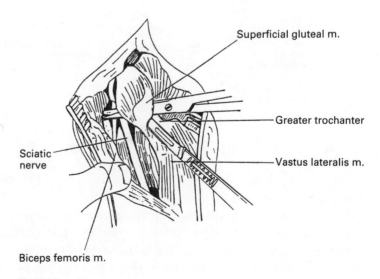

Fig. 5.36

(Fig. 5.37a). These muscles are reflected and the dislocated femoral head is retracted cranial to the acetabulum with bone-holding forceps applied to the proximal femoral shaft. Torn joint capsule is trimmed back and the acetabulum is cleared of haematoma or granulation tissue. When a pseudo-arthrosis has formed in a long-standing dislocation, thickened joint capsule must be removed and adhesions between the femoral head and dorsal rim of the acetabulum broken down before reduction of the dislocation can be achieved.

Once the acetabulum has been debrided, a tunnel is drilled through the acetabular fossa using a 3/16ths drill bit (Fig. 5.37b). Artery forceps are used to guide the toggle into the tunnel then the blunt end of the 7/64ths drill bit is used to push the toggle completely through the acetabulum. Traction is applied to the braided nylon round ligament prosthesis to ensure that the toggle rotates and engages firmly on the medial side of the acetabulum (Fig. 5.37b).

The femoral head is rotated in a caudolateral direction. The blade of a Hohmann retractor is inserted between the caudal border of the gluteal muscles and the femoral neck. The retractor is used to elevate the femoral head out of the incision and remnants of the round ligament are removed. A second Hohmann retractor may be necessary to depress the biceps femoris muscle while a tunnel is drilled using a 7/64ths bit from the fovea capitis through the femoral head and neck to emerge just ventral to the greater trochanter (Figs 5.37c and d). A second tunnel is drilled through the greater trochanter (Fig. 5.37d). Wire loops are placed through both tunnels. The braided nylon is drawn through the femoral tunnel using a loop. Traction is maintained on the nylon while the dislocation is reduced. Half the nylon is drawn through the trochanteric tunnel using the remaining wire loop and the free ends of the prosthesis are tightly tied. Reduction and stability of the hip should be checked before cutting off the excess nylon. Once reduction is complete, the obturator and gemellus muscle are no longer easily accessible and are left unsutured. The transected superficial gluteal muscle is repaired using horizontal mattress sutures of linen or fine monofilament nylon. The fascia lata and biceps femoris, the subcutaneous fascia and skin are coapted in layers in routine fashion.

Post-operative care
The leg is strapped in flexion for 5 days and skin sutures are generally removed after 8 days. Exercise is severely

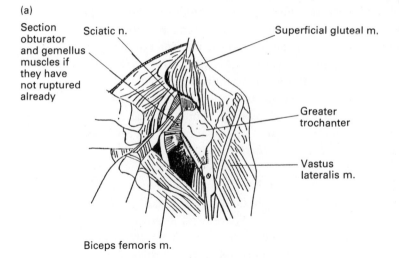

(a)

Section obturator and gemellus muscles if they have not ruptured already

Sciatic n.

Superficial gluteal m.

Greater trochanter

Vastus lateralis m.

Biceps femoris m.

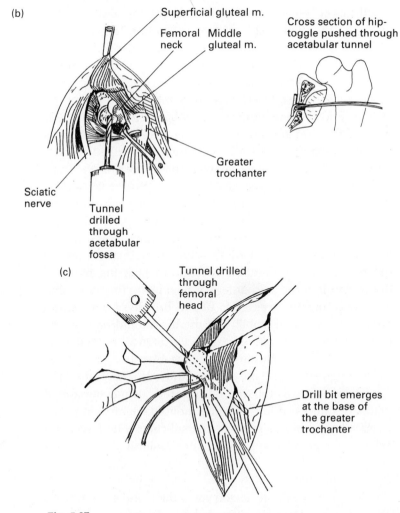

(b)

Superficial gluteal m.

Femoral neck   Middle gluteal m.

Greater trochanter

Sciatic nerve

Tunnel drilled through acetabular fossa

Cross section of hip-toggle pushed through acetabular tunnel

(c)

Tunnel drilled through femoral head

Drill bit emerges at the base of the greater trochanter

Fig. 5.37

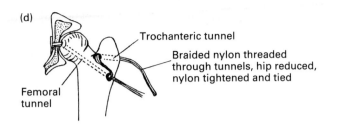

(d)

Trochanteric tunnel

Braided nylon threaded
through tunnels, hip reduced,
nylon tightened and tied

Femoral
tunnel

restricted for 4 weeks post-operatively. The progress is usually good and 84% of cases will regain full limb function. In the remainder varying degrees of lameness persist.

Post-operative complications
1 Redislocation with rupture of the braided nylon round ligament prosthesis. Factors predisposing to premature breakage of the prosthesis include overactivity in the recovery period, hip dysplasia and muscle contraction in long-standing dislocations. The hip joint may be salvaged by excision of the femoral head.
2 If dislocation occurs in an immature dog before closure of the proximal femoral growth plate, then rupture of the joint capsule may lead to ischaemic necrosis of the femoral head. When this complication arises following the hip toggle procedure, excision arthroplasty should be carried out.
3 Osteo-arthritis — this is a possible complication of any joint injury.

HIP DISLOCATIONS IN THE CAT
Dislocations of the hip in the cat are often associated with gross displacement of the femoral head. Although it may be possible to do a closed reduction it is often difficult to maintain reduction even with the application of an Ehmer sling and some 60% of cases redislocate.

Fortunately many cats compensate well to neglected dislocations of the hip and form a satisfactory functional pseudo-arthrosis. However the range of hip movement remains limited and some animals are left with an awkward gait. Therefore if the femoral head cannot be retained in its normal position following closed reduction, open reduction and stabilization should be recommended. At this clinic the hip toggle procedure is used in both dogs and cats. In the cat the toggle is constructed from 18 gauge wire and Polydioxanone (PDS) or braided nylon is used as the round ligament prosthesis. The other options are:

1 Suture the joint capsule followed by application of a flexion bandage.

2 Use pre-articular stabilization using mattress sutures. See 5, p. 322.

3 Use a transarticular pin for fixation. The pin is removed after 3–4 weeks.

4 Excision arthroplasty can be used as a salvage procedure.

Fractures of the femoral head and neck

Fractures of the femoral head and neck can be divided into two types: intracapsular, those occurring within the joint capsule, and extracapsular, those occurring outside the joint capsule. Ninety per cent of these fractures occur during the first year of life and the majority of cases are presented between 4 and 6 months of age. If the blood supply to the femoral head is examined in puppies and kittens (see p. 304), it would be reasonable to assume that the main complication of intracapsular fractures in immature animals would be ischaemic necrosis of the femoral head. Although this is a common complication of such fractures in children it does not appear to be a problem in cats and dogs provided that internal fixation is carried out soon after the accident, preferably within 48 hours and certainly within a week. Two methods of fixation are commonly employed:

1 Lag screw fixation used in conjunction with a Kirschner wire (Fig. 5.38) (Hulse *et al*. 1974).

2 Three diverging Kirschner wires (Fig. 5.38b). This method is used particularly for separations or fracture separations of the capital femoral epiphysis in dogs. The method is also used in cats for fractures of either the femoral head or neck (0.8 and 1 mm wires). Excellent results were achieved

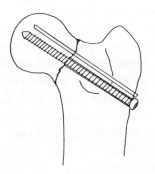

Fig. 5.38a

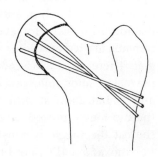

Fig. 5.38b

with this method in a series of 15 cats described by Jeffery (1989).

In young dogs with separation or fracture separation of the capital femoral epiphysis lysis of the dorsal aspect of the femoral neck is often seen on follow-up radiographs taken 4–6 weeks after surgery. This is probably due to a local disturbance in blood supply. The zone subsequently revascularizes and remodels.

Fracture of the capital epiphysis is sometimes accompanied by separation of the greater trochanter (Denny 1971). The latter may be missed on radiograph of the hips but should be obvious on a lateral view. The trochanteric separation provides a ready-made dorsal approach for either excision or fixation of the femoral head. The trochanter is then reattached with a lag screw, or wire tension band.

LONG-STANDING OR NEGLECTED FRACTURES OF
THE FEMORAL HEAD AND NECK
Intracapsular fractures in the dog, if untreated, invariably result in non-union with osteolysis of the femoral neck. The condition causes severe hip pain and lameness. Excision arthroplasty is the best treatment option. The same fracture in the cat will also result in non-union but the functional end results are often surprisingly good with the cat showing very little evidence of hip pain or lameness 6–8 weeks after the accident. If lameness is a problem then excision arthroplasty can always be used to salvage the situation. So is it necessary to treat fractures of the femoral head and neck in cats? The answer should be yes in most cases; certainly treatment by Kirschner wire fixation is the best method and will give the cat a much more rapid recovery with the best chance of normal hip function. Early excision arthroplasty is the second best option and should give a more rapid recovery than conservative treatment.

COMMINUTED FRACTURES OF THE PROXIMAL
FEMUR INVOLVING FEMORAL NECK AND
GREATER TROCHANTER
These fractures are usually treated by plate fixation (Figs 5.38c, d and e). Initial fixation of the femoral neck fracture is achieved with a Kirschner wire. A lag screw is then placed parallel with the Kirschner wire. The screw is often placed through the plate. The plate functions as a buttress to support the other fragments.

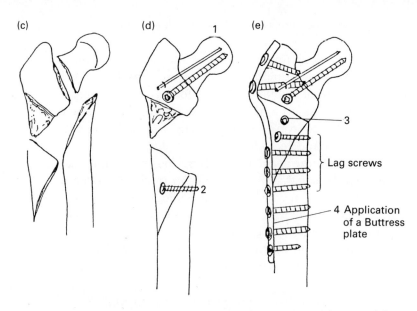

Fig. 5.38c,d,e Stages in reconstruction of a comminuted fracture of the proximal femur (1–4).

FRACTURES OF THE SHAFT OF THE FEMUR

Fractures of the femur are common. Simple transverse fractures of the shaft in young dogs and cats are best treated by intramedullar fixation (see p. 81, Figs 2.6–2.9), while plate and screw fixation is used for comminuted and oblique fractures especially in large dogs. The plate is usually applied to the lateral aspect of the shaft.

The femur is exposed by a lateral skin incision extending from the greater trochanter to the stifle. The attachment between the tensor fascia lata and the biceps femoris is cut and blunt dissection between the vastus lateralis and biceps femoris will reveal the femoral shaft (Figs 5.39 and 5.40). The incision can be extended into the joint capsule of the stifle to complete exposure of the distal femur as necessary. Exposure of the proximal shaft is achieved by subperiosteal elevation and cranial reflection of the origin of the vastus lateralis muscle (Fig. 5.40).

Figs 5.41–5.45 illustrate the stages in the repair of a comminuted fracture of the femur using lag screws and a plate. Soft tissue attachments to the fragments are retained where possible. Ideally lag screws are inserted in a craniocaudal or caudocranial direction so that they do not interfere with the application of a plate to the lateral surface of the

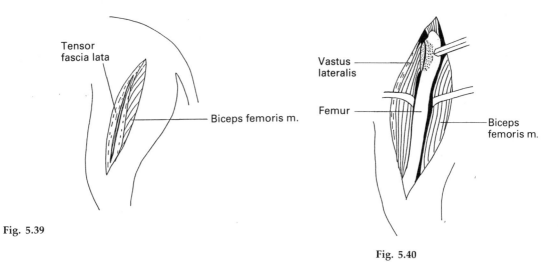

Tensor fascia lata

Biceps femoris m.

Fig. 5.39

Vastus lateralis

Femur

Biceps femoris m.

Fig. 5.40

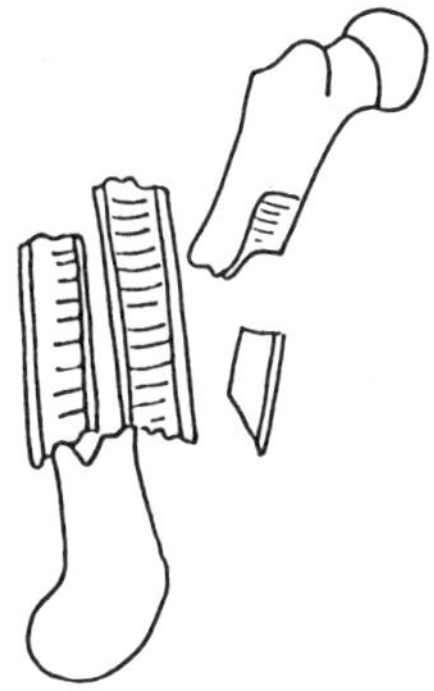

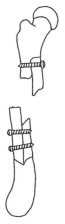

Fig. 5.41

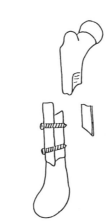

Fig. 5.42

Fig. 5.43

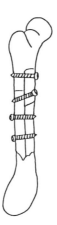

Fig. 5.44

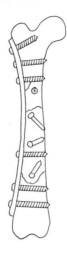

Fig. 5.45 Antero-posterior view.

femur. However, due to the plane of the fracture it is sometimes necessary to place the lag screws in a latero-medial direction. Under these circumstances temporary reduction of the fragments can be achieved with a cerclage wire (Fig. 5.46). The plate is applied and screws inserted through the plate are used to lag the fragments together (Fig. 5.46). The cerclage wire can be removed before the screws are finally tightened or can be left *in situ* to provide extra stability.

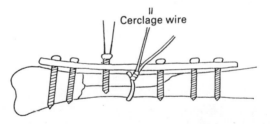

Fig. 5.46

Segmental fractures of the femur (Fig. 5.47) are sometimes encountered. Although these may be stabilized with an intramedullary pin there is a risk of rotation at one or other of the fracture sites. The dynamic compression plate is an ideal method of fixation and permits axial compression of both fracture sites (Fig. 5.48).

The treatment of femoral shaft fractures in puppies deserves a short mention. An intramedullary pin can be used for fixation in most instances. However reduction should be undertaken with a minimum of soft tissue trauma as a common complication of the fracture is the formation of

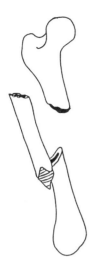

Fig. 5.47

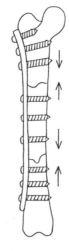

Fig. 5.48

adhesions between the quadriceps and femur which result in rigid extension of the stifle (see p. 334).

If a pin is broken off flush below the level of the greater trochanter, rapid longitudinal growth of the femur in the puppy usually results in the pin becoming sealed within the medullary cavity and prevents its retrieval. Consequently if removal of an intramedullary pin is contemplated radiographs should always be taken to check its position.

External fixator and femoral shaft fractures

The external fixator can only be applied to the lateral side of the femur. The pins penetrate large muscles and premature loosening is said to occur in 50% of cases (Brinker *et al.* 1990). If the external fixator is used as the only method of fixation it should be reserved for femoral shaft fractures in young, small breeds of dog and cats (Brinker *et al.* 1990). However the external fixator does provide a useful method of improving stability in larger dogs when used in conjunction with an intramedullary pin (Fig. 2.5c).

Femoral shaft fractures in cats

As a general rule virtually all types of fracture, even the severely comminuted fractures of the femoral shaft, in cats, can be successfully treated by the use of intramedullary fixation used in conjunction with cerclage wires as necessary. If the fragments are too small for reconstruction using cerclage wires then they are just left *in situ* and a plate applied to maintain length and alignment (Fig. 5.49). Alternatively an external fixator can be used in the same manner.

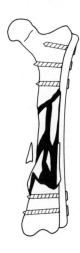

Fig. 5.49 Cat-comminuted fracture of the femoral shaft stabilized with a buttress plate.

CONTRACTURE OF THE QUADRICEPS FEMORIS MUSCLES (Vaughan 1979)

Quadriceps contracture can occur as a congenital deformity or a complication of femoral shaft fractures in puppies. The latter is seen most frequently. Splints or casts which fit tightly round the mid-thigh may cause muscle ischaemia leading to contracture. Alternatively internal fixation of shaft fractures may be followed by adhesion of the quadriceps to the fracture site.

The clinical features of quadriceps contracture are:

1 Rigid extension of the stifle.

2 Hyperextension of the hock.

3 The foot tends to be dragged, giving excoriation of the dorsum.

4 Quadriceps become fibrous and taut.

A lateral radiograph of the stifle shows the patella riding high in the femoral trochlea. Congenital contracture leads to genu recurvatum, with deformity of the distal femur, proximal tibia and a patella riding some distance proximal to the trochlea (Fig. 5.50).

Treatment

If adhesions have formed between the quadriceps and femur, then surgical release and vigorous physiotherapy may improve the range of stifle movement. Quadriceps-plasty — section of each of the quadriceps muscles — is used for congenital or ischaemic contractures. The leg is then maintained in semi-flexion with a splint or bandage for 2 weeks to encourage lengthening of the quadriceps during the healing process and an improved leg posture.

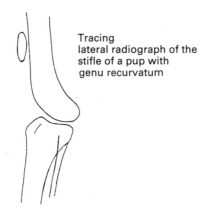

Tracing
lateral radiograph of the
stifle of a pup with
genu recurvatum

Fig. 5.50

The prognosis is not good however and a recurrence of contracture frequently occurs despite these procedures.

RUPTURE OF THE GRACILIS MUSCLE
(Bateman 1960; Sanders 1962; Bateman 1964; Davis 1967; Vaughan 1969; Hickman 1975)

Rupture of the gracilis muscle is seen in the racing Greyhound. The right hindleg is most frequently affected and injury to the muscle is usually accompanied by haematoma formation. Tears of the muscle occur in a number of positions, through the belly of the muscle, the musculotendinous junction and at the conjoined tendon of insertion with the sartorius and semitendinosis muscle. The caudal border of the muscle is most frequently involved.

Hickman (1975) recommends that in recent cases treatment should be directed towards a radical surgical repair rather than conservative treatment (cold applications, pressure bandages and aspiration to limit the size of the haematoma). Surgical exposure of the medial aspect of the thigh allows inspection of the damaged tissues. The haematoma can be drained and haemorrhage controlled but more important accurate anatomical reconstruction of the torn muscle may be carried out using a series of mattress sutures. Consequently, after repair the torn muscles should heal with a minimum of fibrous tissue formation and not impede the animal's future racing potential.

Conservative treatment invariably leads to excessive fibrous tissue formation which may require surgical release (Bateman 1964) to improve the dog's action.

CONTRACTURE OF THE GRACILIS MUSCLE IN THE GERMAN SHEPHERD
(Vaughan 1979)

Contracture of the gracilis muscle in German Shepherd dogs causes a characteristic alteration in gait. The condition has been recorded in dogs between 3 and 7 years of age and affected animals have generally led extremely active lives. Gait changes suddenly and deteriorates over a period of 6 weeks and then remains static. When walking, the affected leg is raised in a jerky fashion with the hock hyperflexed and rotated outwards while the foot is turned inwards. The gracilis muscle can be palpated as a taut band on the medial aspect of the thigh.

Section of the gracilis tendon gives immediate relief but recurrence of the gait defect usually occurs 3–5 months after surgery. Dogs continue to lead an active life despite the condition. In the German Shepherd, contracture involves the tendon of insertion of the gracilis muscle, unlike the Greyhound where the muscle belly is affected.

THE CANINE STIFLE: DEVELOPMENTAL LESIONS

The stifle is a complex joint both anatomically (Figs 5.51–5.53) and functionally. Although its primary motion is hinge-like, the menisci allow the femoral condyles to slide

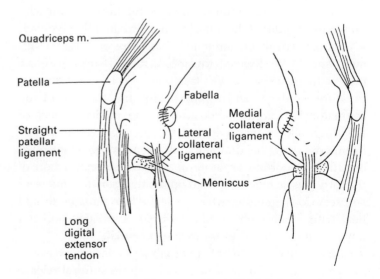

Fig. 5.51 Lateral view of stifle.   **Fig. 5.52** Medial view of stifle.

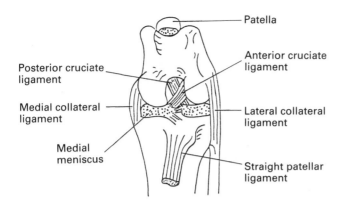

Posterior cruciate ligament

Medial collateral ligament

Medial meniscus

Patella

Anterior cruciate ligament

Lateral collateral ligament

Straight patellar ligament

Fig. 5.53 Anterior view of stifle.

during movement so that the axis of rotation of the femur relative to the tibia varies according to the degree of flexion (Arnoczky & Marshall 1977). Medial and lateral rotation of the tibia are also possible.

Congenital medial luxation of the patella and rupture of the anterior cruciate ligament are the main indications for surgery of the stifle but a variety of less common developmental and traumatic conditions also causes lameness. Developmental lesions of the stifle include:
1 Congenital medial luxation of the patella.
2 Congenital lateral luxation of the patella.
3 Genu valgum.
4 Osteochondritis dissecans.
5 Genu recurvatum.

Congenital medial luxation of the patella
Cavalier King Charles Spaniels, Yorkshire Terriers, Chihuahuas and Papillons are the breeds most frequently affected with medial luxation of the patella. The majority of cases are under a year old with a peak incidence at 5 months at the onset of lameness.

The normal conformation of the hip and stifle is illustrated in Fig. 5.54. The femoral neck angle should be approximately 145°. The pull of the quadriceps muscle group is directed straight down the cranial aspect of the femur to the patella, straight patella ligament and tibial crest. In the dog with medial luxation of the patella, radiographic examination of the hips (Fig. 5.55) will generally show evidence of coxa vara, that is a femoral neck angle of less than 140°, and as a result the femur bows laterally and the pull of the quadriceps is directed medially rotating the tibial crest in this direction and causing medial luxation of the patella. Singleton's

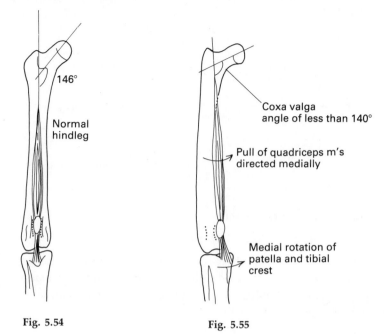

Fig. 5.54   Fig. 5.55

(1969) classification is useful to assess the degree of deformity associated with luxation and the type of treatment required. He divided animals into four grades:

Grade 1 Intermittent patella luxation causes the leg to be carried occasionally. The patella can be easily luxated manually but returns to its normal position when pressure is released. There is minimal medial deviation of the tibial crest.

Grade 2 Frequent luxation of the patella associated with 15–30° medial deviation of the tibial crest.

Grade 3 Permanent medial luxation of the patella associated with 30–60° medial deviation of the tibial crest. The trochlea is usually shallow.

Grade 4 Permanent medial luxation of the patella associated with 60–90° medial deviation of the tibial crest. The trochlea is absent or convex.

Permanent medial luxation of the patella causes a crouching hindleg action with lateral bowing of the stifle. The luxation seldom causes pain or degenerative joint disease in small breeds. Lameness is mechanical, the dog being unable to extend the stifle fully while the patella is luxated. The condition is regarded as an inherited defect and affected animals should not be bred from. Dogs with grade 1 luxation or traumatic dislocation of the patella are treated by lateral capsular overlap (Campbell & Pond 1972), while those with grade 2–4 luxations are treated by tibial crest transplantation.

TECHNIQUE FOR LATERAL CAPSULAR OVERLAP
A lateral parapatellar skin incision is made. The lateral aspect of the joint capsule is incised parallel to the patella and the lateral joint capsule is then overlapped with two layers of nylon mattress sutures as shown in Figs 5.56 and 5.57.

(a)   (b)

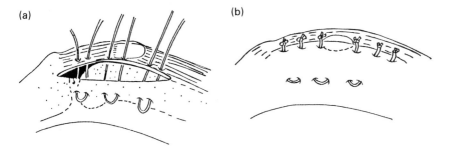

Fig. 5.56

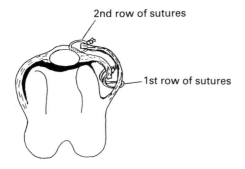

2nd row of sutures

1st row of sutures

Fig. 5.57

TIBIAL CREST TRANSPLANTATION
The following procedure is based on that described by De Angelis & Hohn (1970). A skin incision is made over the anterolateral aspect of the stifle. The joint capsule is incised lateral to the patella and reflected to allow inspection of the trochlea (Fig. 5.58). If the trochlea is shallow or absent, it is deepened. The new groove is carved through the cartilage into the subchondral bone with a scalpel blade and smoothed off with a Putti type rasp (Fig. 5.59). The groove should be large enough to retain the patella and allowance should be made for some infilling which will occur as the defect in the subchondral bone becomes lined by fibro-cartilage during healing.

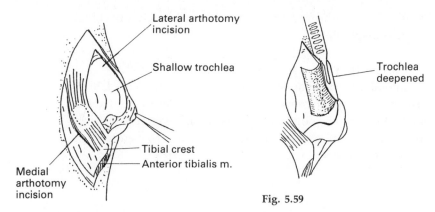

Fig. 5.58

Fig. 5.59

The origin of the anterior tibialis muscle is reflected from the lateral side of the tibial crest. The joint capsule is incised medial to the straight patella ligament (Fig. 5.58). The blade of Liston bone cutting forceps is slid beneath the straight patellar ligament, the blades are closed on either side of the tibial crest and it is cut free proximally but a periosteal attachment is retained distally (Fig. 5.60). The crest is levered laterally with a Hohmann retractor to bring it into line with the trochlea and the patella luxation is reduced (Fig. 5.61a).

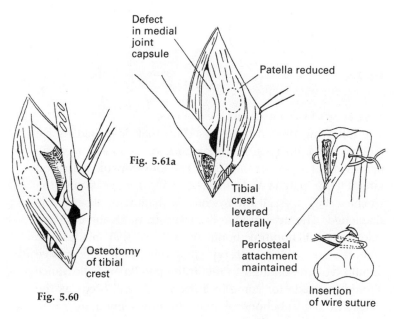

Fig. 5.61a

Fig. 5.60

Fig. 5.61b

A tunnel is drilled through the tibial crest and proximal tibia from lateral to medial, using a 1.5 or 2 mm drill bit. A length of 24 or 20 gauge wire is passed through the tunnel. A second tunnel is drilled from the medial side of the proximal tibia; this does not penetrate the tibial crest but merges just caudal to it (Fig. 5.61b). The medial end of the wire is passed back through this tunnel and the free ends of the wire are twisted tight drawing the tibial crest down firmly in its new lateral position. The medial and lateral arthrotomy incisions are closed next. Excess joint capsule on the lateral side of the patella is overlapped with a double row of sutures while the defect in the medial joint capsule (Fig. 5.61a) is covered with a layer of subcutaneous fascia. The anterior tibialis muscle is secured to the straight patella ligament or adjacent joint capsule with mattress sutures. The subcutaneous tissues and skin are closed in routine fashion.

Post-operative care
A support bandage is applied for a week post-operatively. Antibiotic cover is given for 5 days and skin sutures are removed at 10 days. Exercise is restricted for 4 weeks and then gradually increased. In dogs with bilateral patella luxation, an interval of 2 months is left between operations on each stifle.

Complications
1 Re-luxation of the patella may result from:
(a) Failure to transplant the tibial crest in normal alignment with the trochlea.
(b) Failure to adequately immobilize the tibial crest in its new position.
(c) Failure to provide a trochlea of sufficient depth.
2 Inability to fully extend the stifle joint. This complication is generally seen in dogs with grade 4 medial luxation when surgical correction has been attempted towards the end of growth or after 1 year of age. Ideally, surgical correction should be undertaken at 4−5 months of age, before contracture of the caudal muscles of the stifle has resulted in permanent joint deformity with inability to extend the stifle.

Further modifications to the tibial crest transplant operation

Trochlear chondroplasty (deepening the trochlea). Although the functional end results of trochlear chondroplasty using a rasp are satisfactory, especially in small breeds of dog, the technique does involve removal of existing articular cartilage. The defect that is produced heals by fibrocartilage formation only. An alternative method of trochlear chondroplasty is the recession wedge technique (Boone *et al.* 1983) which permits the trochlea to be deepened while preserving the normal articular surface. This technique (Fig. 5.61c) is recommended in larger breeds of dog. The wedge is retained in position by tension of the patella and the quadriceps muscle group. Healing is rapid and normal limb function is quickly regained following surgery.

Fixation of the tibial crest. One or two Kirschner wires can be used for fixation (Fig. 5.61d) instead of the wire suture illustrated in Fig. 5.61b.

CONGENITAL PATELLAR LUXATION IN CATS
There are few references to patellar luxation in the cat in the veterinary literature. These were reviewed by Davies &

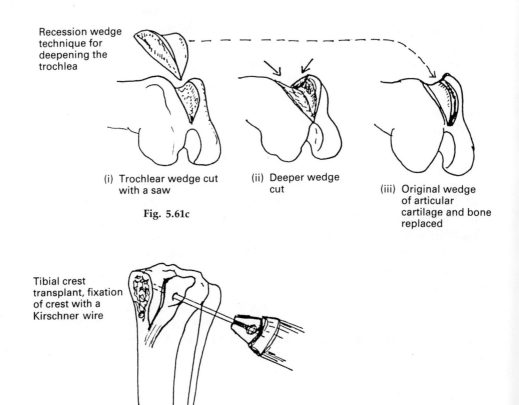

Recession wedge technique for deepening the trochlea

(i) Trochlear wedge cut with a saw

(ii) Deeper wedge cut

(iii) Original wedge of articular cartilage and bone replaced

Fig. 5.61c

Tibial crest transplant, fixation of crest with a Kirschner wire

Fig. 5.61d

Gill (1987) and they described congenital bilateral medial patellar luxation (grade 4) in littermate British shorthaired cats. These cats had already been allowed to mate and had produced two litters, and it was concluded from examination of these litters that there was little genetic component to the patellar luxation. However in a series of Devon Rex cats examined by Flecknell & Gruyffydd-Jones (1979), 34 out of the 37 cats were considered to have patellar instability and a genetic predisposition to the condition was postulated. Congenital medial luxation of the patella has also been found in the Siamese cat and a variety of crossbreeds. Traumatic luxations also occur.

Only about 30% of cats with patellar luxation exhibit lameness and consequently the true incidence of the condition is probably higher than is generally thought. The principles of treating congenital and acquired traumatic dislocation of the patella are the same as in the dog. The prognosis for a return of normal limb function following corrective surgery is usually good in the cat.

Congenital lateral luxation of the patella

This condition is uncommon but tends to be seen in larger breeds of dog, particularly the Flatcoat Retriever. Cases are presented at 5–6 months of age with severe disability caused by the luxation. They have 'knock knees' (genu valgum) and cow hocks. The patellar luxation is usually reducible. Management is similar to medial luxation of the patella except that the capsular overlap is performed on the medial side of the stifle and tibial crest transplantation, if necessary, is directed medially instead of laterally.

LATERAL LUXATION OF THE PATELLA IN
TOY POODLES

Spontaneous lateral luxation of the patella is recognized as a serious cause of lameness in older poodles (8–9 years of age). The condition is often bilateral and carries a poor prognosis. A collagen disorder is the most likely cause. Cases are treated by medial capsular overlap (alignment of the tibial crest is usually normal). Although patella stability may be good initially, recurrence of the luxation frequently occurs within a few weeks of surgery. The risk of recurrence can be minimized by immobilizing the stifle in a cast for 4 weeks following surgery.

GENU VALGUM (Vaughan 1976)

The commonest growth disturbance affecting the distal femur and proximal tibia is known as genu valgum. The condition is seen in giant breeds of dog especially Great Danes, Irish Wolfhounds, English Mastiffs and St Bernards. Average age at the onset is 5 months and the condition is often bilateral. There is medial bowing of the distal femur so the stifles tend to knock together and the lower leg is turned out. We say these dogs have 'knock knees' and 'cow hocks'. There is often a tendency for the patella to luxate laterally. Genu valgum is usually the result of a distal femoral growth plate disturbance; the medial side grows more rapidly than the lateral producing medial bowing of the distal femur. The proximal tibial growth plate can also be involved and in some cases the main site of deformity appears to be the proximal tibia. The deformity can be corrected by stapling provided the pup still has plenty of growth potential left. It is important to place the staple in the correct position so that it bridges the medial side of the growth plate. To aid in positioning the staple, the leg is first prepared for surgery, and two or three 19 gauge needles are placed on the medial side of the stifle. A radiograph is taken. These needles serve as landmarks to locate the growth plate while the staple is being inserted (Figs 5.61e and f). The staple temporarily impedes growth on the medial side of the growth plate while continued growth on the lateral side gradually straightens the leg in 4–6 weeks. The staple(s) are removed as soon as the leg is straight.

A method of correcting angular limb deformities which is used very successfully in foals and has limited application in the dog is the periosteal strip procedure (Auer *et al.* 1982). Unlike stapling, which temporarily impedes growth, the periosteal strip procedure stimulates bone growth. Consequently it is done on the lateral or concave side. A transverse inverted 'T'-shaped incision is made through the periosteum just proximal to the growth plate and the periosteum is elevated (Fig. 5.61g). The leg should straighten within 4–8 weeks.

DEGENERATIVE JOINT DISEASE IN THE STIFLE ASSOCIATED WITH A PROXIMAL TIBIAL GROWTH PLATE DISTURBANCE

In 1982 Read & Robins described several cases of degener-

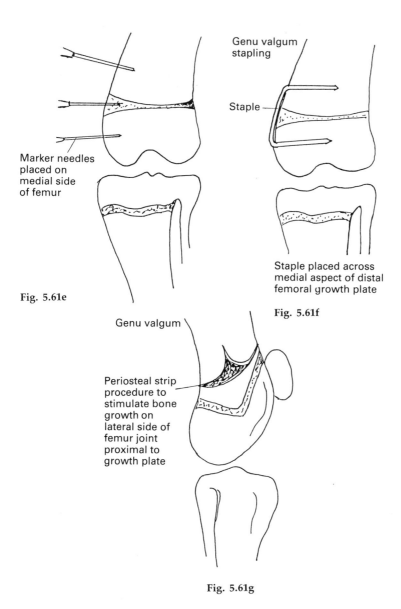

Genu valgum
stapling

Staple

Marker needles
placed on
medial side
of femur

Fig. 5.61e

Staple placed across
medial aspect of distal
femoral growth plate

Fig. 5.61f

Genu valgum

Periosteal strip
procedure to
stimulate bone
growth on
lateral side of
femur joint
proximal to
growth plate

Fig. 5.61g

ative joint disease in the stifle associated with a proximal tibial growth disturbance.

In the normal dog the tibial angle formed between the proximal tibial plateaux and the long axis of the tibial shaft is 69.5° (Fig. 5.61h). If the tibial angle is less than this then anterior tibial thrust on the anterior cruciate ligament (as described by Slocum & Devine 1984) is increased resulting in early breakdown of the ligament and degenerative joint disease in the stifle. An abnormal tibial angle results from overgrowth of the cranial half of the tibial growth plate and premature closure of the caudal half of the tibial growth plate and is probably the result of trauma. The result is dogs with cranial bowing of the tibia, with anterior cruciate ligament rupture and degenerative joint disease. Surgical treatment of the cruciate ligament rupture gives poor results in these cases. At Bristol a series of five cases were seen with this problem: one Greyhound, one Springer Spaniel, two Golden Retrievers and one Border Collie. The case details of two of these are summarized in Table 5.1. The dogs were treated by wedge osteotomy of the proximal tibia to correct the abnormal tibial angle. The osteotomy was stabilized with a dynamic compression plate (3.5 DCP). Following surgery there was a rapid improvement in the dogs' actions with normal function at 3 months. Follow-up radiographs showed remodelling of peri-articular osteophytes.

Table 5.1 Case details of two dogs with proximal tibial growth plate disturbances

Breed	Age (years)	Duration of lameness (years)	Degree of DJD	Tibial angle	Progress/follow-up period
Greyhound	6	2	Advanced leg carried	50°	Arthrotomy and removal of osteophytes. No change Osteotomy — rapid improvement Full function — 3 months Follow up — 15 months
Welsh Springer Spaniel	5	4½	Moderate	42°	Rapid improvement Sound. Follow-up period — 5 months

Genu recurvatum (Vaughan 1979)

Genu recurvatum (Fig. 5.50) is a stifle deformity which results from contracture of the quadriceps muscles. The condition can occur as a congenital deformity or as a complication of femoral shaft fractures in puppies. The clinical features include:

1 Rigid extension of the stifle.
2 Hypertension of the hock.
3 The foot tends to be dragged, giving excoriation of the dorsum.
4 The quadriceps muscles become fibrous and taut.

The prognosis is poor and the response to physiotherapy, surgical release of adhesions or section of the quadriceps is generally disappointing.

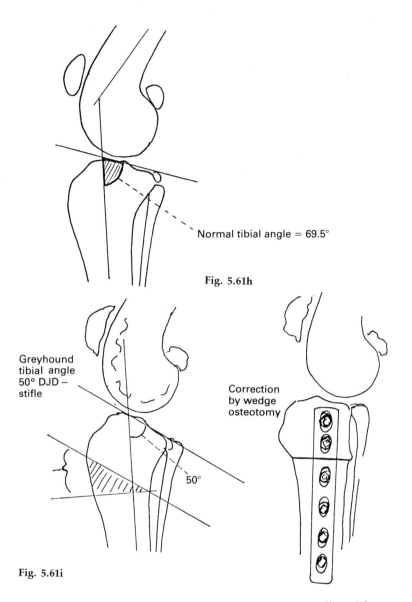

Normal tibial angle = 69.5°

Fig. 5.61h

Greyhound
tibial angle
50° DJD –
stifle

50°

Correction
by wedge
osteotomy

Fig. 5.61i

Fig. 5.61j

Osteochondritis dissecans (Denny & Gibbs 1980)
Osteochondritis dissecans (OCD) is a fairly uncommon
cause of stifle lameness. The OCD lesion is found in either
the medial or lateral condyle of the femur. The breed
incidence in decreasing order of frequency is: Wolfhound,
Labrador, Staffordshire Bull Terrier, German Shepherds,
Golden Retriever, Standard Poodle and Chow. Male dogs
are more frequently affected than females. There is a gradual
onset of lameness at approximately 5 months of age. Cases

with bilateral lesions have a crouching action and difficulty in rising. There is discomfort and crepitus on manipulation of the stifle but no instability. OCD is generally associated with synovial effusion and joint swelling which may be appreciated on palpation.

In the radiographic examination the craniocaudal view of the stifle is the most useful to demonstrate the OCD lesion in the femoral condyle (Fig. 5.61k and l).

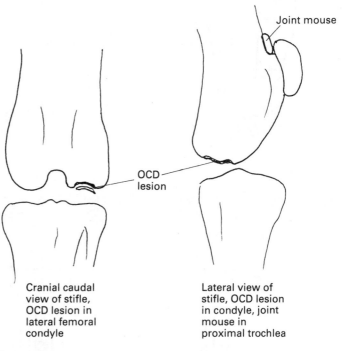

Joint mouse

OCD lesion

Cranial caudal view of stifle, OCD lesion in lateral femoral condyle

Lateral view of stifle, OCD lesion in condyle, joint mouse in proximal trochlea

Fig. 5.61k   **Fig. 5.61l**

In the lateral view calcified fragments may be seen within the joint. Occasionally a fragment will find its way into the proximal trochlea beneath the patellar tendon and cause intermittent bouts of quite severe lameness. Surgical treatment is recommended in most cases with removal of the cartilaginous flap or joint mouse and curettage of the underlying erosion. However the stifle, like the shoulder, has a large joint space to accommodate loose fragments of cartilage and dogs with OCD affecting either of these joints will eventually recover with conservative treatment although lameness may persist for several months. In a series of 40 cases of stifle OCD treated at Bristol University, 23 were treated surgically. Twenty of these became sound and three remained lame, while of the 17 cases treated conservatively (rest + NSAIDs), 12 became sound and five remained lame.

THE CANINE STIFLE: TRAUMATIC CONDITIONS

Traumatic conditions of the stifle can be broadly divided into:
1 Fractures.
2 Ligament injuries.
3 Muscle and tendon injuries.

Fractures
The specific fractures include:
1 Supracondylar and condylar fractures of the femur.
2 Patellar fractures.
3 Fractures of the fabellae (see avulsion of the gastrocnemius muscle).
4 Fractures of the proximal epiphyses of the tibia.

SUPRACONDYLAR AND CONDYLAR FRACTURES OF THE FEMUR

Supracondylar fractures of the femur are common. The injury tends to be seen in pups between 3 and 10 months old and typically trauma causes separation or fracture separation of the distal femoral epiphysis. There is pain and crepitus on manipulation but gross instability is not always a feature and such fractures can sometimes be missed in a cursory examination. The fracture however is obvious on radiographic examination (Fig. 5.62).

Open reduction is essential to prevent caudal rotation of the femoral condyles and malunion. In puppies and kittens under 6 months old crossed Kirschner wires are used for fixation (Sumner-Smith & Dingwall 1973) (Fig. 5.63). This method should have minimal effect on longitudinal growth of the bone. Care should be taken during reduction to

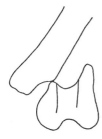

Fig. 5.62

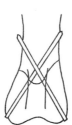

Fig. 5.63

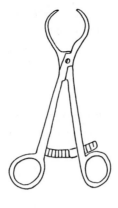

Fig. 5.64 Small reduction forceps
(Straumann, Great Britain Ltd).

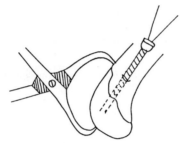

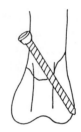

Fig. 5.65

Fig. 5.66

protect the germinal cells of the growth plate by avoiding leverage on the epiphyseal side of the fracture. In pups over 7 months old, with limited growth potential left, a single lag screw (Fig. 5.66) provides optimal stability (Knight 1956; Hinko 1974). If this method is used in younger pups the screw should be removed after 3–4 weeks to prevent premature closure of the distal femoral growth plate.

The fracture is exposed through a lateral parapatellar skin incision, the lateral aspect of the joint capsule is incised and the patella if it has not already been displaced is reflected to reveal the fracture site. Reduction is not always easy. An ideal pair of bone-holding forceps for gripping the distal epiphysis of the femur is shown in Fig. 5.64. These forceps are also useful to maintain reduction of the fracture (Fig. 5.65) while the implants are inserted.

Failure to treat a supracondylar fracture by internal fixation usually results in ankylosis of the stifle joint. Because the condyles rotate caudally, the distal shaft of the femur is displaced anteriorly and the patella becomes involved in a mass of callus at the fracture site.

Single condylar fractures of the distal femur
These fractures are relatively uncommon in dogs and cats.

Carmichael *et al.* (1990) described a series of nine cases in dogs. The medial condyle fractured in eight of these. The fracture is caused by trauma. Seven of the cases described had 'been caught and suspended by the affected leg and had then struggled to free themselves. Diagnosis is confirmed by radiography; the lateral view is the most useful to demonstrate caudal displacement of the fractured condyle. Early open reduction and fixation of the condyle using a combination of lag screw plus Kirschner wire is recommended. The prognosis is good provided accurate reduction and rigid fixation is achieved. The same technique is used for the repair of single condylar fractures in the cat (Fig. 5.67).

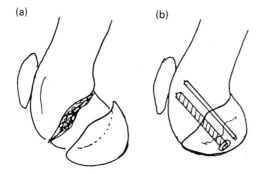

Fig. 5.67 (a) Cat: fracture of medial femoral condyle; (b) fixation with Kirschner wire and lag screws.

Fractures of both femoral condyles, 'T' fracture
This is an uncommon injury in both the cat and the dog. The condyles are lagged together with a screw used in combination with a Kirschner wire to prevent rotation. The condyles are attached to the femoral shaft with crossed Kirschner wires (Fig. 5.68).

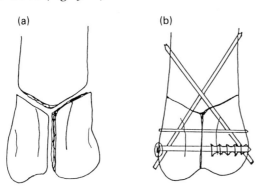

Fig. 5.68 (a) 'T' fracture of the distal femur; (b) reconstruction with transcondylar lag screw and Kirschner wires.

FRACTURES OF THE PATELLA, OR AVULSION
OF THE STRAIGHT PATELLAR LIGAMENT
(Denny 1975; Betts & Walker 1975)

Fracture of the patella is rare. The injury is caused by direct violence and results in a variety of fractures, transverse, longitudinal or comminuted. Transverse fracture of the patella (Fig. 5.69) or an avulsion of the straight patellar ligament (Fig. 5.70) results in inability to fully extend the stifle. On palpation the straight patellar ligament feels slack and the patella rides 'high' in the trochlea. A lateral radiograph of the stifle will confirm the diagnosis. Another useful radiographic view to demonstrate the number of fragments is a sky-line view of the patella (Figs 5.71 and 5.72). A transverse fracture is repaired by the use of a wire suture and wire tension band (see Fig. 2.48).

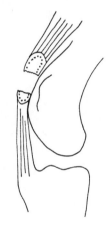

Fig. 5.69a

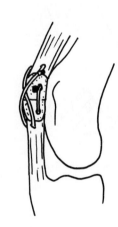

Fig. 5.69b

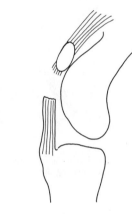

Fig. 5.70

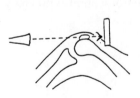

Fig. 5.71

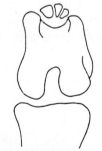

Fig. 5.72

If avulsion of the straight patellar ligament has occurred, small fragments of bone are removed from the end of the ligament. A Bunnell tendon suture of wire is inserted (Fig. 5.73) and used to reattach the ligament to the patella. The

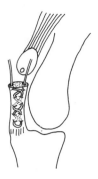

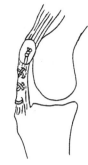

Fig. 5.73   Fig. 5.74

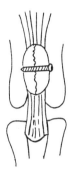

Fig. 5.75

wire is anchored to the patella through a transverse tunnel (Figs 5.74 and 5.75). Longitudinal fractures of the patella can be stabilized with a lag screw (Fig. 5.75).

Comminuted fractures of the patella are a problem; if the fragments are large enough they may be screwed or wired together. In some cases this is a technical impossibility and under these circumstances patellectomy is performed. This could be followed by a homogeneous patella transplant. This operation has been successfully undertaken in experimental dogs (Vaughan & Formston 1973) (see Fig. 1.34h, Chapter 1).

Patellar fracture in the cat
The basic principles of treating patellar fractures in the cat are the same as in the dog. Occasionally transverse fractures of the patella are found as an incidental radiographic finding in cats without any associated clinical signs.

AVULSION OF THE TIBIAL TUBEROSITY (Dingwall & Sumner-Smith 1971; Pettit & Slatter 1973; Denny 1975; Withrow *et al.* 1976)
Fractures of the tibial tuberosity (Fig. 5.76) are avulsion fractures. The fragment is distracted by the pull of the quadriceps on the patella and straight patella ligament. The fracture is usually associated with a fall or jumping and is seen in dogs between 4 and 8 months of age. Treatment of the fracture is by open reduction and fixation using Kirschner wires and a wire tension band (Fig. 5.76a and b). In growing animals the implants should be removed as soon as healing is complete (4−6 weeks) otherwise the tibial tuberosity becomes prematurely fused with the metaphysis and comes to lie further distally than normal because of continued growth from the proximal tibial growth plate. Although the radiographic appearance of this type of de-

(a)   (b)

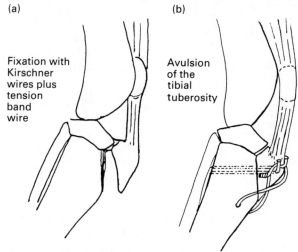

Fixation with
Kirschner
wires plus
tension
band
wire

Avulsion
of the
tibial
tuberosity

Fig. 5.76

formity (Fig. 5.77) can be a little alarming there is generally no effect on limb function.

AVULSION OF THE TIBIAL TUBEROSITY AND FRACTURE OF SEPARATION OF THE PROXIMAL EPIPHYSIS OF THE TIBIA

Fracture through the proximal growth plate of the tibia is seen in immature dogs occasionally and results in caudal displacement of the epiphysis (Fig. 5.78). Treatment is by

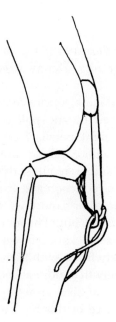

Fig. 5.77 Failure to remove implants results in premature fusion of the tuberosity with the metaphysis of the tibia and distal migration of the tuberosity.

open reduction and fixation is achieved by two transfixion pins inserted down through the medial and lateral side of the proximal tibial epiphysis into the metaphysis (Figs 5.79 and 5.80). The tibial tuberosity is then stabilized with a wire tension band (Fig. 5.81).

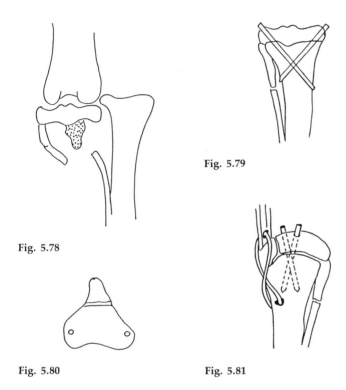

Fig. 5.79

Fig. 5.78

Fig. 5.80   Fig. 5.81

Rupture of the anterior cruciate ligament

Rupture of the anterior cruciate ligament is the main indication for surgery of the stifle joint. The clinical features and recent trends in treatment are summarized below.

CLINICAL FEATURES

Rupture of the anterior cruciate ligament can occur in any breed of dog. The peak incidence is at 6 years old, with a lesser peak at 2 years. In the younger dog there is usually a sudden onset of lameness at exercise or through the dog catching its leg in a fence or other obstacle. In the older dog, lameness is often more insidious in onset and perhaps this is related to degenerative change in the ligament before rupture. The typical clinical features include:

1 Sudden onset of lameness.
2 The leg is carried with the stifle slightly flexed.

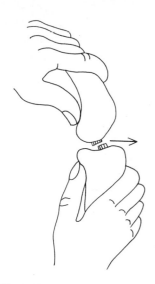

Fig. 5.82

3 After 7−10 days, the dog uses the leg when walking but at rest stands with the toe just touching the ground.

4 The thigh muscles atrophy.

5 'Clicking' noises may be heard when the dog is walking due to the femoral condyles slipping in and out of their normal position on the menisci.

6 Normally the anterior cruciate ligament prevents cranial displacement of the tibia on the femur. Abnormal movement in this direction is diagnostic of anterior cruciate ligament rupture and is known as the anterior draw sign (Fig. 5.82).

7 Joint instability leads to degenerative joint disease. In the larger breeds of dog, weighing 15 kg or more, this is characterized by peri-articular osteophyte formation. In the small breeds of dog, minimal osteophytic reaction occurs.

8 The stifle gradually restabilizes by peri-articular fibrosis which is particularly marked over the medial side of the joint.

9 Restabilization occurs within 6−8 weeks and the lameness may resolve during this period, especially in small breeds. In larger breeds, varying degrees of lameness tend to persist because of the osteo-arthritic changes which have occurred during restabilization.

TREATMENT

Small breeds of dog with anterior cruciate ligament rupture are treated conservatively with 6−8 weeks rest. If lameness has not resolved during this period and the stifle is still unstable, surgical replacement of the ligament is undertaken. In larger breeds of dog, early surgical stabilization of the stifle is recommended to prevent the development of osteo-arthritis. The fact that numerous techniques have been described since Paatsama's original work on anterior cruciate ligament rupture in 1952 suggests perhaps that none is entirely satisfactory but the description by Arnoczky *et al.* (1979) of the 'over the top' procedure for anterior cruciate ligament replacement represented a major advance.

A graft consisting of the medial third of the straight patellar ligament, a wedge of the patella, patellar tendon and fascia lata is passed through the stifle joint along the path of the original anterior cruciate ligament (Fig. 5.83a). The free end of the graft is pulled over the top of the lateral condyle of the femur where it is sutured to the periosteum (Fig. 5.83b). The graft overlies the origin of the anterior cruciate ligament and at no time during flexion or extension of the stifle is it subjected to excessive tension. In most

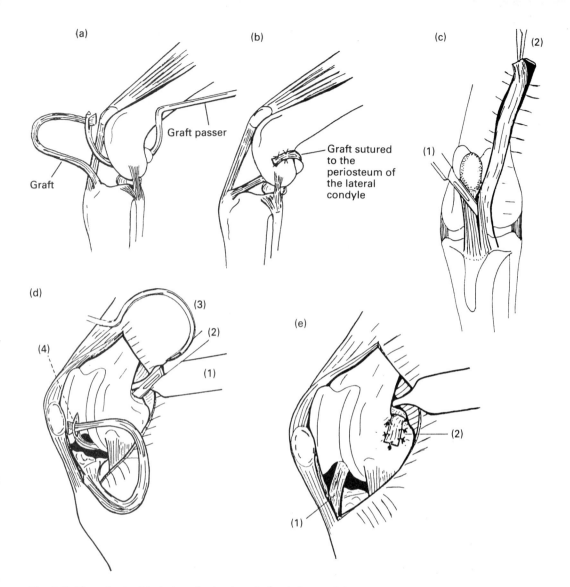

Fig. 5.83 'Over the top' technique for treatment of anterior cruciate ligament rupture. (a) Passage of the graft through the joint using the graft passer. (b) Graft passed through the stifle over the origin of the original anterior cruciate ligament and the lateral condyle of the femur. (c) Cruciate replacement using the lateral third of the straight patellar ligament (1) and fascia lata (2) as a graft. Preparation of the graft. (d) Passage of graft through the stifle. (1) Lateral joint capsule retracted with Hohmann retractor to reveal lateral femoral condyle. (2) Incision in femoro-fabellar ligament. (3) Graft passer introduced through incision (2). (4) Graft passed through 'eye' of graft passer. (e) (1) Graft *in situ*. (2) Free end of graft sutured to femoro-fabellar ligament and periosteum of lateral condyle. (Denny & Barr 1984.)

other intra-articular techniques, particularly those in which a prosthesis or graft is passed through bone tunnels, it is difficult to replicate the origin of the anterior cruciate ligament accurately. This leads to excessive tension on the replacement ligament as the stifle is flexed and results in excessive wear and early breakdown. The 'over the top' techniques offer a distinct advantage in this respect. It has been demonstrated in experimental dogs that the patellar ligament graft is revascularized within 20 weeks, and at 1 year the vascular and histological appearance of the graft resembles that of a normal anterior cruciate ligament (Arnoczky *et al.* 1982).

Biomechanically, the 'over the top' technique has many advantages over the other methods of anterior cruciate ligament replacement and gives excellent results, particularly in large and giant breeds of dog. However, the operation in its original form presents some technical difficulties, particularly in the preparation of the patellar segment of the graft and passage of the graft through the joint.

A much simpler 'over the top' technique was described by Hulse *et al.* (1980) in which the lateral third of the patellar ligament and fascia lata was used as a graft. A biomechanical analysis of the method was subsequently reported (Butler *et al.* 1983; Hulse *et al.* 1983); the results were encouraging with a gradual reduction in joint instability and an increase in the stiffness and strength of the graft.

However, even at 26 weeks following surgery, the material properties of the graft were considerably weaker than those of the normal anterior cruciate ligament. Nevertheless no mechanical failures of the graft were seen in *in vivo* laboratory tests, and in a series of 38 operations in clinical cases 93% of animals regained normal limb function (Shires *et al.* 1984). Similar results in clinical cases have been reported by Denny & Barr (1984, 1987).

'OVER THE TOP' PROCEDURE USING THE LATERAL THIRD OF THE STRAIGHT PATELLAR LIGAMENT AND FASCIA LATA AS A GRAFT

The fascia lata, patella and straight patellar ligament are exposed through a lateral parapatellar skin incision. A graft consisting of the lateral third of the straight patellar ligament and fascia lata is prepared (Fig. 5.83c). Starting from the tibial crest the straight patellar ligament is split with a scalpel longitudinally through the lateral third. The incision is curved laterally just before reaching the patella and is then extended proximally into the fascia lata. A parallel incision is made in the fascia lata caudal to the first, and a strip 1–1.5 cm wide is prepared. The strip is reflected ventrally but the attachments to the tibial crest are retained (Fig. 5.83c). A lateral arthrotomy incision is made and the patella is dislocated medially. The stifle is inspected; torn ligament remnants, torn meniscal tissues and accessible peri-articular osteophytes are removed as necessary.

The lateral joint capsule is reflected with a Hohmann retractor (Straumann, Great Britain Ltd) to reveal the lateral femoral condyle and fabella (Fig. 5.83d). A small vertical incision is made through the femoro-fabellar ligament into the posterior compartment of the joint. The stifle is flexed and a graft passer (graft passer can be constructed from a 4 mm diameter Steinmann pin) (Oosterom, 1982) is inserted through this incision into the intercondylar fossa and directed into the anterior aspect of the joint (Fig. 5.83d). The graft is threaded through the 'eye' of the graft passer and the instrument is used to draw the graft through the stifle.

The patella is replaced, the graft is pulled tight over the lateral condyle and the free end is sutured to the femoro-fabellar fascia using monofilament nylon sutures (Fig. 5.83e). For optimal stability a ligament staple (Veterinary Instrumentation) is used to fix the graft to the femoral condyle. The position of the joint during suturing is not critical as there is even tension on the graft through the whole range of stifle movement. Nylon or Polydioxanone (PDS) sutures are used to close the joint capsule and fascia lata. The rest of the wound closure is routine and a Robert Jones bandage is applied for 7 days. Skin sutures are removed at 10 days. Exercise is restricted to walking on a leash for 12 weeks and then gradually increased. Dogs carry the affected leg for an average of 3 weeks (range 1–12 weeks) following surgery. There is then a gradual improvement in limb function with recovery in 12 weeks in most animals.

PARTIAL RUPTURE OF THE ANTERIOR
CRUCIATE LIGAMENT

The clinical features of partial rupture of the anterior cruciate ligament (ACL) were described by Strom (1990) and the relevant publications on the condition reviewed. It is said that partial rupture of the ACL is rare in dogs but in fact the condition is being diagnosed with increasing frequency at referral clinics particularly in young Rottweilers. In a series of 80 dogs treated by the author in 1990/91 for ACL injury using the 'over the top' technique, 15 had partial rupture of the ACL.

The ACL consists of two main ligament bundles or bands: the caudolateral band (CLB) which is taut in extension and loose in flexion, and a craniomedial band (CMB) which is taut at all angles. One of the problems of diagnosing a partial rupture of the ACL is the lack of an anterior drawer movement, and yet the dog presents with a typical history and signs suggestive of cruciate ligament injury: a sudden onset of lameness, stifle pain, and synovial effusion. Rupture of the craniomedial band of the ACL occurs most frequently, and with this injury it is possible to elicit an anterior drawer movement when the stifle is flexed but not when the joint is in extension. Rupture of the caudolateral band of the ACL does not cause any stifle instability and it is impossible to elicit an anterior drawer movement with the joint in flexion or extension. Despite the lack of instability partial cruciate ligament ruptures do cause pain and persistent lameness. There may be concurrent damage to the medial meniscus and untreated cases may gradually progress to complete rupture of the ACL. Initially it is difficult to differentiate a partial ACL rupture from a stifle sprain. Initial treatment tends to be 6 weeks rest and administration of non-steroidal anti-inflammatories. If lameness does not resolve in this period and radiographs show evidence of early osteo-arthrosis (loss of infrapatellar fat pad outline, joint effusion, peri-articular osteophyte formation) then arthrotomy should be recommended to confirm the diagnosis of partial cruciate ligament rupture. The torn band of the ACL is resected and the remaining band is augmented with a graft of the lateral third of the straight patellar ligament and fascia lata using the 'over the top' technique for ACL replacement. The medial meniscus should be checked for damage and partial meniscectomy performed if necessary. The prognosis is good following surgery with a successful outcome in 80% of cases.

COMPLICATIONS FOLLOWING REPLACEMENT OF THE ANTERIOR CRUCIATE LIGAMENT
1 Prolonged recovery time. The average time before maximum limb function is regained following an 'over the top' (OTT) cruciate ligament replacement is 3 months (Denny & Barr 1987). However in large and giant breeds the recovery period can be considerably longer and it is not unusual for 6 months to elapse before full function is regained.

2 Persistent lameness beyond the usual recovery period. This can be associated with several factors:

(a) The presence of osteo-arthrosis at the time of surgery although this does not necessarily preclude a successful outcome.

(b) Failure to recognize and deal with a medial meniscal injury.

(c) Persistent instability.

(d) Wasting of the quadriceps muscle group.

Try and improve limb function by encouraging the dog to exercise with lots of short frequent walks and the use of non-steroidal anti-inflammatories (see Chapter 1). The aim is to build up the quadriceps. If severe lameness and instability persist then further surgery should be undertaken with meniscectomy if necessary, removal of peri-articular osteophytes and restabilization of the stifle by an extra-capsular retinacular imbrication technique.

3 A recurrence of stifle lameness. The same factors as listed in **2** can account for this problem. A degree of stifle instability following cruciate ligament replacement is not unusual and does not necessarily result in persistent lameness. If there is a sudden recurrence of lameness with pain and instability then manage the dog conservatively initially; restrict exercise to short walks on a leash only (10 minutes maximum) for 6 weeks. A 4-week course of sodium pentosan polysulphate (Cartrophen Vet, Univet) often seems to help dampen down the lameness. In most cases the lameness will eventually resolve again and fortunately repeat operations are not necessary too often (surgical management is as described in **2** above).

RETINACULAR IMBRICATION TECHNIQUE (Flo 1975)
This is an extracapsular technique (Fig. 5.84a) used to stabilize the stifle following rupture of the anterior cruciate ligament. The technique involves the use of single imbrication sutures on the medial as well as the lateral aspect of the stifle. A heavy non-absorbable suture material is used (7 M, braided polyester, Ethibond, Ethicon Ltd). The sutures are placed around the fabellae and through a drill hole in the tibial crest. The stifle is placed in slight flexion and the lateral imbrication suture is always tied first, followed by the medial suture. One or two lateral imbrication sutures are usually placed around the fabella to the mid-portion of the straight patella ligament. The retinacular technique is usually combined with an arthrotomy to allow inspection of the intra-articular structures particularly the medial

meniscus. Following surgery a Robert Jones bandage is applied for 2 weeks. Exercise should be restricted for 6 weeks.

MENISCAL INJURIES

Meniscal injuries occurred as a complication of rupture of the anterior cruciate ligament in 53% of a series of 113 dogs described by Flo & De Young (1978) who have classified meniscal tears and described the technique for medial meniscectomy. The medial meniscus is injured more frequently than the lateral because of its more rigid ligamentous attachments.

Meniscal injuries are a problem of the large and giant breeds of dog. The injury is seldom encountered in small dogs following cruciate rupture presumably because the leg tends to be carried. It is invariably the medial meniscus which is damaged and it is associated with partial or complete rupture of the anterior cruciate ligament. Meniscal damage without concurrent cruciate ligament injury is extremely rare.

During the anterior draw movement the medial meniscus moves forward with the tibia and the femoral condyles crush its caudal horn. Repeated crushing can cause meniscal tearing and detachment which in turn cause erosion of the femoral condyle. The meniscal parenchyma has poor healing

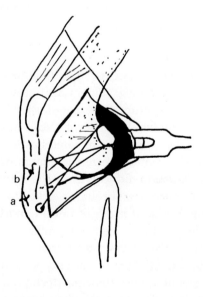

Fig. 5.84a Retinacular imbrication; a, b, sutures placed between patella, tibial crest and straight patellar ligament.

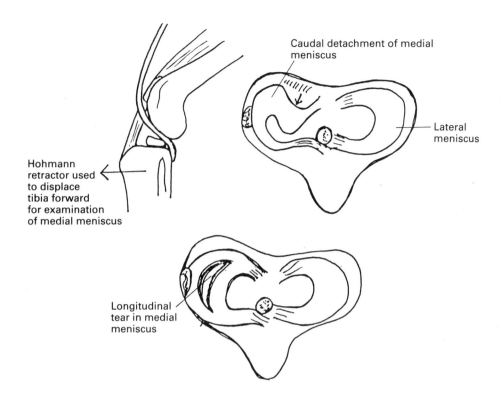

Fig. 5.84b Meniscal injuries.

properties (Pearson 1971) and this has led to the development of techniques for partial or total meniscectomy. At arthrotomy the meniscus is exposed by fully flexing the stifle. The tip of a narrow Hohmann retractor is placed on the caudal aspect of the proximal tibia and the tibia and used to displace the tibia forward to complete exposure (Fig. 5.84b).

Meniscal injuries are summarized in Fig. 5.84b. The two commonest are:

1 Caudal detachment of the medial meniscus with folding of the caudal horn and anterior displacement.

2 Single ('bucket handle') or multiple longitudinal tears.

When dealing with a meniscal injury only the damaged portion of the meniscus should be removed (partial meniscectomy). Total meniscectomy should be avoided if possible unless there is extensive damage to the structure. (Total medial meniscectomy has been used as a method of causing osteo-arthritis in experimental dogs (Cox *et al.* 1975).)

RUPTURE OF THE ANTERIOR CRUCIATE LIGAMENT IN CATS

Rupture of the anterior cruciate ligament in cats is usually associated with gross stifle instability. There is often concurrent injury to the posterior cruciate ligament. Matis & Kostlin (1978) summarized 17 cases of cruciate ligament injury in cats. Eight cases involved the anterior cruciate ligament alone and in nine both the anterior and the posterior cruciate ligaments were involved. In five of these the ligaments were totally ruptured with consequent dislocation of the stifle. The majority of cases in this series were treated by prosthetic replacement of the anterior cruciate ligament and meniscectomy (see Fig. 5.88).

The 'over the top' technique (Fig. 5.83) using the lateral third of the straight patellar ligament and fascia lata as a graft to replace the anterior cruciate ligament is also readily applicable in the cat and is the author's preferred method of treatment. The cat should be confined for 6 weeks following surgery.

Rupture of the posterior cruciate ligament in dogs

The posterior cruciate ligament (PCL) stabilizes the stifle by limiting caudal subluxation and internal rotation of the tibia. The PCL is well protected by the adjacent ligaments and joint structures. Rupture is uncommon and usually occurs with a concurrent rupture of the anterior cruciate ligament (ACL). Nevertheless solitary ruptures of the posterior cruciate ligament do occasionally occur and a series of 14 dogs with this injury was described by Johnson & Olmstead (1987). The condition was seen primarily in large young adult dogs and was associated with trauma; six of the dogs had been struck by cars. Stifle instability with a posterior drawer sign is the main diagnostic feature of PCL rupture, however most cases are initially misdiagnosed as ACL ruptures and the diagnosis of PCL rupture is only confirmed at surgery. None of the dogs reported by Johnson & Olmstead had meniscal damage. Extracapsular imbrication techniques to stabilize the joint are favoured by most surgeons and the results are good.

Some doubt is cast on the necessity to stabilize the joint following PCL rupture by the results of experimental transection of this ligament in dogs (Harari *et al.* 1987). Six months after transection and partial excision of the ligament none of the dogs were lame although there was still a posterior drawer movement present. None of the dogs developed radiographic evidence of osteo-arthritis. It was concluded that loss of the PCL has very little affect on gait compared with loss of the ACL.

Collateral ligament rupture (Figs 5.85a and b)
Rupture of the collateral ligament may occur alone or in combination with rupture of the anterior cruciate ligament. Manipulation of the stifle reveals abnormal movement in a medial or lateral direction. If the medial collateral ligament has ruptured the tibia can be displaced laterally in relation to the femur and the medial side of the stifle can be hinged open. The reverse applies if the lateral collateral ligament has ruptured. Traditionally the collateral ligament has been replaced with a figure of eight wire anchored around two screws, one placed at the origin and one at the insertion of the ligament (Fig. 5.85b). This method is satisfactory if the medial ligament is affected but the shape of the proximal

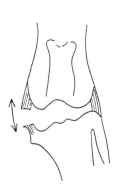

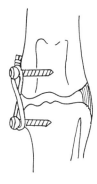

Fig. 5.85b

Fig. 5.85a

tibia and fibula makes it difficult to place a screw accurately at the insertion of the lateral collateral ligament. This problem is simply overcome by anchoring the wire under the head of the fibula (Fig. 5.86). If rupture of the anterior cruciate ligament is complicated by rupture of the collateral ligament then the cruciate ligament is replaced by the 'over the top' technique using a long strip of fascia lata. Having anchored the fascia lata to the lateral condyle of the femur, the free end of the strip is passed under the head of the fibula and sutured to itself (Fig. 5.86b) to create a lateral collateral ligament.

Dislocation of the stifle
Dislocation of the stifle is occasionally encountered in dogs. In a series of five cases recorded by the author (Denny & Minter 1973b), two dogs had rupture of both cruciate liga-

(a)   (b)

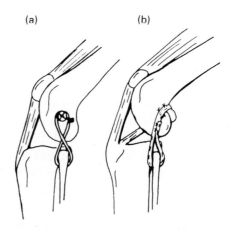

Fig. 5.86 (a) Replacement of the lateral collateral ligament using a screw and wire; (b) replacement of the anterior cruxiate ligament and the lateral collateral ligament using fascia lata.

ments and the medial collateral ligament, one had rupture of both cruciate ligaments and long digital extensor tendon, and a fifth had rupture of both collateral ligaments. The femur was dislocated caudally on the tibia in those cases with cruciate rupture, and medially or laterally depending on which collateral ligament or laterally depending on which collateral ligament was rupture. The joint is stabilized by replacing the anterior cruciate ligament and one of the collateral ligaments. In some cases extra support is given with a plaster cast for 3 weeks.

Dislocation of the stifle in cats has already been mentioned under anterior cruciate ligament rupture. Phillips (1982) described a series of nine cases of stifle dislocation in cats and reviewed the relevant literature. Caudal displacement of the femoral condyles in relation to the tibia was a common feature on lateral radiographs of the stifle (Fig. 5.87). Phillips favoured treatment of these cases using a braided nylon prosthesis (No. 7 braided nylon, Arnolds Veterinary Products) to replace the anterior cruciate ligament. The nylon was placed through double tunnels in the distal femur and proximal tibia as described by Singleton (1969) (Fig. 5.88).

Lateral meniscectomy was necessary in two cases and removal of both medial and lateral menisci in five cases. All cats in this series made excellent recoveries within 4 weeks of surgery.

Avulsion of the tendon of origin of the long digital extensor muscle (Denny & Minter 1973b; Pond 1973)
The long digital extensor muscle arises on the lateral condyle

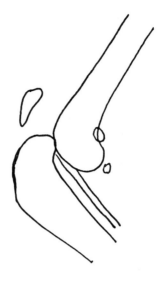

Fig. 5.87 Cat: dislocation of the stifle with caudal displacement of the femur.

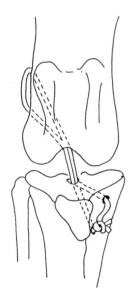

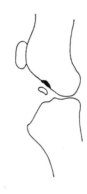

Fig. 5.89

Fig. 5.88

of the distal femur, crosses the femorotibial joint and passes beneath the anterior tibial muscle (Fig. 5.51). Avulsion of the tendon of origin is occasionally encountered in young dogs (average age of recorded cases is 6 months).

There is a sudden onset of lameness, the leg is carried and there is swelling, pain but no instability evident on manipulation of the stifle. After the acute stage has subsided, mild lameness with slight discomfort on palpation persists. A lateral radiograph of the stifle will reveal a radiolucent defect in the anterior aspect of the distal femoral epiphysis with a small fragment of calcified material lying in the joint ventral to the defect (Fig. 5.89). Other conditions to consider in the differential diagnosis are osteochondritis dissecans and avulsion of the anterior cruciate ligament. The latter however, will result in joint instability.

An exploratory arthrotomy will confirm the diagnosis. Surgical reattachment of the tendon is carried out using a lag screw if the fragment is large enough (Pond 1973). Alternatively the fragment is removed and the tendon is sutured to the joint capsule.

Displacement of the tendon of origin of the long digital extensor muscle

Single case reports of caudal displacement of the tendon from the tibial sulcus have been described by Addis (1971) and Bennett & Campbell (1979). The tendon can be retained in the sulcus using a wire suture.

Avulsion of the origin of the popliteus muscle

Single case reports of this injury have been described by Pond & Losowsky (1976) and Eaton-Wells & Plummer (1978). There was a sudden onset of lameness at exercise with stifle swelling and pain but no instability. A lateral radiograph showed a defect at the site of origin of the popliteus with bone fragments and also caudoventral displacement of the popliteal sesamoid bone. The tendon was reattached to the femoral condyle with a screw in one case and sutured to the long digital extensor tendon in the other.

Avulsion of the origin of the lateral head of the gastrocnemius muscle (Chaffee & Knecht 1975; Vaughan 1979; Reinke *et al.* 1982)

There have been four case reports of this injury, which causes swelling and pain over the caudal stifle and hyperextension of the hock. The diagnosis is confirmed radiographically by demonstrating ventral displacement and possibly fracture of the lateral fabella. The head of the gastrocnemius muscle must be reattached to the femur using wire if the dog is to regain normal limb posture.

Stifle arthrodesis

Stifle arthrodesis is only occasionally necessary and is used most frequently for the relief of pain associated with severe degenerative joint disease.

The stifle is exposed through a craniolateral skin incision. Osteotomy of the tibial crest with dorsal reflection of the quadriceps allows a wide exposure of the joint. Ostectomies of the distal articular surface of the femur and proximal tibia are planned to allow the stifle to be fixed at an angle of 140°. A saw or osteotome is used to remove the articular surfaces together with the intra-articular structures. The stifle is stabilized temporarily with crossed Kirschner wires while a DCP is contoured and applied to the cranial aspect of the distal femur and proximal tibia (Fig. 5.90). The tibial crest is reattached on the medial side of the tibia using a lag screw.

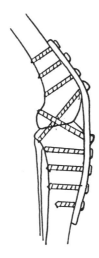

Fig. 5.90 Stifle arthrodesis.

Dogs and cats accommodate to the arthrodesis well although there may be a tendency to knuckle at the digits for the first 3–4 weeks. Exercise should be restricted for at least 8 weeks following surgery. Plate removal 6–9 months after surgery is recommended to minimize risk of tibial fracture at the distal end of the plate.

FRACTURES OF THE TIBIA

Fractures of the proximal tibia are described under surgery of the stifle joint while those involving the distal tibia are described under surgery of the hock.

Mid-shaft fractures are usually oblique or spiral and the fibula is invariably fractured also. As there is little soft tissue cover on the medial aspect of the tibia the fractures are often compound. Stable fractures can be treated by external support with a cast, however in the majority of cases internal fixation is favoured. In dogs, particularly the larger breeds, application of a plate to the medial aspect of the tibia is the preferred method of treatment. The plate Minter 1973b), two dogs had rupture of both cruciate liga-

must be carefully contoured to the shape of the tibia to prevent malalignment of the fracture and abnormal hock posture (Fig. 5.91a−c). The medial aspect of the tibia is exposed through an anteromedial skin incision and the skin flap is then reflected to expose the medial aspect of the tibia. The reason for the skin flap is to avoid having a skin incision directly over the plate.

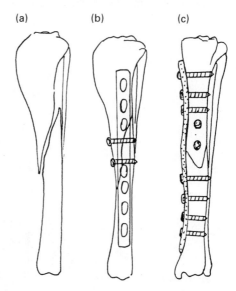

(a)   (b)   (c)

Fig. 5.91 Irish Wolfhound with oblique fracture of the tibia (a) stabilized with two lag screws (b) and application of a broad 4.5 DCP as a neutralization plate (c).

Intramedullary pinning

An intramedullary pin can be used for fixation of transverse or short oblique fractures of the tibia in small dogs and cats. The diameter and length of the pin required are assessed from the pre-operative radiographs and the pin can be pre-cut so that it is readily broken off just above the tibial plateau after insertion (Fig. 5.92). The fracture is reduced through a small medial incision over the fracture site. The pin should be introduced from the proximal end of the tibia. The stifle is held in flexion and the pin is inserted through the skin along the medial border of the straight patellar ligament so that it enters the tibia just caudal to the tibial crest. The pin is then driven down the tibial shaft with the Jacobs chuck and the distal end should be well seated in the cancellous bone of the distal shaft of the tibia. The pin is then broken off through the precut area just proximal to the tibial plateau leaving sufficient pin just protruding for removal once the fracture has healed.

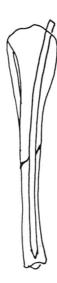

Fig. 5.92 Intramedullary pin fixation of tibial shaft fracture.

If the pin does not appear to provide adequate stability then supplement it with a wire suture (Fig. 5.93) or an external fixator on the medial aspect of the tibia with one half pin in each fragment to prevent rotation (Fig. 2.5a, p. 78).

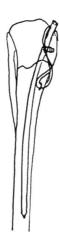

Fig. 5.93 For fractures of the proximal metaphyseal region additional stability can be achieved with a tension band wire placed over the cranial aspect of the fracture.

External fixator

The external fixator is an extremely versatile method of fixation and can be used to stabilize practically all fractures of the tibial shaft together with corrective osteotomies, delayed unions and non-unions. The external fixator is applied to the medial aspect of the tibia (see Fig. 2.5a, p. 78).

Growth disturbances of the tibia are usually traumatic in origin and include the following:

1 Uneven closure of the proximal tibial growth plate causing genu valgum (see p. 344).

2 Uneven closure of the proximal tibial growth plate causing breakdown of the anterior cruciate ligament and degenerative joint disease (see p. 347).

3 Distal displacement of the tibial crest as a complication of tension band wiring (see p. 354).

4 Valgus deformity of the hock associated with premature closure of the distal tibial growth plate.

5 Short tibia associated with premature closure of the distal tibial growth plate.

Valgus deformity of the hock
Most distal tibial growth plate disturbances result in a valgus deformity of the hock. Over 50% of cases presented with this deformity are Rough Collies or Shelties. Average age at presentation is 8 months and the condition is bilateral in 50% of cases. The valgus deformity results from premature closure of the lateral half of the distal tibial growth plate. This growth disturbance presents some problems with regard to management:

1 The dogs tend to be presented towards the end of growth for treatment, so there is little growth potential left to allow use of the usual methods of correcting angular deformities, i.e. staples, periosteal strip procedures.

2 Even if the dogs were presented earlier the small size and shape of the distal tibial epiphysis makes stapling an awkward procedure. An alternative is to bridge the medial side of the distal tibial growth plate with a tension band wire. Continued growth on the lateral side of the growth plate should straighten the leg in 4–8 weeks. The other approach is a periosteal strip procedure to stimulate bone growth. This would have to be done on the lateral side of the tibia just proximal to the growth plate, but of course the fibula gets in the way.

Because of these problems the usual plan of treatment is to wait until the dog is at least 9 months of age and then do a corrective wedge osteotomy of the distal tibia which is stabilized with a dynamic compression plate applied to the medial aspect of the tibia (Fig. 5.94). If necessary the surgery is done on both legs with a 6–8 week interval between operations.

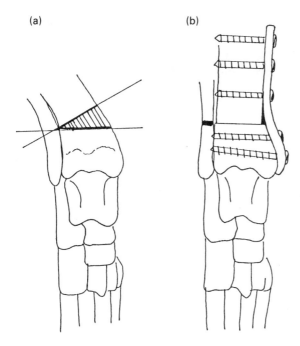

(a)   (b)

Fig. 5.94 Collie; (a) distal tibial growth disturbance with valgus deformity of the hock, (b) corrected by osteotomy and plate fixation.

Short tibia with compensatory overgrowth of the femur in dogs

Overgrowth of the ipsilateral femur to compensate for tibial shortening has been reported in two puppies (Denny 1989). The case details are presented here.

A labrador puppy aged 3 months and a Rough Collie aged 4 months were referred to the clinic for treatment of angular limb deformities associated with premature closure of the distal tibial growth plate (the case details are summarized in Table 5.2). The deformities were corrected by

Table 5.2 Case details

Breed and age in months	Tibial length (cm)		Femoral length (cm)		Femoral neck angle	
	Left	Right	Left	Right	Left	Right
Labrador						
3	11	14	—	—	—	—
7	15	19	—	—	—	—
13	15	19.5	22.5	20	150°	137°
Rough Collie						
4	18	14	17.2	18.2	—	—
9	20.5	16.5	20.5	22	—	—

wedge osteotomy and plate fixation. A considerable deficit in tibial length persisted, but a compensatory increase in the length of the ipsilateral femur which was directly proportional to the tibial deficit enabled the pups to reach maturity without obvious limb shortening or lameness.

ACHILLES TENDON INJURY

The Achilles tendon consists of the tendons of the gastrocnemius muscle and the superficial digital flexor muscle (Fig. 5.95). The gastrocnemius tendon inserts on the tuber calcis while the superficial digital flexor tendon curves over the tip of the os calcis as a broad flat band. A bursa lies between the tendon and the tip of the os calcis.

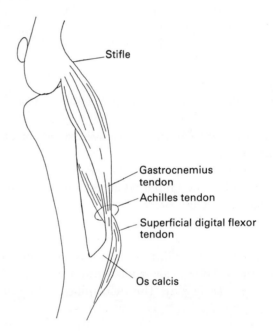

Fig. 5.95

Displacement of the tendon of the superficial digital flexor muscle (Bernard 1977; Bennett & Campbell 1979; Vaughan 1979)

Displacement of the tendon of the superficial digital flexor occurs spontaneously or through direct trauma. Rupture of the medial retinaculum allows the tendon to displace in a lateral direction in most cases. There is a sudden onset of lameness, swelling and pain over the point of the hock and the tendon can be easily returned to its normal position. In untreated cases, extensive fibrosis and tenosynovitis occur.

A curved incision is made over the medial side of the os calcis, the tendon is reduced and the torn retinacular attachments repaired with single interrupted sutures of fine monofilament nylon. In chronic cases, the stretched and fibrosed medial retinaculum is incised parallel with the tendon and overlapped with two layers of sutures in a similar way to the capsular overlap procedure described on p. 339 for patellar luxation. Post-operatively, the hock is immobilized with a Robert Jones bandage for 2 weeks and exercise should be restricted for 4 weeks.

Rupture of the Achilles tendon
(Bloomberg *et al.* 1976; Vaughan 1979)
Rupture of the Achilles tendon usually occurs through direct trauma, the dog striking its leg on a piece of sharp metal for example. Often there is a small skin wound just proximal to the os calcis. However, rupture of the tendon produces an obvious postural deformity; the hock is 'dropped' and a plantigrade stance occurs if the dog attempts to bear weight on the leg. The hock can be hyperflexed and the Achilles tendon remains flaccid instead of becoming taut. Often the cut ends of the tendon can be palpated subcutaneously some distance from the original site of injury.

SURGICAL REPAIR OF THE ACHILLES TENDON
Before suturing the tendon, the hock should be fixed in extension; this facilitates the repair and avoids undue tension on the sutures during the healing process. A skin incision is made over the lateral aspect of the Achilles tendon and extended down over the os calcis. An incision is made in the lateral retinaculum of the superficial digital flexor tendon to allow medial displacement of the tendon and exposure of the caudal surface of the os calcis. The hock is fully extended and a screw is driven through the os calcis into the distal tibia (Fig. 5.96). The lag screw principle is used, the hole in the os calcis being overdrilled so that the screw thread grips in the tibia only. It is important to retract and protect the soft tissues between the os calcis and caudal tibia during preparation of the screw hole and insertion of the screw. The severed ends of the gastrocnemius and superficial digital flexor tendons are identified and each tendon is repaired separately using monofilament nylon. Two types of tendon suture patterns are commonly used—Bunnells' pattern described in 1940 has stood the test of time (see Fig. 5.97) while the locking loop tendon/ligament suture (Figs 5.98 and 5.99) (Pennington 1979) is

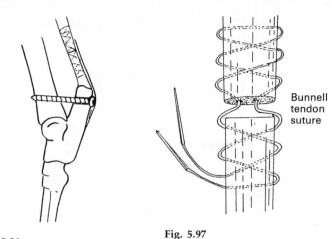

Fig. 5.96

Fig. 5.97

Bunnell
tendon
suture

easier to apply and allows more accurate apposition of the tendon ends (Figs 5.98 and 5.99).

The lateral attachments of the superficial digital flexor tendon to the os calcis are repaired with interrupted sutures of monofilament nylon. The rest of the wound closure is routine. A Robert Jones bandage is then applied for 10 days post-operatively. Exercise is restricted until the lag screw is removed at 4 weeks and is then gradually increased.

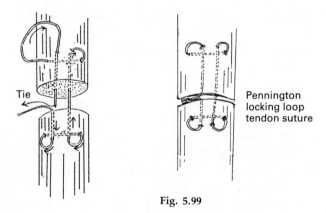

Tie

Pennington
locking loop
tendon suture

Fig. 5.99

Fig. 5.98

MANAGEMENT OF LONG-STANDING ACHILLES TENDON RUPTURE

The principles of treatment are the same as for recent injuries. However contracture of the tendons will have occurred which often prevents complete apposition of the ends. If a defect exists, this should be bridged with carbon fibre (Johnson & Johnson) which acts as a scaffold and induces collagen formation across the defect (Jenkins *et al.* 1977).

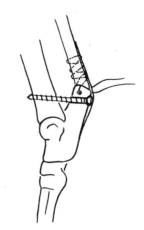

Fig. 5.100

AVULSION OF THE TENDON OF INSERTION OF THE GASTROCNEMIUS MUSCLE

The presenting signs are the same as for rupture of the Achilles tendon but there is no wound, just a swelling over the os calcis. A radiograph may show that the tendon has been avulsed with a small fragment of bone. The hock is fixed in extension with a lag screw as described under Achilles tendon rupture. A Bunnell suture of monofilament wire is inserted into the gastrocnemius tendon, the ends of the wire are passed through a transverse drill hole in the os calcis and then tightened (Fig. 5.100).

Chronic Achilles tendon avulsion

Chronic Achilles tendon avulsion injuries are seen especially in middle-aged overweight Dobermanns. The condition is often bilateral, there is extensive fibrous thickening around the proximal end of the os calcis, there may be pain on palpation of this area, the hock tends to be 'dropped' and the dog may have difficulty in extending the toes. Radiographs demonstrate extensive soft tissue thickening around the insertion of the Achilles tendon on the os calcis and there are often areas of calcification within the swelling. When there is an acute flare up of lameness the hock should be fixed in extension with a screw placed through the os calcis and distal tibia (Fig. 5.100). This will ease tension on the avulsed tendon and allow healing to occur. Healing can be stimulated by splitting the distal end of the tendon longitudinally, laying filamentous carbon fibre or polyester in the tendon and over the proximal end of the os calcis. The implanted material is sutured in place and serves as a scaffold for growth of collagenous tissue. The screw is removed after 6 weeks. Exercise should be restricted to short walks on a leash for 3 months following the initial surgery.

SURGERY OF THE HOCK

The hock is a composite joint consisting of seven tarsal bones and their related soft tissues. The tarsal bones are arranged in three irregular rows (Figs 5.101 and 5.102). The tibiotarsal articulation is ginglymus and it is here that most motion occurs. The intertarsal and tarso-metatarsal

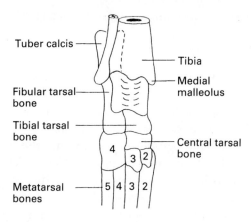

Fig. 5.101 Cranial view right hock.

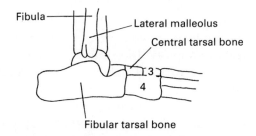

Fig. 5.102 Lateral view right hock.

articulations are arthrodia and normally movement between them is minimal.

The clinical signs of injuries to the canine hock are well recognized, particularly in the racing Greyhound. Injury to the hock may result in:

1 Fractures.

(a) Fracture of the distal epiphysis of the tibia.

(b) Malleolar fractures.

(c) Fracture of the tuber calcis of the fibular tarsal bone.

(d) Fracture of the central tarsal bone.

(e) Occasional fractures of the other tarsal bones.

2 Dislocations and subluxations.

(a) Tibio-tarsal dislocation, often associated with a malleolar fracture.

(b) Intertarsal subluxation.

(c) Tarso-metatarsal subluxation or dislocation.

Fracture of the distal epiphysis of the tibia

Closed reduction and external fixation of this fracture is difficult owing to the small size of the distal fragment. The fracture is therefore usually treated by open reduction. A medial or lateral approach is used depending on the direction of displacement of the fragments. Fixation may be obtained with crossed Kirschner wires. These wires are inserted up through the malleoli (Fig. 5.103). Rush pins may be used in a similar way in larger dogs. Usually further external support is necessary until the fracture has healed.

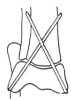

Fig. 5.103

Fig. 5.104

Malleolar fractures
Fracture of a malleolus is often associated with dislocation or subluxation of the tibio-tarsal joint. The malleolus is the point of origin of the collateral ligament and this ligament causes distraction of the fragments. The fracture is therefore treated by open reduction and internal fixation using either a screw (Fig. 5.104) (Leighton 1957; Holt 1976), Rush pin (Lawson 1958) or wire tension band.

Fracture of the os calcis of the fibular tarsal bone
The pull of the gastrocnemius muscle results in marked distraction of the fragments. The fracture is treated by open reduction using a caudolateral approach.

Fixation is achieved using a Steinmann pin or Kirschner wires in combination with a tension band wire (Fig. 5.105).

Sagittal fractures of the distal end of the fibular tarsal bone
These fractures are usually complicated by other hock injuries, for example luxation of the adjacent tibial tarsal bone (Fig. 5.106a–d), or fracture of the central tarsal bone. Lag screw fixation is used for the management of these injuries.

Fractures of the tibial tarsal bone

TROCHLEAR RIDGE FRACTURE
If the trochlear ridge of the tibial tarsal bone is fractured exposure is achieved by osteotomy of the adjacent mal-

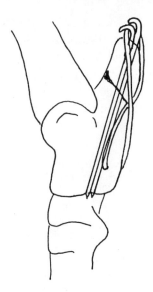

Fig. 5.105 Fracture of the os calcis fixation with two Kirschner wires and a tension band wire.

leolus. If the fragments are large enough they are retained *in situ* with countersunk Kirschner wires. Very small fragments are removed. The malleolar osteotomy is repaired with a lag screw or Kirschner wire plus tension band wire.

FRACTURE OF THE NECK OF THE TIBIAL TARSAL BONE

A lag screw placed from medial to lateral across the fracture line is used for fixation (Fig. 5.107a and b). External support with a cast or splint should be provided for 4 weeks following surgery.

Central tarsal bone fractures

Central tarsal bone fractures are a common injury in the racing Greyhound. It is invariably the right hock that is involved. The reason for this is that the dog runs anticlockwise when racing; during cornering the medial side of the right hock is under compression with the central tarsal bone acting as a buttress which may fracture when subjected to extreme stresses. In managing central tarsal bone fractures joint motion is not important. The aim is to maintain bone space and prevent collapse of the medial side of the hock. Dorsal and medial slab fractures of the central tarsal bone are seen most often. Most of these are best managed by lag screw fixation. Fusion of the adjacent intertarsal joints is often seen during fracture healing but should not compromise the dog's chances of racing again as there is normally very little movement in these joints.

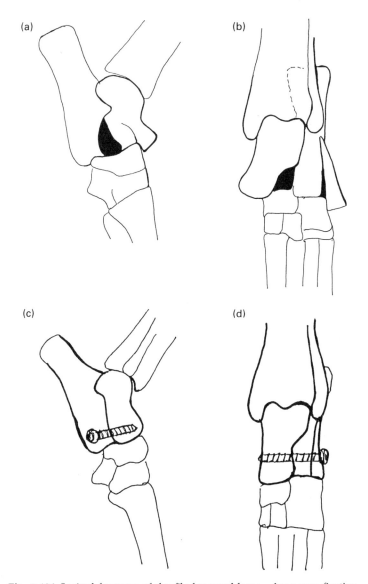

Fig. 5.106 Sagittal fractures of the fibular tarsal bone —lag screw fixation.

The treatment of fractures of the central tarsal bone was described by Bateman in 1958.

In a more recent publication (Dee *et al.* 1976) a classification of fractures of the central tarsal bone was presented together with treatment and prognosis. The fractures were grouped into five types:

Type 1 An anterior slab fracture with no displacement is treated by external fixation.

Type 2 An anterior slab fracture with anterior and proximal displacement is treated by open reduction and fixation with a single lag screw (Fig. 5.108a and b).

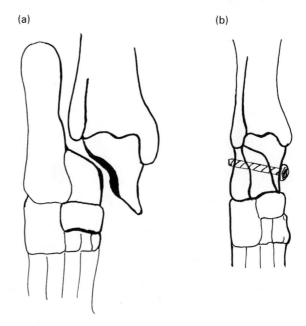

Fig. 5.107 (a) Fracture of the neck of the tibial tarsal bone; (b) lag screw fixation.

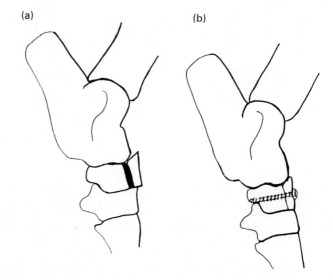

Fig. 5.108 (a) Fracture of central tarsal bone (Type 2); (b) lag screw fixation.

Type 3 A fracture in the sagittal plane with or without anterior displacement of the medial fragment is treated by open reduction and fixation with a single lag screw.

Type 4 This fracture is a combination of types 2 and 3, in which there is anterior displacement of a slab, in conjunction with a larger medially displaced fragment. The fracture is treated by open reduction and fixation with two lag screws.

Type 5 The central tarsal bone is severely comminuted and displaced. Treatment is by closed reduction and external support.

The prognosis for types 1 and 2 fractures is good, for types 3 and 4, fair to good and type 5, poor. External support is provided in all cases treated by internal fixation.

Tibio-tarsal dislocation

Treatment of this injury when associated with fracture of a malleolus has already been described.

The tibia most commonly luxates medially due to rupture of the lateral collateral ligament. Closed reduction and immobilization in a plaster cast may be carried out. However, if the joint is unstable or irreducible, following open reduction it may be stabilized by replacing the collateral ligament with a wire prosthesis. A screw is placed at the origin and insertion of the collateral ligament and a wire figure of eight suture placed around them (Fig. 5.109b).

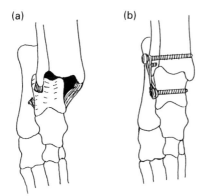

(a)   (b)

Fig. 5.109

Dislocation of the hock may occur as a complication of severe abrasive injury, for example, the dog which has been dragged along the road by a car. The soft tissues of the lateral hock and foot and varying degrees of bone are planed away as a result (Fig. 5.110). Initial debridement is carried out and the foot protected with a Robert Jones bandage. The bandage is changed once every 2 or 3 days. Once discharge has ceased and the wound is beginning to fill with healthy granulation tissue, a cast is applied from the toes to just below the stifle. It is surprising how well some of these wounds heal just with the protection afforded by the cast. If hock instability persists, then replacement of the collateral ligament can be carried out using screws and

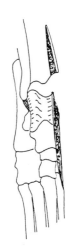

Fig. 5.110

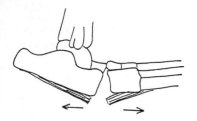

Fig. 5.111a

a figure of eight wire but this should not be done until the wound has almost healed.

Intertarsal joint arthrodesis

Luxation of the intertarsal joint is a common problem in overweight, middle-aged Shelties and Collies. The luxation is associated with rupture of the plantar ligaments (Fig. 5.111a) and the standard method of treatment is arthrodesis of the joint. A caudolateral approach is used. The intertarsal joint is readily identified because of the abnormal movement at the site. Scar tissue, joint capsule and remnants of the plantar ligament are trimmed from the caudolateral side of the joint. The joint is hinged open and a very thorough removal of the articular cartilage undertaken. A 2 mm drill bit is used to prepare two holes. One is placed through the proximal end of the lateral metatarsal bone and the second is drilled transversely through the os calcis (Fig. 5.111b). These holes are subsequently used to anchor a wire tension band after an intramedullary pin, or preferably a lag screw (if the dog is big enough), has been driven down through the os calcis and across the intertarsal joint (Fig. 5.111b). Cancellous bone is collected from the proximal humerus and packed around the joint space and finally a wire tension band of 18 or 20 gauge wire is placed over the caudolateral aspect of the hock. External support should also be provided with a gutter splint for 6 weeks following surgery.

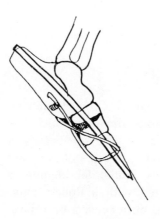

Fig. 5.111b Arthrodesis of the intertarsal joint using a Steinmann pin and tension band wire.

The most common complication of intertarsal arthrodesis is implant failure with loss of stability before fusion is complete. Incomplete removal of articular cartilage, failure to use a bone graft, strong tension band or external support all predispose to this complication.

Tarso-metatarsal subluxations and dislocations

Conservative treatment with a cast or splint is seldom successful in these cases and primary arthrodesis is the treatment of choice. This is most readily achieved by application of a plate to the lateral aspect of the hock having removed articular cartilage from the tarso-metatarsal joints and packed the joint space with a cancellous bone graft. A five or six hole plate is usually used; the proximal two screws are placed in the fourth tarsal, central tarsal and distal tarsal bones, while the distal three or four screws are placed in the lateral two metatarsal bones. External support with a splint should be provided for 4 weeks following surgery.

Osteochondritis dissecans of the hock joint

(Olsson 1975; Mason & Lavelle 1979; Denny 1981)

Osteochondritis dissecans of the hock joint has been recognized as a cause of lameness with increasing frequency during the past few years. The onset is between 4 and 10 months of age. The lesion is located in the articular surface of the medial ridge of the tibial tarsal bone (Fig. 5.112) and the condition is often bilateral. Occasionally, however, the lateral ridge of the tibial tarsal bone is affected (Robins *et al.* 1983). The condition is seen most frequently in Labradors, Retrievers, Rottweilers and Irish Wolfhounds.

Trauma is thought to play a part in the aetiology of osteochondritis dissecans as lesions are invariably found in areas of articular cartilage which are particularly prone to concussion. It has been suggested (Mason & Lavelle 1979) that a straight hindleg conformation predisposes to concussion of the joint surface and osteochondritis dissecans in the hock. However, the straight hock noticed in clinical cases may simply reflect the posture adopted to reduce joint pain.

The main clinical findings are restricted flexion of the joint and pain. A craniocaudal radiograph of the tibial tarsal joint will reveal an increase in the medial joint space and erosion in the articular surface of the tibial tarsal bone. Later flattening of the medial ridge of the tibial tarsal bone occurs and a free fragment may be seen within the joint (Fig. 5.113). In long-standing cases secondary changes occur with marked periarticular osteophyte formation.

The prognosis is dependent on early recognition of the disease and surgical excision of the cartilaginous flap before secondary changes occur.

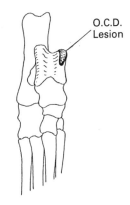

O.C.D. Lesion

Fig. 5.112

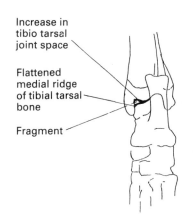

Increase in tibio tarsal joint space

Flattened medial ridge of tibial tarsal bone

Fragment

Fig. 5.113

CAUDOMEDIAL ARTHROTOMY

The osteochondritis dessicans lesion can usually be satisfactorily exposed by a caudomedial approach to the hock. A curved skin incision is made just caudal to the medial malleolus of the tibia (Fig. 5.114). The joint capsule is usually distended and thickened and is incised close to the caudal border of the tibia. Care should be taken to avoid the flexor hallucis longus tendon, the tibial nerve and plantar branches of the saphenous artery and vein which lie caudally (Fig. 5.115). The joint is flexed to reveal the trochlea of the tibial tarsal bone; additional exposure can be achieved by cutting the joint capsule transversely towards the collateral ligament. The cartilaginous flap is easily identified in the medial ridge of the trochlea and once the flap has been removed the underlying erosion in the subchondral bone is curetted. The joint capsule is closed with simple interrupted sutures of 2/o BP vicryl. The remainder of the closure is routine and a support bandage is applied before removal of the tourniquet. The operation is then carried out on the other hock if the dog has bilateral lesions. Exercise is restricted for 4 weeks post-operatively.

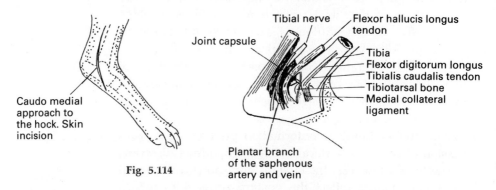

Caudo medial approach to the hock. Skin incision

Fig. 5.114

Joint capsule
Tibial nerve
Flexor hallucis longus tendon
Tibia
Flexor digitorum longus
Tibialis caudalis tendon
Tibiotarsal bone
Medial collateral ligament
Plantar branch of the saphenous artery and vein

Fig. 5.115

Tibio-tarsal joint arthrodesis

The most common indication for arthrodesis of the tibio-tarsal joint is fracture dislocation associated with bone loss. A craniolateral approach is used to expose the joint and the extensor tendons are reflected medially. The articular surface of the distal tibia and the adjacent surface of the tibial tarsal bone are removed leaving two flat surfaces which can be apposed at an angle of between 135° and 145° in the dog. In the cat the tibiotarsal joint is fused at an angle of 115–125°. Fixation is achieved with a DCP applied to the cranial aspect of the distal tibia, hock and third metatarsal bone (Fig. 5.116). External support should be provided with a splint for 6 weeks following surgery.

A simpler method of arthrodesis is currently being evaluated at this clinic. It was noticed when managing dogs with Achilles tendon injuries that the placement of a lag screw through the os calcis and distal tibia (Fig. 5.96) was a very satisfactory method of fixing the hock in extension. These screws were generally left *in situ* for 6 weeks and there was no evidence of loosening during this period.

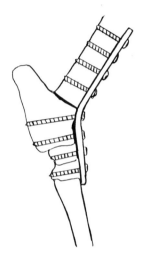

Fig. 5.116 Arthrodesis of tibiotarsal joint using a DCP.

The fixation was rigid but part of this stability was of course dependent on the integrity of the collateral ligaments. It seemed logical therefore that a dog or cat requiring hock arthrodesis for relief of pain associated with degenerative joint disease could be simply treated by the permanent placement of a lag screw through the os calcis and distal tibia. After the screw has been placed several drill holes are made across the articular surfaces of the tibial tarsal joint from the lateral side taking care to avoid the collateral ligament, the aim being promotion of bone fusion across the joint. The procedure has been used successfully in several dogs including a Dobermann in which the operation was performed bilaterally. Exercise should be restricted for 8 weeks following surgery. One case fractured its screw between the tibia and os calcis at 4 weeks; fortunately the tip of the screw was protruding through the cranial cortex of the tibia so that it could be grasped and twisted out. The proximal half of the screw was then removed and another AO cortical screw placed in the original position. There were no further complications.

AMPUTATION OF THE HINDLEG

The indications for amputation of a limb have already been described on p. 278. Amputation of the hindlimb is performed through the proximal third of the femur. A semi-circular skin incision is made on the lateral aspect of the leg extending from the distal third of the thigh to the stifle joint. The leg is lifted by an assistant and a similar skin incision is made on the medial aspect of the thigh. The medial skin flap is reflected and the femoral artery and vein identified just cranial to the pectineus muscle. Both vessels are ligated. Early ligation of these vessels reduces haemorrhage during the subsequent amputation. The limb is then lowered. The biceps femoris, semi-membranosus and semi-tendinosus muscles are sectioned just proximal to the stifle together with the sciatic nerve and distal femoral artery. The sartorius muscle and quadriceps are sectioned to complete exposure of the distal femur. The muscle bellies are bluntly reflected from the femur with a swab and exposure of the proximal shaft completed by elevation of the adductor muscle. The amputation is completed by section of the femur through the proximal third of the shaft with a saw. Wound closure is as described under amputation of the forelimb.

REFERENCES

Addis F. (1971) Nuove concoscenze sulla palologia del muscolo extensore digitorum longus del cane. *Folia veterinaria* 1, 630.

Allen S.W. & Chambers J.N. (1986) Extracapsular suture stabilization of canine coxofemoral luxation, *Compendium of Continuing Education* 8(7), 457−61.

Arnoczky S.P. & Marshall J.L. (1977) The cruciate ligaments of the canine stifle: an anatomical and functional analysis. *Am. J. Vet. Res.* 11, 1807.

Arnoczky S.P., Tarvin G.B., Marshall J.L. & Saltzman B. (1979) The over-the-top procedure: a technique for anterior cruciate ligament substitution in the dog. *J. Am. Anim. Hosp. Assoc.* 15, 283.

Arnoczky S.P., Tarvin G.B. & Marshall J.L. (1982) Anterior cruciate ligament replacement using patellar tendon: an evaluation of graft revascularization in the dog. *J. Bone Joint Surg.* 64A, 217.

Auer J.A., Martens R.J. & Williams E.H. (1982) Periosteal transections for correction of angular limb deformities in foals. *J. Am. Vet. Med. Assoc.* 181, 459.

Bardens J. & Hardwick H. (1968) New observations on the diagnosis and causes of hip dysplasia. *Vet. Med./Small Anim. Clin.* 63, 238.

Barr A.R.S., Denny H.R. & Gibbs C. (1987) Clinical hip dysplasia in growing dogs; the long term results of conservative treatment. *J. Small Anim. Pract.* 28, 243−52.

Bateman J.K. (1958) Broken hock in the Greyhound: repair methods and the plastic scaphoid. *Vet. Rec.* 70, 621.

Bateman J.K. (1960) The racing Greyhound. *Vet. Rec.* **72**, 893.

Bateman J.K. (1964) Dropped thigh muscle in the racing Greyhound. *Vet. Rec.* **76**, 201.

Bennett D. & Campbell J.R. (1979) Unusual soft tissue orthopaedic problems in the dog. *J. Small Anim. Pract.* **20**, 27.

Bennett D. & Duff S.R. (1980) Transarticular pinning as a treatment for hip luxation in the dog and cat. *J. Small Anim. Pract.* **21**, 373–9.

Bernard M.A. (1977) Superficial digital flexor tendon injury in the dog. *Can. Vet. J.* **18**, 105.

Betts C.W. & Walker M. (1975) Lag screw fixation of a patellar fracture. *J. Small Anim. Pract.* **16**, 21.

Bloomberg M.S., Hough J.D. & Howard D.R. (1976) Repair of a severed Achilles tendon in a dog: a case report. *J. Am. Anim. Hosp. Assoc.* **12**, 841.

Bowen J.M., Lewis R.E., Kneller S.K., Wilson R.C. & Arnold R.A. (1972) Pectineus myectomy in the dog. *J. Am. Vet. Med. Assoc.* **161**, 899.

Boone E.G., Hohn B.R. & Weisbrode S.E. (1983) Trochlear recession wedge technique for patellar luxation: an experimental study. *J. Am. Anim. Hosp. Assoc.* **19**, 735–42.

Brinker W.O. (1965) *Canine Surgery*, 1st Archibald edn. American Veterinary Medical Publications Inc., Santa Barbara, California.

Brinker W.O. (1971) Corrective osteotomy procedures for treatment of canine hip dysplasia. *Vet. Clin. N. Am.* **1**, 467.

Brinker W.O. (1975) In: Bjorab M.J. (ed.) *Current Techniques in Small Animal Surgery*. Lea & Febiger, Philadelphia.

Brinker W.O., Piermattei D.L. & Flo G.L. (1983) *Handbook of Small Animal Orthopaedics and Fracture Treatment*. 1st edn. W.B. Saunders, Philadelphia.

Brinker W.O., Piermattei D.L. & Flo G.L. (1990) *Handbook of Small Animal Orthopaedics and Fracture Treatment*. 2nd edn. W.B. Saunders, Philadelphia.

Brown G.S. & Biggart J.F. (1975) Plate fixation of iliac shaft fractures in the dog. *J. Am. Vet. Med. Assoc.* **167**, 472.

Bunnell S. (1940) Primary repair of severed tendons. *Am. J. Surg.* **47**, 502.

Butler D.L., Hulse D.A., May M.D., Grood E.S., Shires P.K., D'Ambrosia R. & Shoji H. (1983) Biomechanics of cranial cruciate ligament reconstruction in the dog. II. Mechanical properties. *Vet. Surg.* **12**, 113.

Campbell J.R. & Pond M.J. (1972) The canine stifle joint. II. Medial luxation of the patella. An assessment of lateral capsular overlap and more radical surgery. *J. Small Anim. Pract.* **13**, 11.

Campbell J.R., Bennett D. & Lee R. (1976) Intertarsal and tarsometatarsal subluxation in the dog. *J. Small Anim. Pract.* **17**, 427.

Carmichael S., Wheeler S.J. & Vaughan L.C. (1990) Single condylar fractures of the distal femur. *Eur. J. Compan. Anim. Pract.* **1**, 8–12.

Chaffee V.W. & Knecht C.D. (1975) Avulsion of the medial head of the gastrocnemius in the dog. *Vet. Med. Small Anim. Clin.* **70**, 929.

Cox J.S., Nye C.E., Schaffer W.W. *et al.* (1975) The degenerative effect of partial and total resection of the medial meniscus in dogs' knees. *Clin. Orthop.* **109**, 178.

Davies M. & Gill I. (1987) Congenital patellar luxation in the cat. *Vet. Rec.* **121**, 474–5.

Davis P.E. (1967) *Aust. Vet. J.* **43**, 519.

De Angelis M. & Hohn R.B. (1970) Evaluation of surgical corrections of canine patella luxation in 142 cases. *J. Am. Vet. Med. Assoc.* **156**, 587.

De Angelis M. & Prata R. (1973) Surgical repair of coxofemoral luxation in the dog. *J. Am. Anim. Hosp. Assoc.* **9**, 175–82.

Dee J.F., Dee J. & Piermattei D.C. (1976) *J. Am. Anim. Hosp. Assoc.* **12**, 398.

Denny H.R. (1971) *J. Small Anim. Pract.* **12**, 613.

Denny H.R. (1975) The use of the tension band in treatment of fractures in the dog. *J. Small Anim. Pract.* **16**, 173.

Denny H.R. (1981) Osteochondritis dissecans of the hock joint in the dog. *The Veterinary Annual*, 21st edn. Wright Scientechnica, Bristol, p. 224.

Denny H.R. (1989) Femoral overgrowth to compensate for tibial shortening in the dog. *Vet. Comp. Orthop. Traumatol.* **1**, 47–8.

Denny H.R. & Barr A.R.S. (1984) An evaluation of two 'over the top' techniques for anterior cruciate ligament replacement in the dog. *J. Small Anim. Pract.* **25**, 759.

Denny H.R. & Barr A.R.S. (1987) A further evaluation of the 'over the top' technique for anterior cruciate ligament replacement in the dog. *J. Small Anim. Pract.* **28**, 681–6.

Denny H.R. & Gibbs C. (1980) Osteochondritis, dissecans of the canine stifle joint. *J. Small Anim. Pract.* **21**, 317.

Denny H.R. & Minter H.M. (1973a) Recurrent coxofemoral luxation in the dog. *The Veterinary Annual*, 14th edn. Wright Scientechnica, Bristol, p. 220.

Denny H.R. & Minter H. (1973b) The long term results of surgery of canine stifle disorders. *J. Small Anim. Pract.* **14**, 695–713.

Dingwall J.S. & Sumner Smith G. (1971) A technique for repair of avulsion of the tibial tubercle in the dog. *J. Small Anim. Pract.* **12**, 665.

Dueland R.T., Wagner S.D. & Sooy T.E. (1989) Von Willebrand heterotopic osteochondrofibrosis of Dobermanns (VW Hood), four new cases. *Vet. Surg.* **18**, 77.

Duff R. & Campbell H.M. (1977) Long-term results of excision arthroplasty of the canine hip. *Vet. Rec.* **101**, 181.

Eaton-Wells R.D. & Plummer G.V. (1978) Avulsion of the popliteal muscle in an Afghan hound. *J. Small Anim. Pract.* **19**, 743.

Flecknell P.A. & Gruyffydd-Jones T.J. (1979) *Fel. Pract.* **9**, 8.

Flo G. (1975) Modification of the lateral retinacular imbrication technique for stabilizing cruciate ligament injuries. *J. Am. Anim. Hosp. Assoc.* **11**, 570.

Flo G. & De Young D. (1978) Meniscal injuries and medial meniscectomy in the canine stifle. *J. Am. Anim. Hosp. Assoc.* **14**, 683.

Grondalen J. (1969) Fractura pelvis hos hund. *Nord. Vet. Med.* **21**, 505.

Harari J., Johnson A.L., Stein L.E. *et al.* (1987) Evaluation of experimental transection and partial excision of the posterior cruciate ligament in dogs. *Vet. Surg.* **16**(2), 151–4.

Hauptman J., Hulse D. & Chitwood J. (1976) Indications for stabilization of sacroiliac luxations in the dog and cat. *Vet. Med./Small Anim. Clin.* **20**, 1415.

Henricson B., Ljunggren G. & Olsson S.A. (1972) Canine hip dysplasia in Sweden. Incidence and genetics. *Acta Radiol. Suppl.* **175**, 317.

Henry J.D. (1973) A modified technique for pectineal tenotomy in the dog. *J. Am. Vet. Med. Assoc.* **163**, 465.

Henry W.B. & Wadsworth P. (1975) Pelvic osteotomy in the treatment of subluxation associated with hip dysplasia. *J. Am. Anim. Hosp. Assoc.* **11**, 636.

Herron M. (1990) Pectineus myectomy. Personal communication.

Hickman J. (1975) Rupture of the gracilis muscle in the Greyhound. *J. Small Anim. Pract.* **16**, 455.

Hinko P.J. (1974) Lag screw fixation for distal femoral epiphyseal fractures. *J. Am. Anim. Hosp. Assoc.* **10**, 61.

Hohn R.B. (1982) Pelvic osteotomy. *Proc. Am. Anim. Hosp. Assoc.* **49**, 302.

Hohn R.B. & Janes J.M. (1969) Pelvic osteotomy in the treatment of canine hip dysplasia. *Clin. Orthop. Rel. Res.* **62**, 70.

Holt P.E. (1976) *Vet. Rec.* **99**, 335.

Holt P.E. (1978) Hip dysplasia in a cat. *J. Small Anim. Pract.* **19**, 273–6.

Hulse D.A., Wilson J.W. & Butler H.C. (1974) *J. Am. Anim. Hosp. Assoc.* **10**, 29.

Hulse D.A., Michaelson P., Johnson C. & Abdelbaki Y.Z. (1980) A technique for reconstruction of the anterior cruciate ligament in the dog: preliminary report. *Vet. Surg.* **9**, 135.

Hulse D.A., Butler D.L., Kay M.D., Boyes F.R., Shires P.K., D'Ambrosia R. & Shoji H. (1983) Biomechanics of cranial cruciate ligament reconstruction in the dog. In-vitro laxity testing. *Vet. Surg.* **12**, 109.

Jeffery N.D. (1989) Internal fixation of femoral head and neck fractures in the cat. *J. Small Anim. Pract.* **30**, 647−77.

Jenkins D.H.R., Forster I.W., McKibbin B. & Ralis Z.A. (1977) Induction of tendon and ligament formation by carbon implants. *J. Bone Joint Surg.* **59B**, 53.

Johnson A.L. & Olmstead M.L. (1987) Caudal cruciate ligament rupture: a retrospective analysis of 14 dogs. *Vet. Surg.* **16**(3), 202−6.

Kirkbride L.M. & Carter J.G. (1970) Fracture of the inominate bone in a male mongrel dog. *Vet. Rec.* **87**, 643.

Knight G.L. (1956) The use of transfixion screws for the internal fixation of fractures in small animals. *Vet. Rec.* **68**, 415.

Knowles A.T., Knowles J.O. & Knowles R.P. (1953) *J. Am. Vet. Med. Assoc.* **123**, 508.

Lawson D.D. (1958) Treatment of malleolar fractures. *Vet. Rec.* **70**, 763.

Lawson D.D. (1963) The radiographic diagnosis of hip dysplasia in the dog. *Vet. Rec.* **75**, 445.

Lawson D.D. (1965) Management of canine hip dislocation. *J. Small Anim. Pract.* **6**, 57.

Lee R. (1970) A study of the radiographic and histological changes occurring in Legg−Calvé Perthes disease in the dog. *J. Small Anim. Pract.* **11**, 621.

Lee R. & Fry P.D. (1969) Some observations on the occurrence of Legge−Calvé Perthes disease (coxoplana) in the dog, and an evaluation of excision arthroplasty as a method of treatment. *J. Small Anim. Pract.* **10**, 309.

Leighton R.C. (1957) Malleolar fracture in the dog. *Cornell Vet.* **47**, 396.

Leighton R.L. (1968) The surgical treatment of some pelvic fractures. *J. Am. Vet. Med. Assoc.* **153**, 1739.

Leighton R.L. (1969) Symphysectomy in the cat and use of a steel insert to increase pelvic diameter. *J. Small Anim. Pract.* **10**, 355.

Leighton R. & Ferguson J.R. (1987) Von Willebrand heterotopic osteochondrofibrosis of Dobermanns. *Vet. Surg.* **16**, 21−4.

Leonard E.P. (1971) *Orthopaedic Surgery of the Dog and Cat*, 2nd edn. W.B. Saunders Company, Philadelphia.

Littlewood J.D., Herrtage M.E., Gorman N.J. & McGlennon N.J. (1987) Von Willebrand's disease in dogs in the United Kingdom. *Vet. Rec.* **121**, 463−8.

Ljunggren G. (1966) A comparative study of conservative and surgical treatment of Legg−Perthes' disease in the dog. *J. Am. Anim. Hosp. Assoc.* **2**, 6.

Ljunggren G. (1967) Legge−Perthes' disease. *Acta Orthop. Scand. Suppl.* **95**, 1967.

Lust G., Craig P.H., Ross G.E. & Geary J.C. (1972) *Cornell Vet.* **62**, 628.

Mann F.A., Tangner C.H., Wagner-Mann C. *et al.* (1987) A comparison of standard femoral head and neck excision and femoral head and neck excision using a biceps femoris muscle flap in the dog. *Vet. Surg.* **16**(3), 223−30.

Mason T.A. & Lavelle R.B. (1979) Osteochondritis dissecans of the lateral ridge of the tibial tarsal bone in the dog. *J. Small Anim. Pract.* **20**, 423.

Matis U. & Kostlin R. (1978) Zur Kreuzbandruptur bei der Katze. *Prakt. Tierarzt.* **59**(8), 582.

Mehl N.B. (1988) A new method of surgical treatment of hip dislocation in dogs and cats. *J. Small Anim. Pract.* **29**, 789−95.

Montgomery R.D., Milton J.L., Horne R.D. *et al.* (1987) A retrospective comparison of three techniques for femoral head and neck excision in dogs. *Vet. Surg.* **16**(6), 423–6.

Moore R.W. & Withrow S.J. (1981) Arthrodesis. In: *The Compendium of Continuing Education for the Small Animal Practitioner*, Vol. 3. Veterinary Learning Systems Co., Trenton, N.J. p. 319.

Morris R.E. (1970) Surgical repair of the pelvis in a dog. *Vet. Rec.* **86**, 559.

Muller M.E., Allgower M. & Willenegger H. (1970) *Manual of Internal Fixation.* Springer-Verlag, Berlin.

Newton C.D. (1985) Arthrodesis of the shoulder, elbow and carpus, arthrodesis of the stifle, tarsus, and interphalangeal joints. In: Newton C.D. & Nunamaker D.M. (eds) *Textbook of Small Animal Orthopaedics.* J.B. Lippincott Co., Philadelphia, pp. 565–75.

Nissen K.I. (1971) The rationale of early osteotomy for idiopathic cox-arthrosis (epichondro-osteoarthrosis of the hip). *Clin. Orthop.* **77**, 98.

Olmstead M.L., Hohn R.B., Turner T.T. (1981) Technique for total hip replacement. *Vet. Surg.* **10**, 44.

Olsson S.E. (1975) Lameness in the dog. *Proc. Am. Anim. Hosp. Assoc.* **42**, 363.

Oosterom R.A.A. (1982) Intra-articular graft passer. *Vet. Surg.* **11**, 132.

Paatsama S. (1952) Ligament injuries in the canine stifle joint. Dissertation, University of Helsinki.

Paatsama S., Rissanen P. & Rokkanen P. (1967) Legge Perthes disease in the dog. *J. Small Anim. Pract.* **8**, 215.

Paatsama S., Rissanen P. & Rokkanen P. (1969) Microangiographic changes in Legge Perthes disease in young dogs. *Scand. J. Clin. Lab. Invest.* **23**, Suppl. 108, 95.

Pearson P.T. (1971) Ligamentous and meniscal injuries of the stifle joint. *Vet. Clin. N. Am.* **3**, 489.

Pennington D.G. (1979) The locking loop tendon suture. *Plas. Reconstr. Surg.* **63**, 648.

Pettit G.D. & Slatter D.H. (1973) Tension band wires for fixation of avulsed canine tibial tuberosity. *J. Am. Vet. Med. Assoc.* **163**, 242.

Phillips I.R. (1982) Dislocation of the stifle joint in the cat. *J. Small Anim. Pract.* **23**, 217–21.

Pidduck H. & Webbon P.M. (1978) The genetic control of Perthes' disease in Toy Poodles—a working hypothesis. *J. Small Anim. Pract.* **19**, 729–733.

Piermattei D.C. & Greeley R.G. (1966) *An Atlas of Surgical Approaches to the Bones of the Dog and Cat.* W.B. Saunders Company, Philadelphia.

Pond M.J. (1973) Avulsion of the extensor digitorum longus muscle in the dog: A report of four cases. *J. Small Anim. Pract.* **14**, 785.

Pond M.J. (1975) In: Bjorab M.J. (ed.) *Current Techniques in Small Animal Surgery.* Lea & Febiger, Philadelphia.

Pond M.J. & Losowsky J.M. (1976) Avulsion of the popliteus muscle in the dog. A case report. *J. Am. Anim. Hosp. Assoc.* **12**, 60.

Prieur W.D. (1987) Intertrochanteric osteotomy in the dog: theoretical consideration and opertive technique. *J. Small Anim. Pract.* **28**, 3–20.

Read R.A. & Robins G.M. (1982) Deformity of the proximal tibia in dogs. *Vet. Rec.* **111**, 295–8.

Reinke J.D., Kus S.P. & Owens J.M. (1982) Traumatic avulsion of the lateral head of the gastrocnemius and superficial digital flexor muscles in a dog. *J. Am. Anim. Hosp. Assoc.* **18**, 252.

Riser W.H. (1963) Necrosis of the femoral head. *J. Am. Vet. Med. Assoc.* **142**, 1024.

Riser W.H. (1973) The dysplastic hip joint, its radiographic and histologic development. *J. Am. Vet. Radiol.* **14**, 35.

Robins G.M., Dingwall J.S. & Sumner-Smith G. (1973) The plating of pelvic fractures in the dog. *Vet. Rec.* **93**, 550.

Robins G.M., Read R.A., Carlisle C.H. & Webb S.M. (1983) Osteo-chondritis dissecans of the lateral ridge of the trochlea of the tibial tarsal bone in the dog. *J. Small Anim. Pract.* **24**, 675–85.

Sanders N. (1962) *Aust. Vet. J.* **38**, 239.

Schrader S.C. (1981) Triple osteotomy of the pelvis as a treatment for canine hip dysplasia. *J. Am. Vet. Med. Assoc.* **178**, 39.

Shires P.K., Hulse D.A. & Liu W. (1984) The under-and-over fascial replacement technique for anterior cruciate ligament rupture in dogs: A retrospective study. *J. Am. Anim. Hosp. Assoc.* **20**, 69.

Singleton W.B. (1969) Evaluation of surgical correction of stifle deformities in the dog. *J. Small Anim. Pract.* **10**, 59.

Slocum B. (1984) Pelvic osteotomy. *Proceedings of 2nd International Meeting of Dog Articular Surgery.* Organised by Associated Lyonnaise de Chirurgie Orthopédique Vétérinaire et Comparee Morzine, Avoriaz, France, p. 129.

Slocum B. & Devine T. (1984) Cranial wedge osteotomy: a technique for eliminting cranial tibial thrust in cranial cruciate ligament repair. *J. Am. Vet. Assoc.* **184**, 564.

Smith K.W. (1971) Legg–Perthes' disease. *Vet. Clin. N. Am.* **1**, 479.

Spreull J.S.A. (1961) Excision arthroplasty as a method of treatment of hip joint diseases in the dog. *Vet. Rec.* **13**, 573.

Strande A. (1966) *J. Small Anim. Pract.* **7**, 351.

Strom H. (1990) Partial rupture of the cranial cruciate ligament in dogs. *J. Small Anim. Pract.* **31**, 137–40.

Sumner-Smith G. & Dingwall J.C. (1973) A technique for repair of fractures of the distal femoral epiphysis in the dog and cat. *J. Am. Anim. Hosp. Assoc.* **9**, 171.

Vaughan L.C. (1963) *Vet. Rec.* **75**, 537.

Vaughan L.C. (1969) *J. Small Anim. Pract.* **10**, 363.

Vaughan L.C. (1976) Growth plate defects in dogs. *Vet. Rec.* **98**, 185.

Vaughan L.C. (1979) Muscle and tendon injuries in dogs. *J. Small Anim. Pract.* **20**, 711.

Vaughan L.C. & Formston C. (1973) Experimental transplantation of the patella in dogs. *J. Small Anim. Pract.* **14**, 267.

Vaughan L.C., Clayton Jones D.G. & Lane J.G. (1975) Pectineus muscle resection as a treatment for hip dysplasia in dogs. *Vet. Rec.* **96**, 145.

Wallace L.J. (1971) Pectineus tendonectomy or tenotomy for treating canine hip dysplasia. *Vet. Clin. N. Am.* **1**, 455.

Ward G.W. (1967) Pelvic symphysiotomy in the cat: A steel insert to increase the pelvic diameter. *Can. Vet. J.* **8**, 81.

Wheaton L.G., Hohn R.B. & Harrison J.W. (1973) The surgical treatment of acetabular fractures in the dog. *J. Am. Vet. Med. Assoc.* **162**, 385.

Whittick W.G. (1974) *Canine Orthopaedics.* Lea & Febiger, Philadelphia.

Withrow S., De Angelis M., Arnoczky S. & Rosen H. (1976) Tibial crest avulsion. *J. Am. Vet. Med. Assoc.* **168**, 132.

Zakiewicz M. (1967) *Vet. Rec.* **81**, 538.

Index